Diffusion Weighted Imaging of the Genitourinary System

Deniz Akata · Nikolaos Papanikolaou
Editors

Diffusion Weighted Imaging of the Genitourinary System

Techniques and Clinical Applications

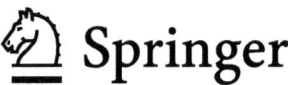 Springer

Editors
Deniz Akata
Professor and Chair, Radiology Department
Hacettepe University School of Medicine
Radiology Department
Ankara, Turkey

Nikolaos Papanikolaou
Head of Computational Clinical Imaging
Group
Centre for the Unknown, Champalimaud
Foundation
Lisbon, Portugal

ISBN 978-3-030-09898-8   ISBN 978-3-319-69575-4   (eBook)
https://doi.org/10.1007/978-3-319-69575-4

Printed on acid-free paper

This Springer imprint is published by Springer Nature
The registered company is Springer International Publishing AG
The registered company address is: Gewerbestrasse 11, 6330 Cham, Switzerland

Preface

Ultrasound was the imaging modality of choice for many decades in evaluating the neoplasms of the female pelvis, prostate gland, and the urinary system. Due to the technological developments, MR imaging has taken over in the beginning of this century. Technical advances in gradient performance, radiofrequency coils, and pulse sequences have increased the clinical applications of diffusion weighted imaging (DWI) beyond the central nervous system. As radiology is moving from the pure anatomical imaging techniques to functional-molecular imaging, the use of DWI gained immense importance.

In the era of "imaging safely," DWI acts as an indispensable noninvasive problem solver. Although it does not seem to be a sophisticated method, radiologists should be aware of all the pearls and pitfalls of DWI in specific diseases and conditions. That was the main idea behind writing this book. We aimed to focus on the urogenital applications of DWI in this book, in order to provide comprehensive coverage of all technical and clinical aspects of MR imaging of the urogenital system.

We are fortunate to have the support and contribution of an outstanding group of internationally recognized and renowned authors in this field. Their expertise, cooperation, and effort, which have made this book possible, are greatly appreciated.

Ankara, Turkey   Deniz Akata
Lisbon, Portugal   Nikolaos Papanikolaou

Contents

DW MRI: Techniques, Protocols and Post-processing Aspects

1

Thierry Metens, Charalampos Mpougias, and Nickolas Papanikolaou

1.1 Introduction

Diffusion is the process of random motion of water molecules in a free medium [1, 2]. For human tissues, water mobility can be assessed in the intracellular, extracellular and intravascular spaces. All media have a different degree of structure and thus pose a variant level of difficulty in water mobility that is called "diffusivity". Although diffusion is an old idea, it became popular in the clinical practice with the advent of gradient technology in the last two decades. Diffusion can provide unique information related to microstructure of tissues by means of strong gradient pulses.

A major requirement in diffusion imaging is to select ultrafast pulse sequences that may freeze macroscopic motion in the form of respiration, peristalsis or patient motion in general. For this reason, echo-planar imaging (EPI) sequences modified with the addition of two identical strong diffusion gradients are routinely used to provide diffusion information. The amplitude and duration of the diffusion gradients are represented by the "b value" (measured in s/mm^2), an index used to control the sensitivity of DWI contrast to water mobility.

T. Metens
Department of Radiology, Hôpital Erasme, MRI Clinics, Bruxelles, Belgium

C. Mpougias
Department of Radiology, Chatzikosta Hospital, Ioannina, Greece

N. Papanikolaou (✉)
Champalimaud Foundation, Centre for the Unknown, Lisbon, Portugal
e-mail: nickolas.papanikolaou@research.fchampalimaud.org

© Springer International Publishing AG 2018
D. Akata, N. Papanikolaou (eds.), *Diffusion Weighted Imaging of the Genitourinary System*, https://doi.org/10.1007/978-3-319-69575-4_1

1

1.2   Basic Technical Aspects

Albert Einstein was the first to identify a linear relationship between the mean displacement of water molecules, the diffusion coefficient and the diffusion time t [2]. In living tissues, diffusion is restricted by many other factors like intracellular metabolites, the presence of cell membranes, the extracellular architecture, the relative size of cells and extracellular compartment. Therefore, the measured diffusion coefficient is called apparent diffusion coefficient (ADC). The apparent diffusion coefficient value is in general reduced if cells expand because of cytotoxic oedema or when the cell density is more elevated, like in most malignant tissues. The link between the ADC and tissue cellularity seems quite complex and is still under investigation [3].

In biological tissue, water diffusion can be spatially restricted by the presence of ordered structures; therefore, diffusion becomes anisotropic where the mathematical description requires a diffusion tensor **D** to be introduced. Although there are studies that suggest the presence of diffusion anisotropy in the kidneys and prostate [4, 5], most studies are dealing with the isotropic part of the diffusion tensor, i.e. the average diffusion measured in three orthogonal directions, called the average diffusivity or the mean diffusion. In what follows we shall simply refer to it as the diffusion coefficient.

1.3   The Stejskal-Tanner Sequence

Following the seminal works on MR and diffusion by Carr and Purcell [6], Torrey [7] and Woessner [8], in 1965, Stejskal and Tanner [9] have shown that the MR signal can be made sensitive to diffusion by the addition of supplementary gradients, called diffusion gradients (Fig. 1.1). Diffusing spins travelling at least partially along the direction of the diffusion gradients will accumulate a net dephasing, and this results into a signal attenuation, while stationary spins will be identically

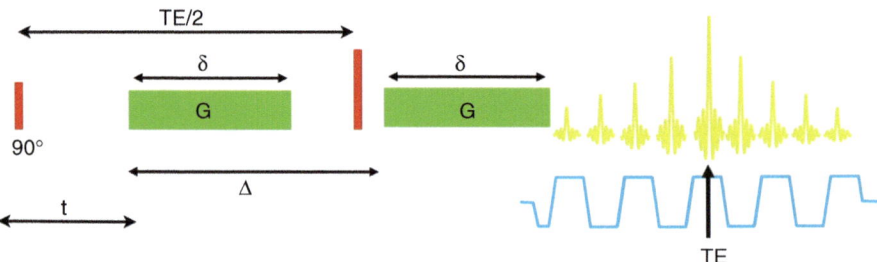

Fig. 1.1 Stejskal-Tanner SE diffusion sequence with EPI reading (only the diffusion-sensitized gradients are shown in green); these gradients are aligned along one spatial direction. G is the gradient amplitude, Δ is the delay between successive diffusion gradients, and δ is the duration of the diffusion gradients; the 90° and 180° RF pulses are used to generate a spin echo in order to minimize T2* effects. Note that after the 180° RF pulse, the effective gradient sign is changed

dephased and rephased with no signal loss. The Stejskal-Tanner gradients are generally used within a spin-echo echo-planar imaging (SE-EPI) sequence, allowing to acquire diffusion-weighted images (DWI). The signal of the SE Stejskal-Tanner sequence can be calculated as

$$S(\text{TE}) = S(\text{TE} = 0, b = 0) e^{-\text{TE}/\text{T2}} e^{-bD} \tag{1.1}$$

with the b value (in s/mm^2)

$$b = (\gamma G d)^2 (\Delta - \delta / 3) \tag{1.2}$$

with γ the proton gyromagnetic ratio, G the gradient amplitude, Δ the delay between successive diffusion gradients and δ the duration of the diffusion gradients. The signal of the Stejskal-Tanner sequence is thus both T2-weighted and diffusion-weighed; the b value controls the diffusion weighting and TE controls the T2 weighting (Fig. 1.2). The product of the two exponential attenuations explains the inherent low signal-to-noise ratio (SNR) of DWI; the spatial resolution is generally kept low to compensate for the otherwise low SNR. Reduction of echo time not only results in less T2-related contamination of the DWI image contrast but also reduces the signal loss related to T2 decay. Equation (1.1) accounts for diffusion in one particular direction in space and shows that increased water mobility results in substantial signal attenuation on diffusion-weighted images. Conversely, water molecules with reduced mobility will present with significantly lower signal attenuation comparing to water molecules with increased mobility leading to a relative higher signal on high b-value images, as shown on Fig. 1.3, where the prostate cancer presents with higher signal to surrounding prostate gland due to reduced water mobility within the lesion. We emphasize that the signal intensity in DW images is not only affected by the b factor and the diffusion of water but also by the T2 and T2*

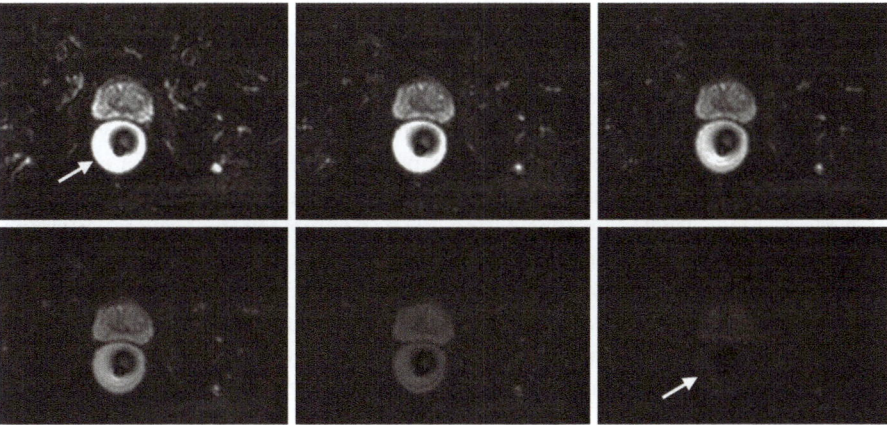

Fig. 1.2 DW images acquired at fixed TE with b = 0, 50, 100, 150, 500 and 1000 s/mm^2 (*starting from upper left*) showing various degrees of diffusion weighting. Notice the increasing attenuation of water signal due to free diffusion (*arrows*)

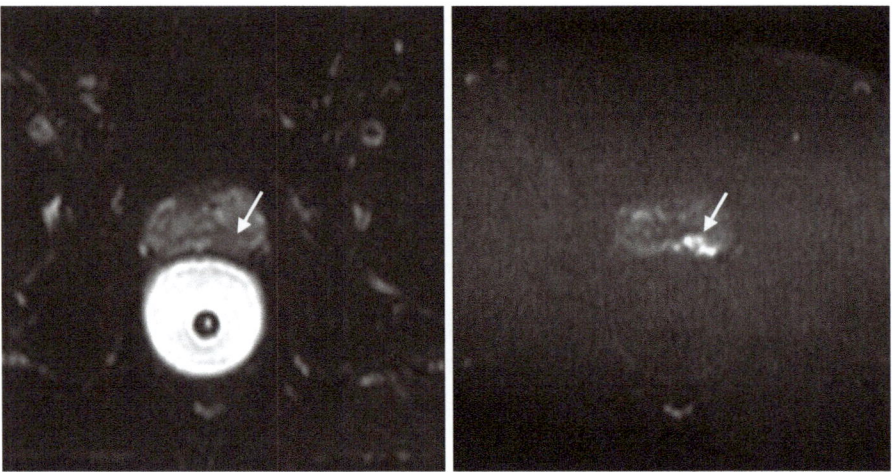

Fig. 1.3 Axial SE-EPI DWI $b = 0$ s/mm^2 (*left*) and 1400.0 s/mm^2 (*right*). Prostate cancer (*arrow*) presents with high signal intensity on the high b-value image (*right*) due to restricted diffusion

relaxation times of the tissues because the Stejskal-Tanner diffusion "carrying sequence" is a SE-EPI. In a tissue with a long T2-relaxation coefficient, a relatively high signal intensity can be maintained mimicking restricted diffusion patterns, the so-called "T2 shine-through" effect. On the contrary, a tissue with a very low T2 value will appear dark, the so-called T2 black-out effect. It is important to avoid such confusion by considering all b-value and possibly T2-weighted images.

In many clinical situations, visual interpretation of DW images is not enough, and further quantification of ADC is considered mandatory. This calculation involves at least the acquisition of two signals S1 and S2 from acquisitions with different b factors, i.e. b_1 and b_2 factors and by computing

$$ADC = \mathrm{Ln}\left(S1 / S2\right)/\left(b_2 - b_1\right) \tag{1.3}$$

If more than two b-value images are involved, a linear regression of the logarithms $\mathrm{Ln}[S(b)/S(0)]$ in function of the b values will provide the ADC value (i.e. slope of the regression line). When this is performed for each pixel, a calculated image of the ADC, called the ADC map, is reconstructed. More generally, the ADC map can be reconstructed by considering one or a combination of several diffusion directions and several b values, while the correct choice of the regression points is influencing the final ADC value. Currently there is no consensus on the optimal b value to use in DWI. Most studies have used b values of 0 and 1000 s/mm^2. Developing DWI into a robust technique, there is a need for standardization of b values. Higher b values may provide better characterization of cancerous lesions due to signal attenuation of non-cancerous tissues. The advantages of using higher b values include increased diffusion weighting (and diminished T2 shine-through), higher contrast-to-noise ratio and—theoretically—higher tumour conspicuity that

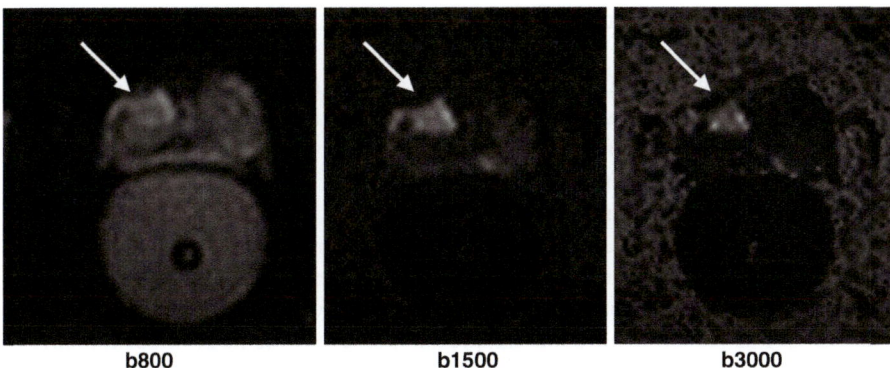

b800   **b1500**   **b3000**

Fig. 1.4 Patient with prostate cancer. In the b800 (*left*) images, the contrast between the lesion (*arrow*) and adjacent tissues is very low. On the contrary, lesion conspicuity is significantly improved on calculated b1500 (*centre*) and b3000 (*right*) images

leads to improved tumour detection. Disadvantages include increased motion and susceptibility artefacts, as well as decreased signal-to-noise ratios. Lower SNR may confound interpretation of different ADC values, as it could be difficult to determine whether the decrease in ADC is due to reduced SNR or true restriction of diffusion. In addition, the ultrahigh *b*-value images can be calculated from images obtained using standard *b* values rather than directly acquired (Fig. 1.4). This process entails no additional acquisition time in comparison with the time required for the acquisition of the standard *b*-value images and is useful if encountering excessive artefacts or insufficient SNR when directly acquiring ultrahigh *b*-value images.

The diffusion sequence must be repeated using diffusion gradients oriented in at least three orthogonal directions. The geometric mean of three orthogonal diffusion-weighted images with the same *b* amplitude gives the isotropic diffusion image (where directional effects have been eliminated):

$$I(b) = S(0)e^{-(^b\mathbf{xx}^D\mathbf{xx}+^b\mathbf{yy}^D\mathbf{yy}+^b\mathbf{zz}^D\mathbf{zz})/3} = S(0)e^{-b(^D\mathbf{xx}+^D\mathbf{yy}+^D\mathbf{zz})/3} = S(0)e^{-b\mathrm{MD}} \quad (1.4)$$

The derivation of Eq. (1.2) is based on the hypothesis that the diffusion is the single source of intravoxel incoherent motion (IVIM). However, in living tissue, micro-perfusion represents another potential source of IVIM; the blood flow appears indeed random as it follows the randomly oriented capillaries and during the diffusion time spins in the capillary blood flow might have changed their direction several times, or different spins will flow along different directions in differently oriented capillaries. This micro-perfusion phenomenon constitutes a pseudo-diffusion movement and will be discussed in detail below. Another complication arises from the fact that the pixel size in DWI is large compared to the various tissue compartments with different diffusivity and partial volume effects might result, again justifying the apparent character of the diffusion coefficient measured in tissue.

1.4 Pulse Sequence Considerations

The Stejskal-Tanner SE-EPI sequence is acquired using a single EPI echo train, providing an image in the so-called "single-shot" mode. In a segmented acquisition (multi-shot mode), the signal phase of the different k-space segments can interfere destructively causing an irremediable signal loss in the final image. This severe segmental dephasing occurs in the strong diffusion gradients because of several physiologic factors like peristalsis respiration and organ movement occurring in-between consecutive k space segment acquisitions. Segmented approaches are possible but require adequate phase corrections that are often difficult to be implemented. The SE-EPI sequence requires fat suppression to avoid the large water-fat shift in the EPI phase-encoding direction. Moreover, T2* image blurring and spatial distortions due to the high EPI echo train length (ETL)-related artefacts are mostly present along the phase-encoding direction. The presence of air in the gastrointestinal tract may result in susceptibility artefacts (Fig. 1.5) that may hamper diagnostic efficacy. Therefore, it is advised to remove rectal air, especially when the examination is performed at 3T systems, with the application of a micro-enema just before the examination.

The spatial resolution of clinical DW imaging is in general relatively lower comparing to that of conventional MRI sequences like T1 or T2. However, multichannel high-performance dedicated coils are nowadays available and do allow the use of parallel imaging with high acceleration factors to minimize geometric distortions and T2* blurring. High *b*-value images suffer from poor SNR, and therefore more averages than in the low *b* values may be acquired to compensate for the limited

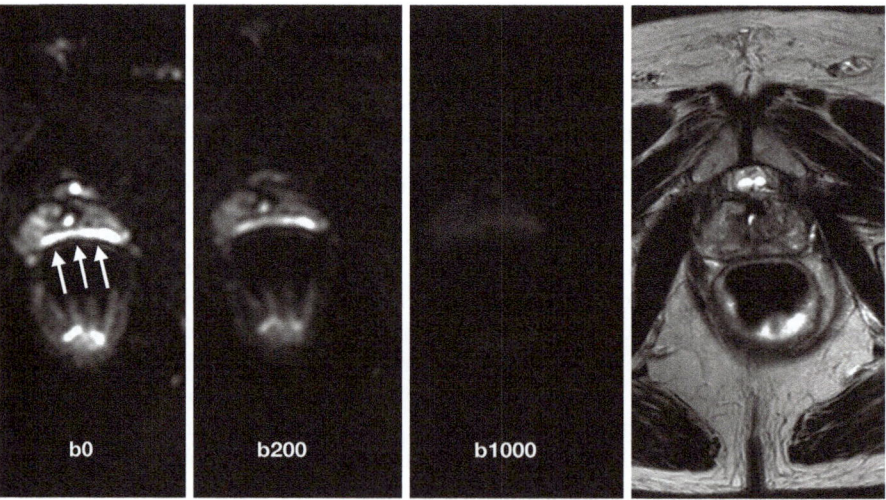

Fig. 1.5 Axial SE-EPI DWI of the prostate acquired with a 3T scanner. The presence of rectal air results to significant geometrical distortions and the formation of susceptibility artefacts (*arrows*). In such cases, it is impossible to diagnose lesions in the peripheral zone. The T2-weighted image (*right*) is shown for reference reasons

signal (Fig. 1.6). Depending on the coil design, the phase-encoding direction, the size and shape of the object of interest, the static magnetic field strength and the image SNR, acceleration factors of 2–4 are used. Recent progress has been provided by the multi-slice simultaneous excitation technique, which allows diffusion-weighted imaging of the liver and pancreas accelerated by a factor two in addition to parallel imaging [8, 9]. Similar studies on the prostate and kidneys are expected to be conducted soon.

The availability of 3T magnets equipped with fast gradient systems makes it possible to acquire high-quality diffusion images avoiding endorectal coils due to the higher SNR that 3T systems offer. Several new DW sequences have been proposed including "Resolve", is a high-resolution DW readout-segmented EPI sequence with two spin echoes (Fig. 1.7). This sequence uses the second echo data from a 2D navigator acquisition to perform a nonlinear phase correction and to control the real-time reacquisition of unusable data that cannot be corrected [10].

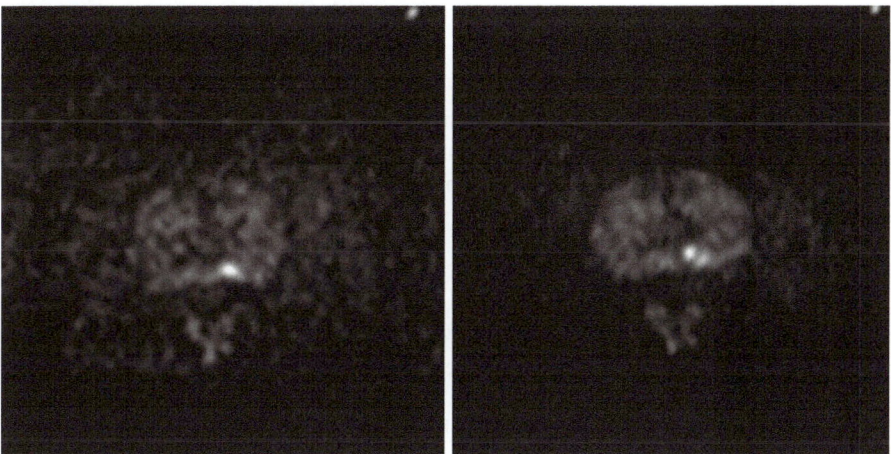

Fig. 1.6 Axial SE-EPI DWI $b = 1000$ s/mm^2, with two (*left*) and four (*right*) averages. The image on the right has significantly higher SNR

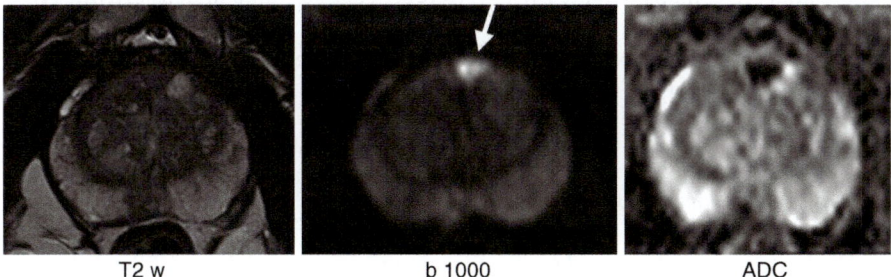

| T2 w | b 1000 | ADC |

Fig. 1.7 Patient with prostate carcinoma in the anterior gland (*arrow*). Multi-shot EPI-based DWI (RESOLVE) results in less geometrical distortion and higher spatial resolution comparing to single-shot EPI DWI

1.5   Diffusion Modelling

Many abdominal organs including the kidneys, prostate and cervix are presented with a strong perfusion component [11–17]. The capillary random movement through the diffusion gradients constitutes an intravoxel incoherent motion, IVIM, dephasing the Stejskal-Tanner signal. An adequate model should thus consider both water diffusion and the pseudo-diffusion from blood capillary flow. One approach is provided by the bi-exponential model:

$$S(b)/S(0) = f e^{-bD^*} + (1-f) e^{-bD} \qquad (1.5)$$

where f is the micro-perfusion fraction, D^* is the pseudo-diffusion coefficient linked to micro-perfusion, and D is the water true diffusion coefficient in the tissue. The major disadvantage that prohibits routine clinical applications of IVIM is that the bi-exponential model is very prone to signal fitting errors. However, fortunately, in general $D^* \gg D$, and there exists a value b^* such that

$$\text{for } b > b^* : e^{-bD^*} \simeq 0 \qquad (1.6)$$

meaning that for $b > b^*$, the attenuation comes from pure diffusion D only. Thus, instead of trying at once to fit the bi-exponential model with three parameters f, D^*, and D, an approximate strategy called "partial fitting" comprises D calculation by fitting a mono-exponential model to the signal of two or more images with b values larger than b^*, typically $b^* = 150$ s/mm^2:

$$\text{Ln}\left[S(b)/S(0) \right] \sim \text{Ln}(1-f) - bD = \beta - bD \qquad (1.7)$$

where β is the intercept of the linear regression and

$$f = 1 - e^{\beta} \qquad (1.8)$$

Alternatively, in a stepwise procedure, the previous approximate values obtained for b and D can be used as initial guessed values of the bi-exponential fit. The bi-exponential character of the prostate apparent diffusion explains why mono-exponential ADC maps obtained with different sets of b-value images provide ADC values that are different.

Some studies have explored other diffusion models, including the stretched exponential model [18]:

$$S(b)/S(0) = \exp-(b\,\text{DDC})^{\alpha} \qquad (1.9)$$

involving the distributed diffusion coefficient (DDC) and the stretching parameter α.

The kurtosis model is based on the non-mono-exponential decay of the diffusion-weighted signal [19]:

$$S(b)/S(0) = \exp-\left(bD + b^2 D^2 K / 6\right) \qquad (1.10)$$

Since diffusion is a process that takes place in four dimensions, we need to utilize a displacement distribution function that will predict the position of each water molecule at a certain time point. In a homogeneous medium, the molecular displacement distribution can be Gaussian, where the width is proportional to the diffusion coefficient. In heterogeneous tissues, the water molecular displacements significantly differ from the true "Brownian motion" defined for free molecules because water molecules bounce, cross and interact with cell membranes and other microstructural components. In the presence of those obstacles, the actual diffusion distance is reduced compared to free water, and the displacement distribution is no longer Gaussian. In other words, while over very short times diffusion reflects the local intrinsic viscosity, at longer diffusion times, the effects of the obstacles become predominant. Typically, the latter effects are presented in a form of signal deviation when using Gaussian models at the ultrahigh b-value (>1000 s/mm^2) area (Fig. 1.8). The number of the b values and the value of the highest b can influence the value of diffusion kurtosis (K) (Fig. 1.9). It is advised to acquire at least three b values, a b0, one lower and one higher than 1000 s/mm^2.

Another more sophisticated model that has been introduced recently, is the VERDICT model that includes three compartments, namely, the intracellular, extracellular and intravascular [20]. The filter exchange imaging is based on a double-pulse gradient spin-echo technique and takes into consideration the water exchange time between two compartments with different diffusion characteristics [21].

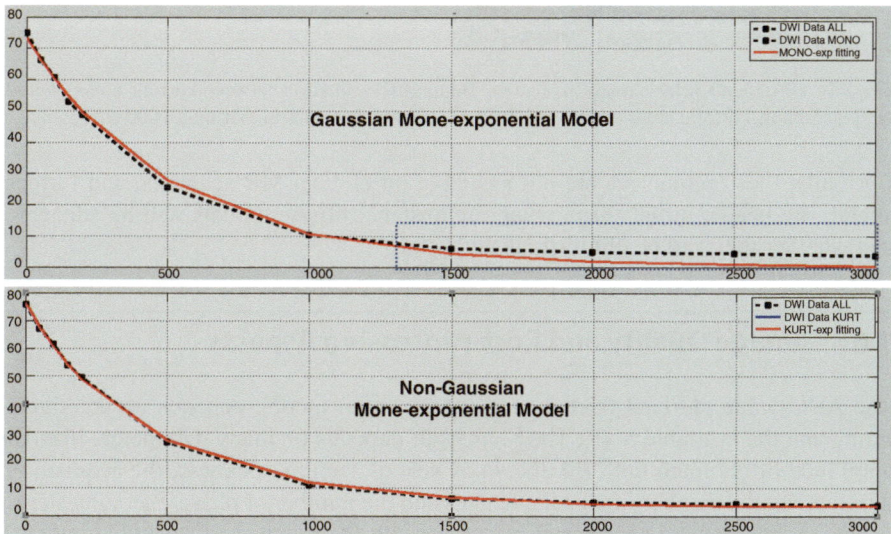

Fig. 1.8 Signal intensity over b-value graphs from prostate carcinoma in the peripheral zone. In the upper graph, a Gaussian mono-exponential model is used where a deviation between the model (*red line*) and the real signal intensities (*dotted black line*) is evident in b values higher than 1000 s/mm^2 (*blue dotted box*). When using non-Gaussian models (*lower graph*), this deviation is minimized (Graphs were made with Diffusion Modeling Tool developed by ICS - FORTH)

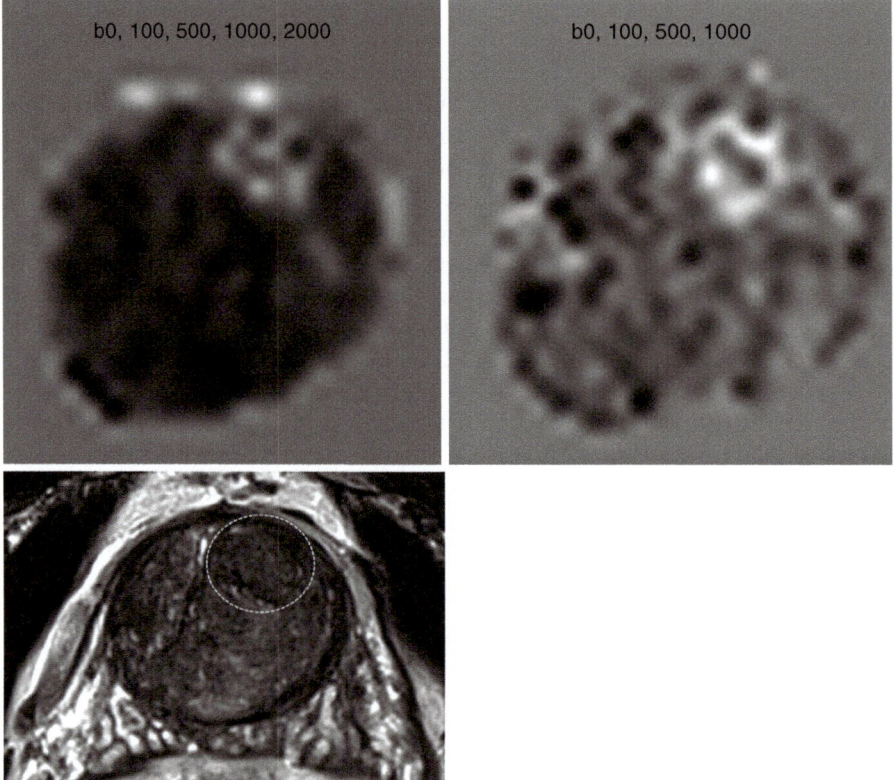

Fig. 1.9 Diffusion Kurtosis maps in prostate. Better discrimination between kurtotic areas (*dotted circle*) and non-kurtotic areas can be achieved when using *b* values higher than 1000 s/mm^2

Currently, these sequences are not available on clinical MR scanners, and further studies are needed to unveil in what circumstances these models will be adequate and whether they can be clinically useful.

1.6 Image Quality and Post-processing Aspects

The ADC value, derived from a mono-exponential model, depends on the signal fitting and the available SNR. The SNR itself depends on many parameters like the amplitude of the main field B0, the voxel size or section thickness, the acquisition duration via the number of signal averages and the number of phase-encoding steps. A high parallel imaging acceleration factor results in less image distortion; however, a too high acceleration factor leads to the failure of the parallel imaging reconstruction and degrades the image quality due to increased noise. In addition, small FOV should be avoided in combination with parallel imaging since they may result in back folding of tissues outside the FOV (Fig. 1.10).

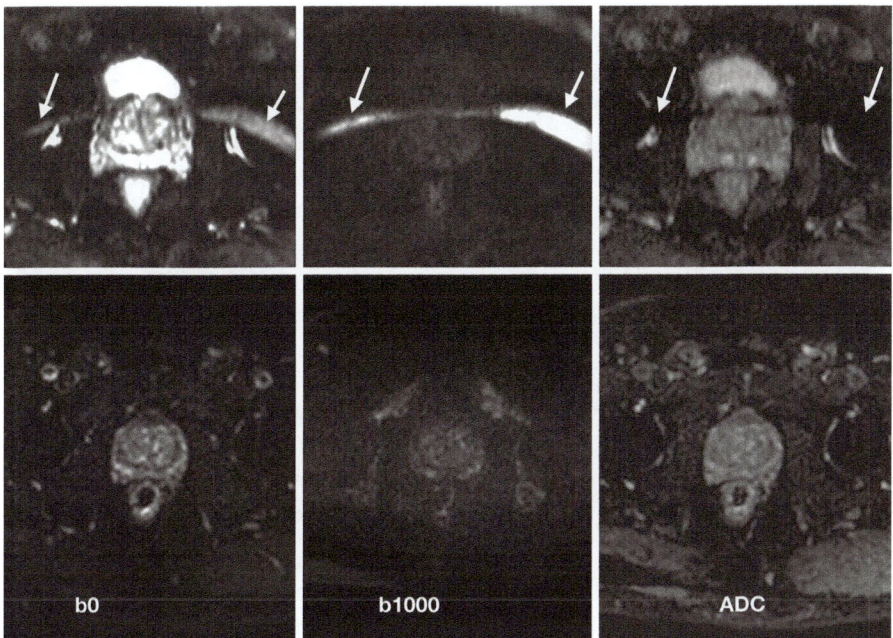

Fig. 1.10 Incomplete fat saturation and utilization of small FOVs together with parallel imaging algorithms may result in tissue back-folding artefacts (*upper row, arrows*). These artefacts can be eliminated by increasing the FOV and acquisition matrix to maintain high resolution (*lower row*)

Artefacts might also significantly influence the fit quality. The slope calculated by the linear regression, giving the ADC, will inevitably be influenced by the signal value measured for each point, especially the points corresponding to the highest b values because these have the most attenuated signal and lowest SNR and therefore are more prone to noise. The fit can be performed pixel by pixel to generate an ADC map but can also be based on ROI signal measurement, and of course the definition of the ROI (size, position, homogeneous region or not) plays a crucial role [22]. In principal, we can expect a better fit quality if an increasing number of b values are used, at the cost of a longer acquisition duration. At fixed b-value and diffusion direction, the acquisition might be repeated, providing an average from a higher number of samples. The number of b values might also be increased at acquisition; the choice of the b values involved in the fit will finally influence the ADC quantification (Fig. 1.11). In the clinical setting, a compromise must be found considering the number of slices, the spatial resolution and the scan time. Of course, a central question is whether the examination aims at lesion detection (ADC map with enough contrast between the lesion and the surrounding tissue) or aims at a precise quantification with low variability, required in the case of a longitudinal study meant to detect a change due to the natural evolution of the disease or being the signature of a response to a treatment.

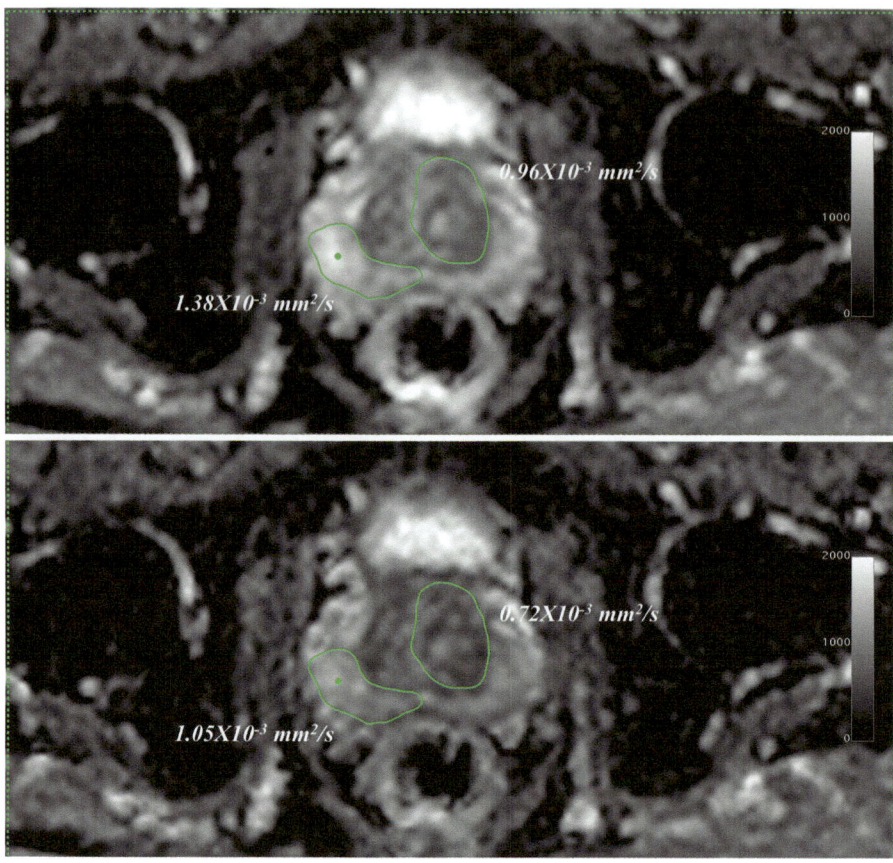

Fig. 1.11 ADC maps generated using b0, 50, 100, 150, 500 and 1000 s/mm² (*lower row*) and b0, 50, 100, 150, 500, 1000 and 1500 s/mm² (*upper row*)

Several studies have suggested the interest of using ADC histograms (Fig. 1.12) as a surrogate marker of treatment response in cancer [22–24] or to differentiate low-grade from high-grade clear-cell renal cell carcinoma [25].

Computer-aided diagnosis (CAD) systems have been proposed and tested for clinical use mainly in prostate with variable results [26–28]. CAD systems provide an integrated environment for the radiologist including lesion segmentation, motion correction, ADC- and DCE-related map generation, image co-registration and fusion between parametric maps and anatomical images (Fig. 1.13). Another more novel approach consists of analysing texture parameters of DWI (Fig. 1.14) or ADC maps [29, 30]. In 1979, Haralick stated that one of the most important sources of an analysed image region could be its texture [31]. Texture analysis studies the spatial relationships between grey levels describing pixels within a predefined region or volume of interest. One of the definitions of texture is the following: texture is a

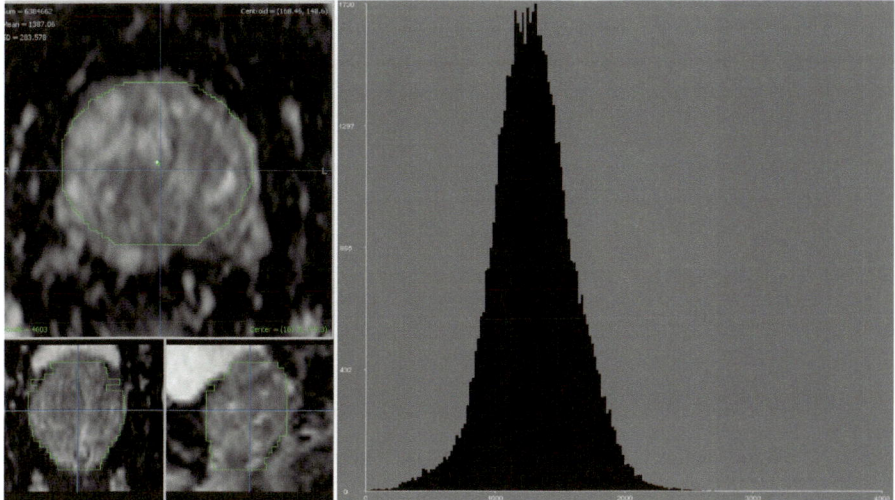

Fig. 1.12 Whole prostate ADC histogram is shown. Apart from visual inspection, it is possible to quantify several histogram metrics including min, max, median, mean, variance, skewness and kurtosis

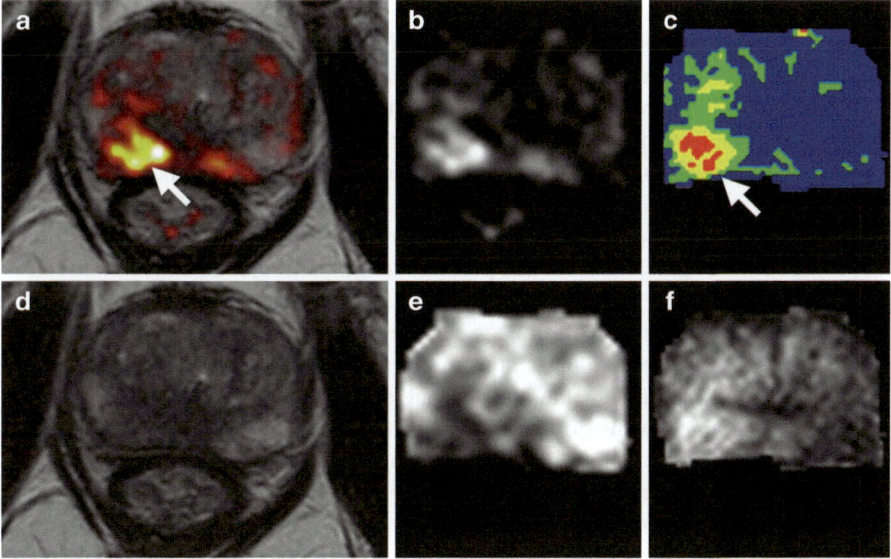

Fig. 1.13 CAD analysis on a patient with prostate cancer located in the right peripheral zone (*arrows*). DWI b1500 (**b**), ADC (**e**), DCE angiomaps (**c**), maximum enhancement (**f**) parametric maps are generated and co-registered with anatomical T2-weighted images (**d**), while image fusion between DWI b1500 and T2-weighted images results in better appreciation of the anatomic location of the lesion (**a**)

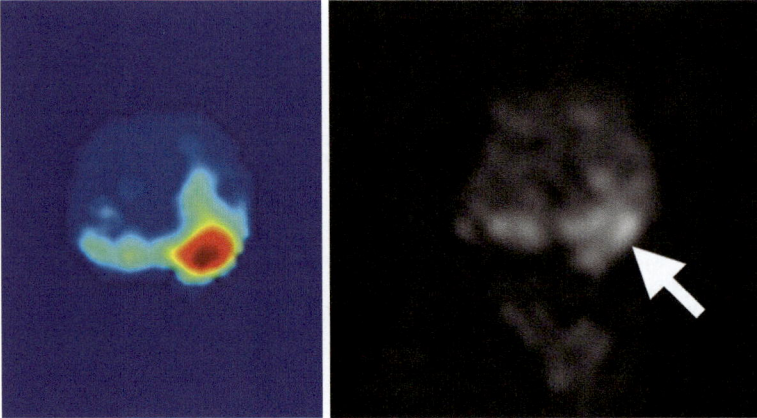

Fig. 1.14 Texture analysis on a patient with prostate cancer in the left peripheral zone (*arrow*). Entropy maps calculated on b1000 diffusion images are presenting the tumour with high values comparing to adjacent tissues (*red colour on the left image*)

regular repetition of an element or pattern on a surface with the characteristics of brightness, colour, size and/or shape. There are several sources of information related to texture including first-order statistics that describe the distribution of voxel intensities within the image region defined by the segmentation mask through commonly used and basic metrics. Among the latter are minimum, maximum, mean, standard deviation, median, skewness, kurtosis and others. Another layer of texture information is related to descriptors of the three-dimensional size and shape of the tumour region. Surface to volume ratio, compactness, elongation and sphericity are among them. Co-occurrence matrices quantify relationships between pairs of voxels. They are usually defined according to a given spatial direction and a given distance between the pairs of voxels. Run-length matrix (RLM) features are based on probabilities of pixel runs of each possible length, arranged in a certain direction [32]. Grey-level difference matrices (GLDM) are constructed with consideration of only the absolute values of differences between the grey levels of pixels, still considered in pairs [33]. Individual texture features or combinations of them are currently under investigation whether they can aid in several clinical problems including accurate lesion characterization, assessment of treatment response or stratification of different tumour subtypes with different prognosis. The combination of machine learning and texture analysis named under the term radiomics is a fast-developing area of research, which translates medical images into mineable data by extracting a large number of quantitative features that objectively define tumour intensity, shape, size and texture in a robust and reproducible way [34].

Conclusions

Diffusion-weighted imaging of the urogenital area is technically challenging due to the presence of physiologic motion (respiration, peristalsis), as well as the presence of air in the GI tract. In addition, the increased vascularity of the kidneys is responsible for ADC contamination with micro-perfusion effects; therefore more complex strategies need to be taken into consideration to minimize these problems. The hardware capabilities of the scanners, namely, the gradient performance and the presence of high-end RF coils, can significantly improve image quality and diagnostic accuracy.

References

1. Paul L. Sur la théorie du mouvement brownien. C R Acad Sci. 1908;146:530–2.
2. Albert E. Über die von der molekularkinetischen Theorie der Wärme geforderte Bewegung von in ruhenden Flüssigkeiten suspendierten Teilchen. Ann Phys. 1905;322(8):549–60.
3. White M, Dale A. Distinct effects of nuclear volume fraction and cell diameter on high b-value diffusion MRI contrast in tumours. Magn Reson Med. 2014;72:1435–43.
4. Gürses B, Kiliçkesmez O, Taşdelen N, Firat Z, Gürmen N. Diffusion tensor imaging of the kidney at 3 Tesla MRI: normative values and repeatability of measurements in healthy volunteers. Diagn Interv Radiol. 2011;17(4):317–22.
5. Quentin M, Pentang G, Schimmöller L, Kott O, Müller-Lutz A, Blondin D, Arsov C, Hiester A, Rabenalt R, Wittsack HJ. Feasibility of diffusional kurtosis tensor imaging in prostate MRI for the assessment of prostate cancer: preliminary results. Magn Reson Imaging. 2014;32(7):880–5.
6. Carr HY, Purcell EM. Effects of diffusion on free precession in nuclear magnetic resonance experiments. Phys Rev. 1954;94:630–8.
7. Torrey HC. Bloch equations with diffusion terms. Phys Rev. 1956;104(3):563–5.
8. Woessner DE. Effects of diffusion in nuclear magnetic resonance spin-echo experiments. J Chem Phys. 1961;34:2057–61.
9. Stejskal EO, Tanner JE. Spin diffusion measurements: spin echoes in the presence of a time-dependent field gradient. J Chem Phys. 1965;42(1):288–92.
10. Porter DA, Heidemann R. High resolution diffusion-weighted imaging using readout-segmented echo-planar imaging, parallel imaging and a two-dimensional navigator-based reacquisition. Magn Reson Med. 2009;62:468–75.
11. Le Bihan D, Breton E, Lallemand D, Aubin ML, Vignaud J, Laval-Jeantet M. Separation of diffusion and perfusion in intravoxel incoherent motion MR imaging. Radiology. 1988;168:497–505.
12. Ahlgren A, Knutsson L, Wirestam R, Nilsson M, Ståhlberg F, Topgaard D, Lasič S. Quantification of microcirculatory parameters by joint analysis of flow-compensated and non-flow-compensated intravoxel incoherent motion (IVIM) data. NMR Biomed. 2016;29:640–9.
13. Lemke A, Stieltjes B, Schad LR, Laun FB. Toward an optimal distribution of b values for intravoxel incoherent motion imaging. Magn Reson Imaging. 2011;29(6):766–76.
14. Wetscherek A, Stieltjes B, Laun FB. Flow-compensated intravoxel incoherent motion diffusion imaging. Magn Reson Med. 2015;74(2):410–9.
15. Döpfert J, Lemke A, Weidner A, Schad LR. Investigation of prostate cancer using diffusion-weighted intravoxel incoherent motion imaging. Magn Reson Imaging. 2011;29(8):1053–8.
16. van Baalen S, Leemans A, Dik P, Lilien MR, Ten Haken B, Froeling M. Intravoxel incoherent motion modeling in the kidneys: comparison of mono-, bi-, and triexponential fit. J Magn Reson Imaging. 2017;46(1):228–39.
17. Winfield JM, Orton MR, Collins DJ, Ind TE, Attygalle A, Hazell S, Morgan VA, deSouza NM. Separation of type and grade in cervical tumours using non-mono-exponential models of diffusion-weighted MRI. Eur Radiol. 2017;27(2):627–36.
18. Bennett KM, Schmainda KM, Bennett RT, Rowe DB, Lu H, Hyde JS. Characterization of continuously distributed cortical water diffusion rates with a stretched-exponential model. Magn Reson Med. 2003;50:727–34.

19. Jensen JH, Helpern JA, Ramani A, Lu H, Kaczynski K. Diffusional kurtosis imaging: the quantification of non-gaussian water diffusion by means of magnetic resonance imaging. Magn Reson Med. 2005;53:1432–40.
20. Panagiotaki E, Walker-Samuel S, Siow B, Johnson SP, Rajkumar V, Pedley RB, Lythgoe MF, Alexander DC. Noninvasive quantification of solid tumor microstructure using VERDICT MRI. Cancer Res. 2014;74(7):1902–12.
21. Nilsson M, Lätt J, van Westen D, Brockstedt S, Lasič S, Ståhlberg F, Topgaard D. Noninvasive mapping of water diffusional exchange in the human brain using filter-exchange imaging. Magn Reson Med. 2013;69(6):1573–81.
22. Kyriazi S, Collins DJ, Messiou C, Pennert K, Davidson RL, Giles SL, Kaye SB, Desouza NM. Metastatic ovarian and primary peritoneal cancer: assessing chemotherapy response with diffusion-weighted MR imaging—value of histogram analysis of apparent diffusion coefficients. Radiology. 2011;261(1):182–92.
23. Ueno Y, Lisbona R, Tamada T, Alaref A, Sugimura K, Reinhold C. Comparison of FDG PET metabolic tumour volume versus ADC histogram: prognostic value of tumour treatment response and survival in patients with locally advanced uterine cervical cancer. Br J Radiol. 2017;90(1075):20170035.
24. Wang F, Wang Y, Zhou Y, Liu C, Xie L, Zhou Z, Liang D, Shen Y, Yao Z, Liu J. Comparison between types I and II epithelial ovarian cancer using histogram analysis of monoexponential, biexponential, and stretched-exponential diffusion models. J Magn Reson Imaging. 2017.
25. Zhang YD, CJ W, Wang Q, Zhang J, Wang XN, Liu XS, Shi HB. Comparison of utility of histogram apparent diffusion coefficient and R2* for differentiation of low-grade from high-grade clear cell renal cell carcinoma. AJR Am J Roentgenol. 2015;205(2):193–201.
26. Rampun A, Zheng L, Malcolm P, Tiddeman B, Zwiggelaar R. Computer-aided detection of prostate cancer in T2-weighted MRI within the peripheral zone. Phys Med Biol. 2016;61(13):4796–825.
27. Giannini V, Mazzetti S, Vignati A, Russo F, Bollito E, Porpiglia F, Stasi M, Regge D. A fully automatic computer aided diagnosis system for peripheral zone prostate cancer detection using multi-parametric magnetic resonance imaging. Comput Med Imaging Graph. 2015;46(Pt 2):219–26.
28. Litjens GJ, Barentsz JO, Karssemeijer N, Huisman HJ. Clinical evaluation of a computer-aided diagnosis system for determining cancer aggressiveness in prostate MRI. Eur Radiol. 2015;25(11):3187–99.
29. Ueno Y, Forghani B, Forghani R, Dohan A, Zeng XZ, Chamming's F, Arseneau J, Fu L, Gilbert L, Gallix B, Reinhold C. Endometrial carcinoma: MR imaging-based texture model for preoperative risk stratification-A preliminary analysis. Radiology. 2017:161950.
30. Rozenberg R, Thornhill RE, Flood TA, Hakim SW, Lim C, Schieda N. Whole-tumor quantitative apparent diffusion coefficient histogram and texture analysis to predict gleason score upgrading in intermediate-risk 3 + 4 = 7 prostate cancer. AJR Am J Roentgenol. 2016;206(4):775–82.
31. Haralick RM, Shanmugam K, Dinstein I. Textural features for image classification. IEEE Trans Syst Man Cybern. 1973;3:610–21.
32. Galloway MM. Texture analysis using gray level run lengths. Comput Vision Graph Image Process. 1975;4(2):172–9.
33. Weszka JS, Dyer CR, Rosenfeld A. A comparative study of texture measures for terrain classification. IEEE Trans Syst Man Cybern. 1976;6:269–85.
34. Gillies RJ, Kinahan PE, Hricak H. Radiomics: images are more than pictures, they are data. Radiology. 2016;278(2):563–77.

Native and Transplanted Kidneys

2

Carlos Nicolau, Carmen Sebastià and Antonio Luna

Key Points
- DW—imaging can help in the early detection and grade of renal parenchymatous disease in CKD patients, having the potential to identify patients who will progress.
- DW—imaging is helpful for the diagnosis and follow-up of acute pyelonephritis with the advantage of the lack of ionising radiation and nephrotoxic contrast agents.
- DW—imaging is a promising tool for noninvasive assessment of allograft dysfunction in patients with renal transplantation.
- DW—imaging acquisition and sequence parameters of the kidneys have to be standardised and implemented, and it is still challenging to perform renal DTI in the clinical setting due to the long acquisition times and artefacts.

2.1 Introduction

Diffusion-weighted (DW) imaging is a magnetic resonance imaging (MRI) technique able to show molecular diffusion, represented by the Brownian motion of the spins in biological tissues [1]. DW imaging provides an indirect estimation of tissue cellularity and cell membrane integrity. In tissues in which the extracellular extravascular space is occupied, the motion of water molecules is restricted compared to

C. Nicolau (✉)
Radiology Department (Urogenital section), Hospital Clinic, Barcelona, Spain
e-mail: cnicolau@clinic.cat

C. Sebastià
Department of Radiology, Hospital Clinic of Barcelona, Barcelona, Spain

A. Luna
Scientific Director, Health Time, Jaén, Spain, Clinical Assistant Professor, Department of Radiology, University Hospitals of Cleveland, Case western Reserve University, Cleveland, OH, USA

© Springer International Publishing AG 2018
D. Akata, N. Papanikolaou (eds.), *Diffusion Weighted Imaging of the Genitourinary System*, https://doi.org/10.1007/978-3-319-69575-4_2

that of normal tissue [2]. DW imaging is measured by means of the apparent diffusion coefficient (ADC), although more advanced methods of analysis have also been applied exploring the non-Gaussian distribution of diffusion signal decay in the kidney [3, 4].

DW imaging has been proposed as an imaging biomarker in several tumour types in the brain and the body, including the kidney [1]. DW imaging and ADC mapping are well-established clinical tools for the characterisation and differentiation between benign and malignant renal masses. Moreover, DW imaging can help in the phenotyping of renal cell carcinoma, differentiating between clear cell, papillary and chromophobic subtypes and defining tumour aggressiveness [5].

DW imaging has also been proposed for the evaluation of diffuse and focal renal diseases. In this scenario, the use of functional MRI is attractive since morphological MRI can only detect advanced stages of disease. With the limited data available, DW imaging has shown a role in the detection and classification of renal impairment in normal and transplanted kidneys [6]. The major advantage of DW imaging in routine clinical practice is that this technique does not require the administration of intravenous contrast material, which is very interesting in patients with chronic kidney disease (CKD). Moreover, DW imaging does not use radiation as compared to other currently available functional techniques, and it can be easily implemented in clinical protocols. However, the use of DW imaging is limited by the lack of standardisation in clinical protocols and the method of quantification, as well as by the variation in ADC of the kidneys in the normal population [1, 6].

This chapter reviews the current knowledge of the application of DW imaging in the assessment of diffuse renal disease, enhancing the different acquisition approaches and quantification models that can be used to analyse diffusion signal decay.

2.2   Technical Aspects

2.2.1   Sequence Design

DW imaging of the kidneys needs to be performed using a surface phased-array coil. The greater the number of elements, the better the improvement in spatial resolution and the shorter the acquisition time. In addition, the use of 3T magnets allows acquisition with an increased SNR and thinner slice thickness [7]. These factors theoretically benefit the quantification of diffusion signal decay by reducing partial volume artefacts. However, 3T magnets increase geometric distortion and susceptibility artefacts, which may be limited with the use of multiple radiofrequency channels and advanced fat suppression techniques, such as gradient reversal.

2.2.2   Optimal *b* Values for Renal DW-MRI

In order to quantify the apparent diffusion coefficient (ADC), it is necessary to obtain at least a low and a high *b* value. The low *b* value is usually $b = 0$ s/mm^2 or

$b = 50$ s/mm^2 if the perfusion effect is to be minimised. The optimal high b value for kidneys is between 750 and 1000 s/mm^2. A higher number of b values acquired improve the fitting of the data for quantification of DW imaging. In order to appropriately calculate ADC in clinical practice, acquisitions are limited to 2–4 b values (i.e., 0, 50, 400 and 800 s/mm^2). The number of b values acquired can be increased if more advanced quantification models are applied. Intravoxel incoherent motion (IVIM) may require better sampling of the initial decay of diffusion signal related to microcirculation, with more b values acquired between 0 and 150 s/mm^2 [2]. In addition, to adequately calculate diffusion kurtosis imaging (DKI), b values >1500 s/mm^2 are necessary [8].

The greater the number of b values acquired, the longer the acquisition time. Therefore, to perform the quantification, the number of b values acquired and adequate fitting of the data must be balanced. It should also be taken into account that the SNR of the b value decreases as the b value increases. In this way, with modern scanners, it is possible to specify a different number of means for each b value. A common strategy is to increase the number of means obtained for b values >500 s/mm^2, with a penalty in acquisition time [5].

There are no standardised protocols for DW imaging of the kidneys. The authors use a six b value protocol (0, 50, 100, 500, 1000 and 1500 s/mm^2) which allows any method of quantification to be applied. With the monoexponential model, only b values between 50 and 1000 s/mm^2 are included in the calculation.

2.2.3   Quantification

Quantification of the diffusion signal is necessary in order to characterise and differentiate normal and pathological tissues. With the use of quantitative biomarkers, the common pitfalls of DW imaging, such as the T2 shine-through effect, can be reduced. Tissues with long T2 values may show high signal intensity with high b values, which do not represent true restriction of free water motion. ADC allows tissues with the T2 shine-through effect to be differentiated from restrictive lesions, as the first show high signal intensity and the latter hypointensity on ADC maps [1, 9]. In addition, ADC can show a reduced signal not representing true restriction of diffusion in tissues with very short T2 or T2* values, as in fibrosis or subacute haemorrhage. This pitfall is known as the T2 blackout effect and occurs in lesions displaying low signal intensities at both high b values and low ADC values related to magnetic susceptibility artefacts [10].

The kidney is a highly perfused organ with a complex microstructure. Although in the clinical setting quantification of DW imaging is usually performed using the monoexponential model, other models that explore the non-Gaussian distribution of diffusion signal have been proposed for better analysis of the diffusion signal in the kidneys [6]. ADC assumes a Gaussian distribution of free water motion, which is not the best approach for in vivo assessment of kidneys, as tissue complexity can hinder water diffusion. Thus, non-Gaussian models such as IVIM, DKI and the stretched-exponential model (SEM), can analyse the in vivo deviation of diffusion signal from the monoexponential model better (Fig. 2.1).

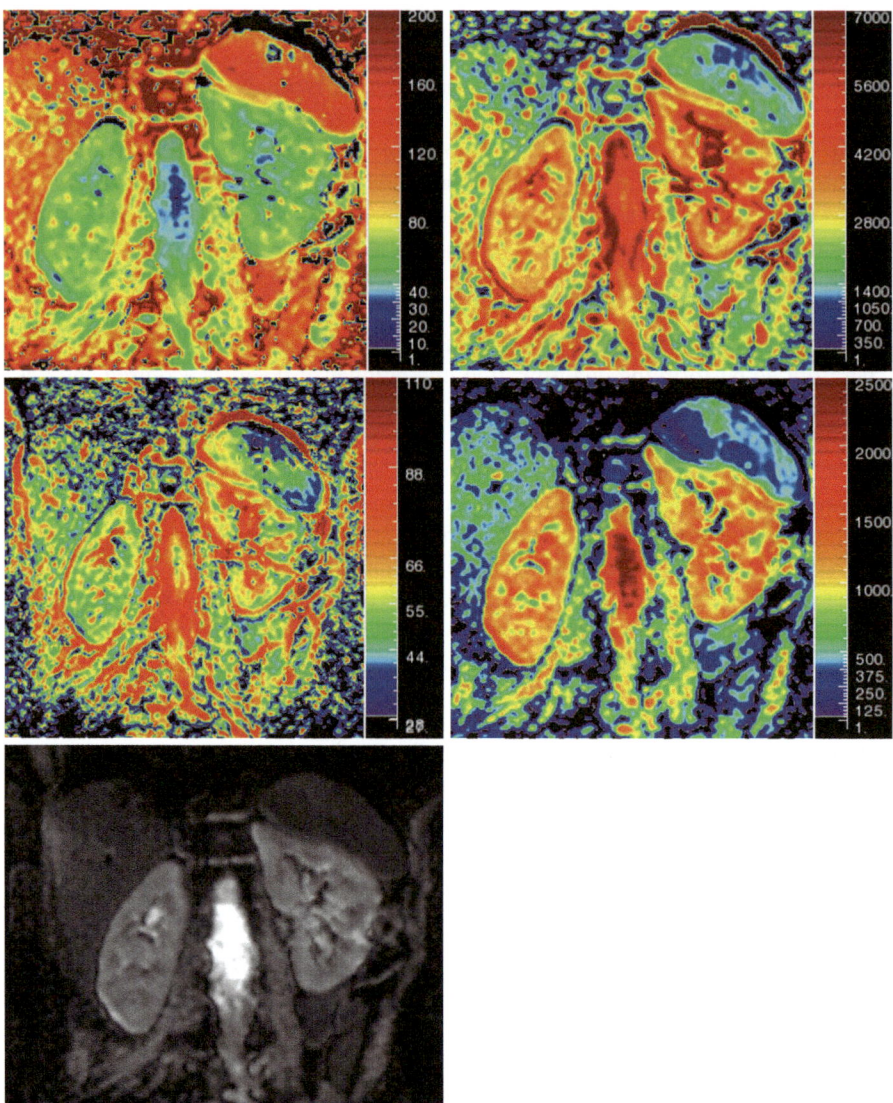

Fig. 2.1 Acquisition and quantification of DW images of normal kidneys. A coronal SS-SE-EPI diffusion-weighted sequence with ten b values between b0 and b1500 s/mm^2 (1) allows differentiation of diffusion signal decay of both the cortex (2) and medulla (3). Different models of quantification can also be applied, such as monoexponential, biexponential and DKI. Parametric maps of the parameters derived are shown as follows: (4) ADC, (5) IVIM-derived D, (6) IVIM-derived perfusion fraction, (7) diffusion kurtosis and (8) kurtosis

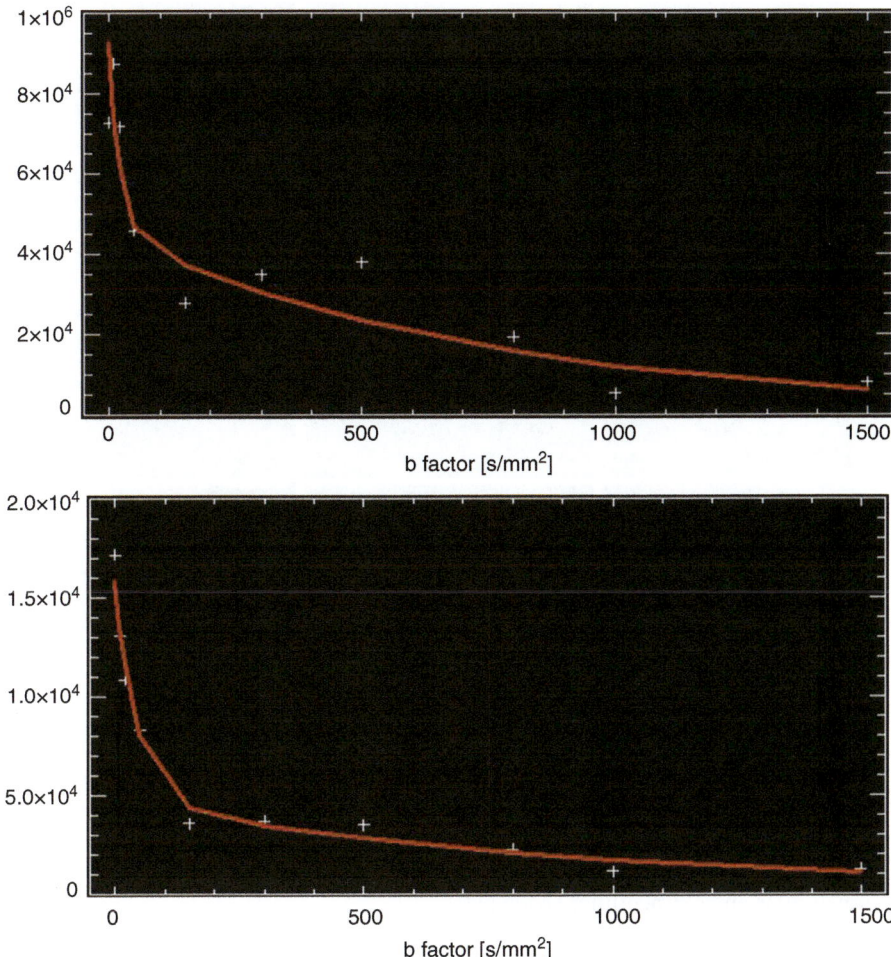

Fig. 2.1 (continued)

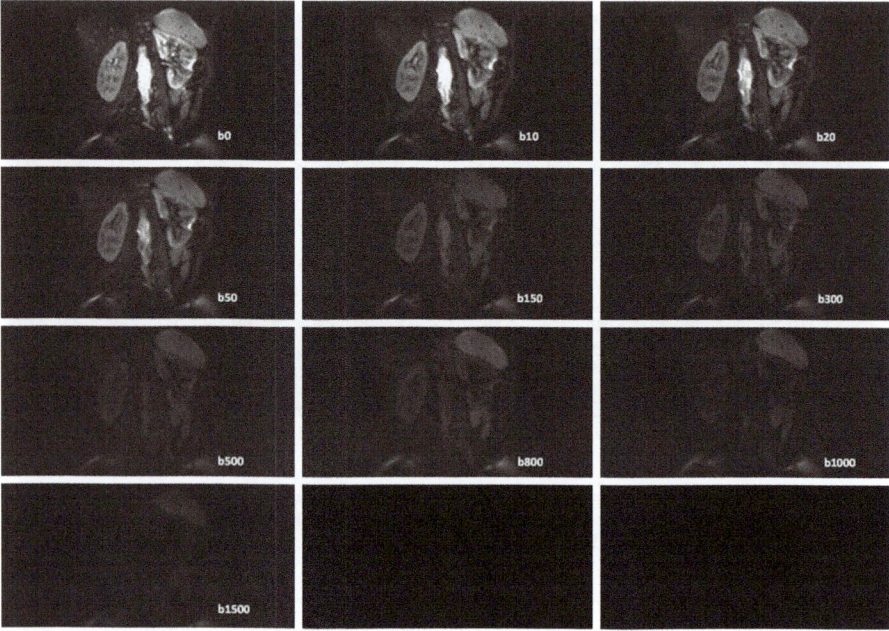

Fig. 2.1 (continued)

Monocompartmental model: By acquiring only one low b value (between 0 and 100 s/mm^2) and one high b value between 800 and 1000 s/mm^2, it is possible to quantify free water movement using ADC. Here, when the b value increases, ADC represents the exponential decay of diffusion, as the average of a single water compartment, which in most tissues corresponds to the movement of free water in the extravascular and extracellular space [1].

ADC represents the absolute line slope of exponential decrease of signal intensities in diffusion images. However, the definition of a threshold value to differentiate normal renal parenchyma and pathological lesions is not possible due to differences in sequence design and the set of b values used for calculation.

Bicompartmental model or IVIM: In well-perfused organs, such as the liver, pancreas, kidney and prostate, diffusion signal decay follows biphasic kinetics. First, there is rapid decay at low b values (between 0 and 150 s/mm^2), which corresponds to microcirculation, and slower decay at higher b values owing to water diffusion inside the tissues. This model was described by Le Bihan, and it assumes that water movements not only occur in the interstitial spaces but also in vascular spaces [11]. In the bicompartmental model, diffusion and perfusion measurements are heavily dependent on the choice of b values. Typically, several b values lower than and greater than 150 s/mm^2 are acquired, although faster methods, involving only three b values, have also been proposed [12].

$$\frac{Sb}{S_0} = (1-f)\exp(-bD) + f\exp\left[-b\left(D+D^*\right)\right]$$

IVIM has shown a potential role in differentiating enhanced from non-enhanced renal lesions with better accuracy than ADC and with a positive correlation of perfusion fraction with a dynamic contrast-enhanced (DCE) MRI-related parameter, known as percent enhancement. These data open the door for the assessment of renal lesion vascularity without the use of gadolinium chelates [4]. IVIM has also been used to assess functional changes in normal kidneys and in renal allografts [13]. In animal models, IVIM has shown promising results in the evaluation of contrast-induced injury and renal fibrosis [14]. Furthermore, interesting results have been obtained in the clinical setting using IVIM to assess kidney function, particularly vascular-derived IVIM parameters [15].

Diffusion kurtosis analysis: This model can assess the non-Gaussian distribution of the diffusion signal, which becomes apparent with high b values >1500 s/mm^2. This effect is due to a new compartment of water with very slow motion, located inside the cells and is also related to the cell membrane [8].

$$\frac{S_b}{S_0} = \exp\left(-bD + \frac{b_2 D^2 K}{6}\right)$$

Kurtosis (K or K^{app}) is a dimensionless parameter representing apparent diffusion kurtosis and does not have a direct biophysical basis. It has been correlated with tissue complexity, due to the interaction of water with membranes and intracellular components, although it is also influenced by other extracellular factors.

DKI has shown to be feasible in the normal human kidney [3, 16], differentiating renal medulla and cortex; however, clinical studies to demonstrate its applications are still lacking.

Stretched-exponential model: This model has recently been introduced in body applications. It allows both Gaussian and non-Gaussian diffusion to be explored by defining a single additional stretching term, which may represent an approximation to either intravoxel diffusion heterogeneity or non-Gaussian diffusion. This model provides new biomarkers such as the distributed diffusion coefficient (DDC) and α, the water heterogeneity index which evaluates the deviation of signal attenuation from the monoexponential behaviour [6]. The stretched-exponential model has been tested in kidney tumour characterisation, showing an advantage over conventional quantitative diffusion parameters in the differentiation between clear cell renal cell carcinoma and minimal fat angiomyolipoma [17].

Texture-based analysis is able to identify imaging texture features, more commonly tactile, which describe and quantify the spatial distribution and heterogeneity of voxel intensities. Initial experiences used histogram analysis of ADC for the assessment of renal tumours [18, 19]. This type of analysis is very promising as it may provide additional quantitative metrics beyond ADC, reflecting tissue heterogeneity.

2.2.4 Diffusion Tensor Imaging (DTI)

Molecular diffusion in a tissue is a three-dimensional process, which can be expressed as a vectorial property depending on the direction of the diffusion gradients applied. If multidirectional (at least six directions) diffusion information is

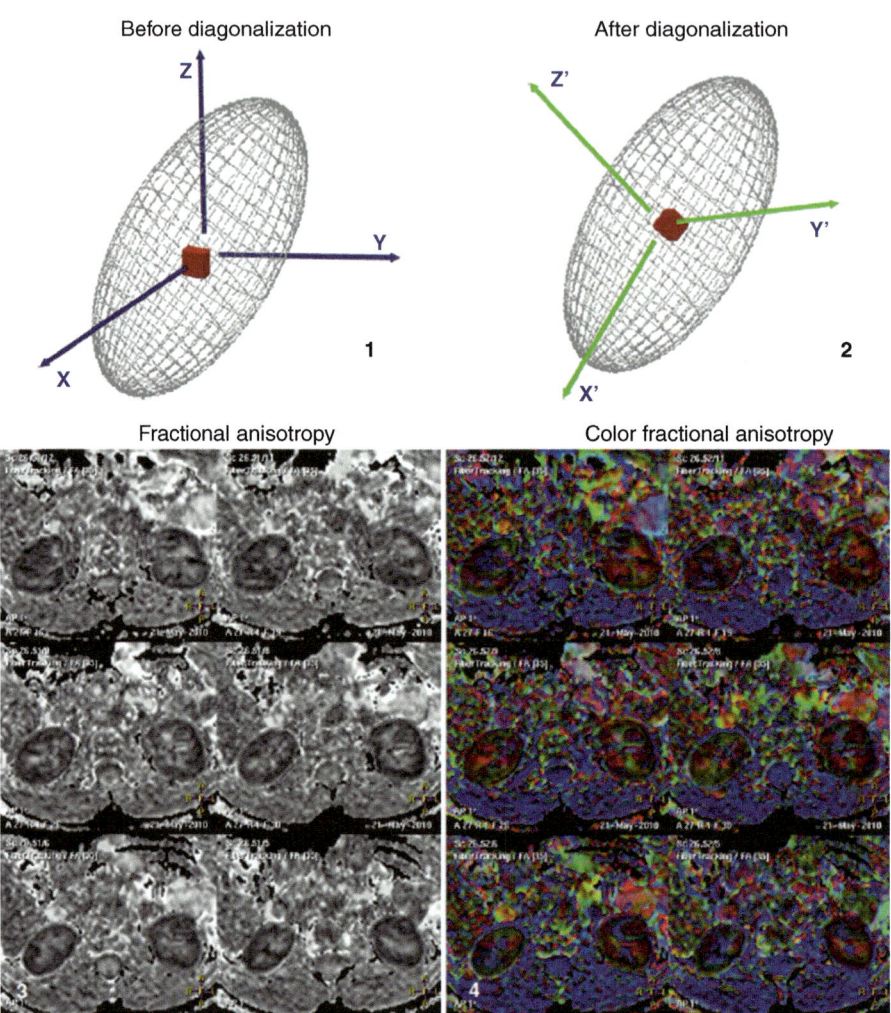

Fig. 2.2 FA and coloured FA. The diffusion signal from a DW imaging study depends on the direction of the diffusion gradients applied. Normally, the diffusion information in one direction is affected by the diffusion information in the other directions. This effect can be seen in the diffusion space as an ellipsoid effect (1), demonstrating the relationship of one diffusion direction with the other directions. If the correlation between different diffusion directions disappears, by means of a diagonalization of the diffusion tensor, a new reference system is obtained (2) in which only three completely independent directions are shown (X′, Y′ and Z′) in the main direction of the axis of the diffusion ellipsoid. These independent directions represent the direction of maximum diffusion. (3) The FA map of an axial acquisition of the kidneys at six different consecutive levels obtained from a DW acquisition with six different diffusion directions is shown as well as (4) a coloured version of this FA map in which the coloured information represents the most important diffusion direction: blue for the FH (foot to head) direction, red for the RL (right to left) direction and green for the AP (anterior to posterior) direction. Reprinted with permission from Sánchez-González J and Luna A. Quantification and postprocessing of DWI. In: Luna A, Ribes R, Soto JA. Diffusion MRI outside the brain. Springer 2012

obtained using DTI, it is possible to obtain detailed information of tissue anisotropy [20, 21], which is related to the microstructure of the kidney [22, 23] (Fig. 2.2). Quantitative-derived biomarkers such as fraction anisotropy (FA), mean diffusivity (MD), axial diffusivity (AD) and radial diffusivity (RD) can be used to differentiate normal and pathological kidneys, reflecting the status of renal function. MD reflects the average of ADC in all three diffusion directions. AD is related to the longitudinal direction of the tensor, and RD reflects the radial direction. All these parameters are related to diffusional anisotropy and FA.

The distribution of extracellular water, particularly at the renal medulla, between tubules, creates an anisotropic water movement that can be evaluated using multiple diffusion directions. Also, DTI tractography can reflect the water pathways in which the water moves easily, thereby reflecting the radial orientation towards the pelvis of tubules, collecting ducts and vessels. In the normal kidney, renal tractography can show the tracks with a radial arrangement and convergence into pyramids, which lose this radial distribution and reduce the number of tracks in cases of disease [22, 23].

DTI has shown promise in the evaluation of the renal microstructure in normal kidney (Fig. 2.3). Furthermore, quantitative-derived biomarkers can reflect the severity of renal function damage.

However, it is still challenging to perform renal DTI in the clinical setting due to the long acquisition times. High-resolution kidney DTI can be carried out using multichannel radiofrequency coils and parallel imaging. Currently, the use of 3T magnets is preferred, as they have shown an improved SNR and CNR in comparison to 1.5T magnets [24]. Moreover, 3T acquisitions allow the acquisition time to be shortened and the number of obtained diffusion directions to be increased.

2.3 Healthy Kidney

MRI demonstrates detailed anatomy of the kidney and urinary tract with the capacity to differentiate distinct intrarenal regions such as the cortex and medulla. The combination of T1- and T2-weighted sequences with DW imaging provides not only morphological but also qualitative and quantitative functional information of the kidney. In T1-weighted images, MRI demonstrates a higher signal intensity of the renal cortex than the medulla. On the contrary, in T2-weighted images, MRI shows poor distinction of corticomedullary contrast.

Several studies have evaluated kidney diffusion in healthy kidneys. In DW imaging sequences and the corresponding ADC map, both healthy kidneys may show symmetrical and almost homogeneous signal parenchyma. However, the ADC of the cortex is higher than that of the medulla [25–28], and there is a positive correlation between the ADCs and split GFR [29]. MRI techniques such as IVIM imaging have been incorporated in the study of the kidney to estimate the contribution of perfusion and diffusion to the total ADC value, and it has been found that the FA value of normal cortex is significantly lower than that of the medulla [25, 26]. Differences between the cortex and medulla can be explained by differences in tissue architecture

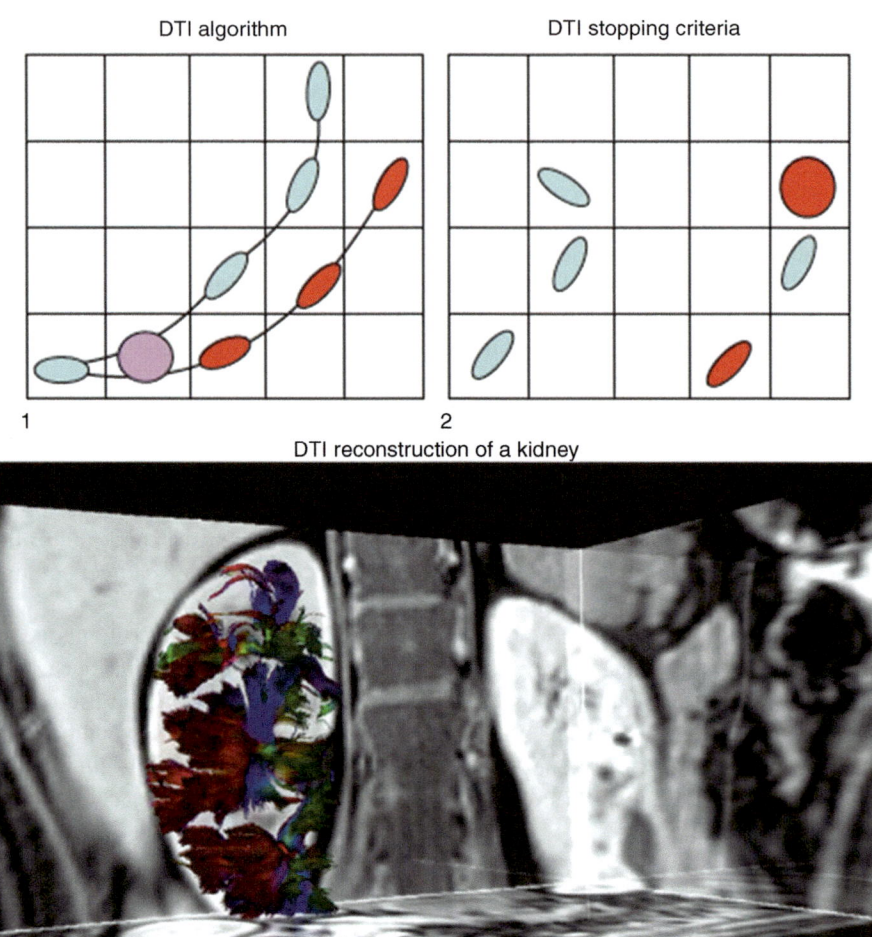

Fig. 2.3 DTI of a normal kidney. Following the ellipsoid description, the main axis of the ellipsoid represents the main diffusion direction in the voxel (coinciding with the direction of the fibres). The eccentricity of the ellipsoid provides information about the degree of anisotropy. In the theoretical case of a tissue with a completely isotropic diffusion, the ellipsoid becomes a perfect sphere. If this ellipsoid is built by all the pixels in an image, then it is possible to link these pixels where the main diffusivity direction is equivalent (1) in order to build the most suitable pathway of a ROI or to link the pixels between two different ROIs. This information among pixels can be linked following some rules (2). It is not possible to establish a pathway with an angular change higher than certain limits, while it is possible to link different consecutive pixels until a non-anisotropic region is reached (3). In the DTI reconstruction of a kidney, the water pathway has been estimated following the theoretical path from the cortex to the medulla, with images representing the pathways of the renal collecting system. The colour of the pathways follows the same code described in the previous coloured FA map. Reprinted with permission from Sánchez-González J and Luna A. Quantification and postprocessing of DWI. In: Luna A, Ribes R, Soto JA. Diffusion MRI outside the brain. Springer 2012

and perfusion, because renal blood flow is high at the cortex to optimise glomerular filtration and reabsorption of solute while blood flow at the medulla is low to enhance urinary concentration [30]. Hydration is one of the physiological conditions that has been shown to increase global ADC [31, 32], but in a recent study by Wang et al., the ADC and FA values in different hydration states did not significantly differ [25]. These discrepancies of data among studies can be explained by the different b values used, as well as the difficulty in differentiating between the cortex and medulla in low-spatial-resolution DW-MRI sequences which results in difficulties in ROI positioning. Up to now, there is no consensus about the normal range of ADCs and the optimum choice of b values for renal studies, with high differences of the b values used and ADCs values between authors ranging from 1.55×10^{-3} mm^2/s to 5.76×10^{-3} mm^2/s [33]. Thoeny et al. suggest the use of ten b values including several low values to allow biexponential fitting with separation of perfusion and diffusion influences [33]. Using this approach they obtained ADC values of 2.03×10^{-3} mm^2/s at the cortex and ADC values of 1.87×10^{-3} mm^2/s at the medulla [26]. Recently, DTI has been described as a useful tool to show the distribution and direction of water molecule diffusion reflecting the integrity of the structure of the renal parenchyma and the differences between the medulla and cortex as the medulla is anisotropic with a radial orientation of the vessels and tubules [34, 35].

2.4   Clinical Applications

Most renal parenchymal diseases including acute and chronic renal failure, renal ischaemia and inflammatory disease are associated with changes in the tissue architecture that can restrict water diffusion. Therefore, qualitative and quantitative parameters of DW-MRI can be used for the diagnosis and follow-up of these renal diseases.

2.4.1   Evaluation of Diffuse Renal Disease

CKD, also known as chronic kidney failure, is a public health problem worldwide, with an increasing incidence and prevalence of CKD patients requiring replacement therapy, with poor outcomes and high cost. CKD is defined as decreased kidney function caused by a long-standing renal parenchymal disease shown by glomerular filtration rate (GFR) of less than 60 mL/min/1.73 m^2 or markers of kidney damage, or both, that is present for 3 or more months, regardless of the underlying cause [36]. Hypertension and diabetes constitute 60% of the cases, but a variety of different diseases such as glomerulonephritis, polycystic kidney disease, obstructive uropathy and pyelonephritis can cause chronic renal damage. The common pathological manifestation of CKD is renal fibrosis which is characterised by the development of tubular atrophy, interstitial fibrosis and glomerulosclerosis due to unsuccessful wound healing of kidney tissue after sustained chronic injury [36]. Fibrotic burden is considered an important predictor of renal outcome [37], and its diagnosis is currently obtained by percutaneous biopsy. However, biopsies have a significant risk of bleeding, and sometimes the biopsy samples are not representative of the real burden of fibrosis due to its possible heterogeneous distribution. Therefore, noninvasive assessment of CKD would be very useful, particularly in early stages of the disease when renal function is not significantly reduced as well as for monitoring the progression of CKD and the effects of novel therapies. The estimated GFR (eGFR) obtained from serum creatinine is the most commonly used indicator of renal function. However, it assesses overall kidney function without providing independent information of each kidney. In addition, it is not considered a good indicator of the early stages of renal dysfunction. Regarding the usefulness of imaging modalities, no specific imaging features for CKD have been described, although several signs including thinning and irregularity of the renal cortex and loss of corticomedullary differentiation (CMD) are well known. Most of these findings are unrelated to the type of underlying disease and can be detected using ultrasound (US), computed tomography (CT) or MRI. However, certain findings may be correlated with the aetiology of kidney disease, including bilaterally small kidneys with thinned cortices suggestive of parenchymatous disease such as glomerulonephritis, unilateral small kidney suggestive of renal arterial disease, clubbed calyces and cortical scars suggestive of reflux with chronic infection or ischaemia and enlarged cystic kidneys suggestive of cystic kidney disease. With MRI, the loss of CMD is secondary to the decrease of signal intensity within the cortex or an increase within the medulla and correlates with the presence of cortical oedema, decreased tubular flow and accumulation of proteinaceous or bloody material in the medulla. Another MRI sign of CKD is delayed and decreased rate of medullary enhancement [38] secondary to the delayed elimination of gadolinium that also correlates with obstruction of tubules by inflammatory debris, oedema or leakage of contrast agent caused by tubular damage.

A variety of DW imaging techniques have been described in the noninvasive assessment of CKD, with promising results, having the potential to identify patients who will progress and who might require kidney replacement therapy in the future [37]. Several studies have evaluated DW-MRI in the evaluation of renal function and as a biomarker in the follow-up of renal disease [26, 29, 39–41]. The majority of studies have shown a reduction of ADC values that can be attributed to reduced water reabsorption or renal fibrosis restricting water diffusion [42–44]. In addition, an inverse correlation has been shown between the degree of renal involvement and ADC values, with ADC values being lower when the disease is worse. This correlation can help in the early detection and grade of renal parenchymatous disease [39, 40]. A few studies have also investigated the usefulness of the IVIM technique (with its ability to separate molecular diffusion from capillary perfusion) and DTI in CKD. Initial data support a reduction of cortical and medullary FA values in patients with CKD in comparison to healthy subjects, demonstrating a positive correlation with the estimated GFR and a negative correlation with tubulointerstitial injury and glomerular lesions [44]. Thus, DTI may be used for early detection of renal damage in patients with glomerulonephritis and diabetic nephropathy [45–48]. In a recent study, Ichikawa et al. found significantly lower cortical ADC, D^* and D values and lower medullary D and D^* in patients with renal dysfunction (with eGFR ranges lower than 80 mL/min) compared to a control group with normal renal function (with eFGR>80 mL/min) [49]. In another recent study, Wang et al. described similar results using DTI with a decrease in ADC and FA values that correlated with the GFR reflecting the severity of renal damage [44]. This positive correlation was also demonstrated by Liu et al. [48]. Interestingly, in patients with CKD, the numbers of radially oriented collecting tubules were shortened and reduced in the DTT maps. However, the study by Wang et al. only allowed the diagnosis of moderate to advanced renal damage, being unable to differentiate between healthy and mild stage CKD kidneys [44]. This limitation was also found in the recent study of Bane et al. who evaluated renal IVIM-DW imaging parameters using 16 b values in a group of 30 patients with liver disease; most patients presented normal kidney function ($n = 26$) or mildly impaired renal function, with an eGFR between 40 mL/min/1.73 m^2 and 60 mL/min/1.73 m^2 ($n = 4$). Cortical ADC and perfusion fraction (PF) were significantly higher than in the medulla. However, none of the IVIM-DW imaging parameters significantly correlated with eGFR [28].

2.4.2 Renal Artery Stenosis

Renal artery stenosis (RAS) is the most common primary renal artery disease with 90% of the cases being secondary to atherosclerosis. Significant RAS compromises renal blood flow, leading to hypoxia, inflammation and microvascular injury, impairing GFR and inducing renovascular hypertension and ischaemic nephropathy. Ischaemic nephropathy is defined as the deterioration of renal function that can arise due to haemodynamically significant RAS in both kidneys or to a solitary functioning kidney or a kidney providing the majority of the GFR. Ischaemic nephropathy is potentially reversible, but without treatment interstitial fibrosis may develop, leading to CKD and being found in approximately 15–20% of patients with CKD older than 50 years of age [50].

CT and MR angiography (MRA) have a good, comparable accuracy in the diagnosis of RAS, being better than Doppler US [51–53]. Nonetheless, MRA has several drawbacks including an overlooking of the degree of stenosis and the presence of artefacts when evaluating stented vessels. Another problem with MRA is the risk of nephrogenic systemic fibrosis in patients with severe kidney failure, although the newer cyclic gadolinium contrast agents are much safer. On the contrary, MRI has some advantages such as non-contrast MRA using rapid sequences that can allow the detection of arterial flow against the tissue without movement or slow venous flow. Indeed, MRI has demonstrated comparable accuracy to that of contrast MRA in the diagnosis of RAS [54, 55]. Moreover, MRI can assess the haemodynamic significance of RAS with time-resolved MRI flow measurements [56].

With respect to treatment, it has been accepted that the blood pressure can be well controlled by medical treatment without the need for revascularization; however, management of ischaemic nephropathy is difficult since only a minority of patients with this disease benefit from revascularization. Therefore, the identification of predictive markers of treatment success or progression of ischaemia is essential. The resistive index (RI) using Doppler US has been postulated as a good predictive marker of treatment success as it has been shown to be an indirect sign of kidney fibrosis or atrophy. There is a direct relationship between the RI and histopathologic changes [57]; an RI > 0.8 is considered a reliable value to identify patients with RAS in whom renal function, blood pressure or kidney survival will not improve following angioplasty or surgery [58]. Other markers such as a reduction of GFR, anatomical progression of RAS, kidney size <9 cm and a renal biopsy with tubulointerstitial atrophy are also predictive factors of ischaemia progression and bad response to revascularization in RAS.

Functional MRI can help in the evaluation of changes secondary to RAS as has been described in a very recent study performed using magnetization transfer MRI in a mice model [59]. In the stenotic kidney, the median magnetization transfer ratio showed progressive increases in the cortex and medulla from baseline to 6 weeks after RAS, respectively, accompanied by a progressive loss in renal volume, blood flow, oxygenation and perfusion demonstrated by arterial spin labelling. There are also indirect signs such as asymmetry of renal enhancement and excretion as well as differences in the degree of renal perfusion and in the degree of medullary oxygenation. Regarding DW imaging, kidneys with RAS show lower ADCs than kidneys without stenosis [60], with a linear correlation between ADCs and the GFR [29]. Ebrahimi et al. evaluated whether IVIM analysis could detect early morphological and functional changes in swine kidneys with RAS [61]. In this study, ADC and the IVIM parameter diffusivity (Dt that is usually linked to morphological changes) correlated inversely with the degree of cortical and medullary fibrosis and directly with GFR. Moreover, the IVIM parameter flow-dependent pseudo-diffusivity (Dp that has shown to be sensitive to both vascular blood and tubular fluid velocities) correlated directly with the histological tubular injury score, which established tubular morphological alterations [61]. Interestingly, morphological and functional alterations could be adequately depicted using the relative simplicity of the analysis of ADC.

DW-MRI has also been described in the evaluation of microvascularization in other kidney diseases, reflecting segmental vascular changes. Mishima et al. described the use of DW-MRI in a patient with segmental renal ischaemia secondary to an occlusion of the renal artery and segmental hypoperfusion [62]. DW-MRI identified cortical areas of restriction correlating with the segmental ischaemia without the administration of contrast media. Another described indication of DW-MRI is sickle cell anaemia which is frequently manifested with a vaso-occlusive crisis secondary to the obstruction of the microcirculation by sickled red blood cells causing ischaemic injury. In a very recent study, the IVIM-DW imaging technique was used to calculate cellular integrity (D) and local perfusion (D^* and F) during a vaso-occlusive crisis, and these three parameters were significantly altered in medullary and cortical areas during these crises [63].

2.4.3 Excretory Tract Obstruction

Dilatation of the collecting system is a common finding in some situations such as pregnancy and renal transplantation. Imaging techniques are used to differentiate a physiologically dilated collecting system and pathological obstruction due to urolithiasis, inflammatory disease or stenosis related to ureteral ischaemia (in the case of transplanted kidneys). Another clinical manifestation of excretory tract obstruction is the presence of acute flank pain with a negative US study that does not necessarily exclude obstruction, since dilatation of the excretory tract secondary to a ureteral lithiasis is not always identified in the early phases of its development. Therefore, functional imaging techniques such as DW imaging have been advocated to determine the functional significance of hydronephrosis.

Regarding DW-MRI, obstructive pyelocaliectasis has not been associated with changes in ADC values. Bozgeyik et al. found no significant differences between the ADC values of early phases of kidney obstruction compared to normal kidneys in a group of 26 patients with acute dilatation of the pelvicalyceal system due to uroli- thiasis (Fig. 2.4) [64]. This finding is in concordance with the study by Thoeny et al. in which no significant differences were observed between ADC values in either the medulla or the cortex in obstructed and non-obstructed kidneys [65]. However, dif- ferences were found on separating the contribution of microperfusion and diffusion

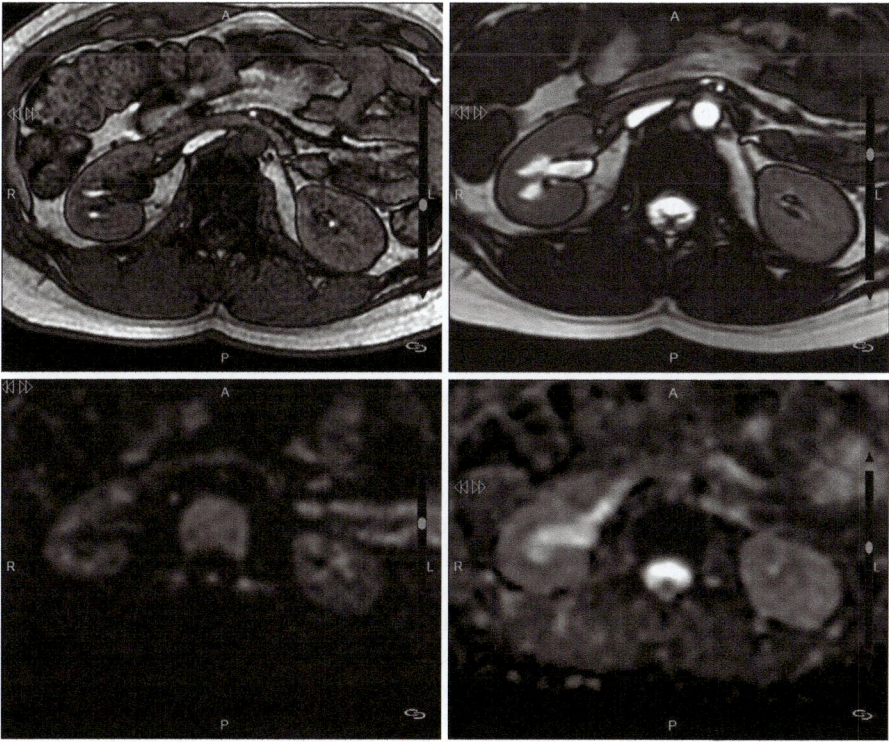

Fig. 2.4 Calculus in the right distal ureter of a 22-year-old woman (not shown). Transverse T1 (1), T2 (2), DWI with high b value = 1000 (3) and ADC map estimated (4) in the midpole of the kid- neys. Morphological sequences and ADC map showed mild dilatation of the right side of the excretory tract; however, there was no visible difference in the renal parenchyma intensity between the two kidneys

to total diffusion. In this way, the ADC D values (the diffusion coefficient) in the medulla of both the obstructed and the non-obstructed kidneys were significantly higher compared with those in control subjects. In addition, the PF of the obstructed kidneys was significantly lower in the cortex and slightly lower in the medulla.

Another important clinical problem is the differentiation between pyonephrosis and hydronephrosis as the first requires urgent drainage. In this scenario, DW-MRI can help in the differentiation, with pyonephrotic kidneys presenting lower ADC values than hydronephrotic kidneys [66, 67].

2.4.4   Renal Infection

Acute pyelonephritis is a bacterial or fungal infection resulting in inflammation of the renal parenchyma and collecting system. Imaging studies are indicated in patients in whom conventional treatment has failed (patients who remain febrile after 72 h of appropriate antibiotic therapy), those who have recurrent or unusually severe symptoms or certain groups of patients with a high risk of complications. Imaging techniques to study pyelonephritis usually require the administration of contrast agents that allow the detection of linear bands of alternating hyper- and hypoattenuation orientated parallel to the axes of the tubules and collecting ducts, secondary to alternation of normal and obstructed tubules with inflammatory cells and debris. In septic patients, decreased renal perfusion is considered to play a major role in the pathogenesis of acute kidney injury but also other mechanisms such as the response of the tubular cells to an injurious inflammatory signal [68] and microvascular dysfunction and heterogeneity in local renal blood flow [69] resulting in areas of hypoperfusion and hypoxia. In addition, enhanced imaging allows the detection of renal and perirenal abscesses that present as non-enhancing fluid collections that may show an enhanced rim. DW-MRI offers the possibility to achieve the diagnosis of pyelonephritis without using ionising radiation or contrast media [70–73]. The regions affected by pyelonephritis present higher signal intensity in images with high b values, whereas the corresponding ADC maps show areas of low signal intensity. Rathod SB et al. showed that DW-MRI had a higher sensitivity of 95.3% compared to that of non-contrast (66.7%) and contrast-enhanced CT (88.1%) in the diagnosis of pyelonephritis [74]. Areas of nephritis had significantly lower ADCs ($P < 0.001$) than the normal renal cortical parenchyma. In addition, renal abscesses had significantly lower ADCs ($P < 0.001$) than areas of nephritis. These results are in concordance with the study of Faletti et al. that found agreement of 94.3% between contrast-enhanced MRI and DW imaging in the diagnosis of acute pyelonephritis [75]. Due to its high accuracy, of also close to 95% in the study by De Pascale et al. [70] and lack of radiation, DWI is recommended not only for the diagnosis but also for the follow-up of pyelonephritis (Fig. 2.5) and should be considered the second-line imaging modality for pregnant and paediatric patients after US.

Novel potential applications of the IVIM model include the prediction of renal damage related to vesicoureteral reflux in children with urinary tract infection and assessment of cortical defects in the same type of patients [76, 77].

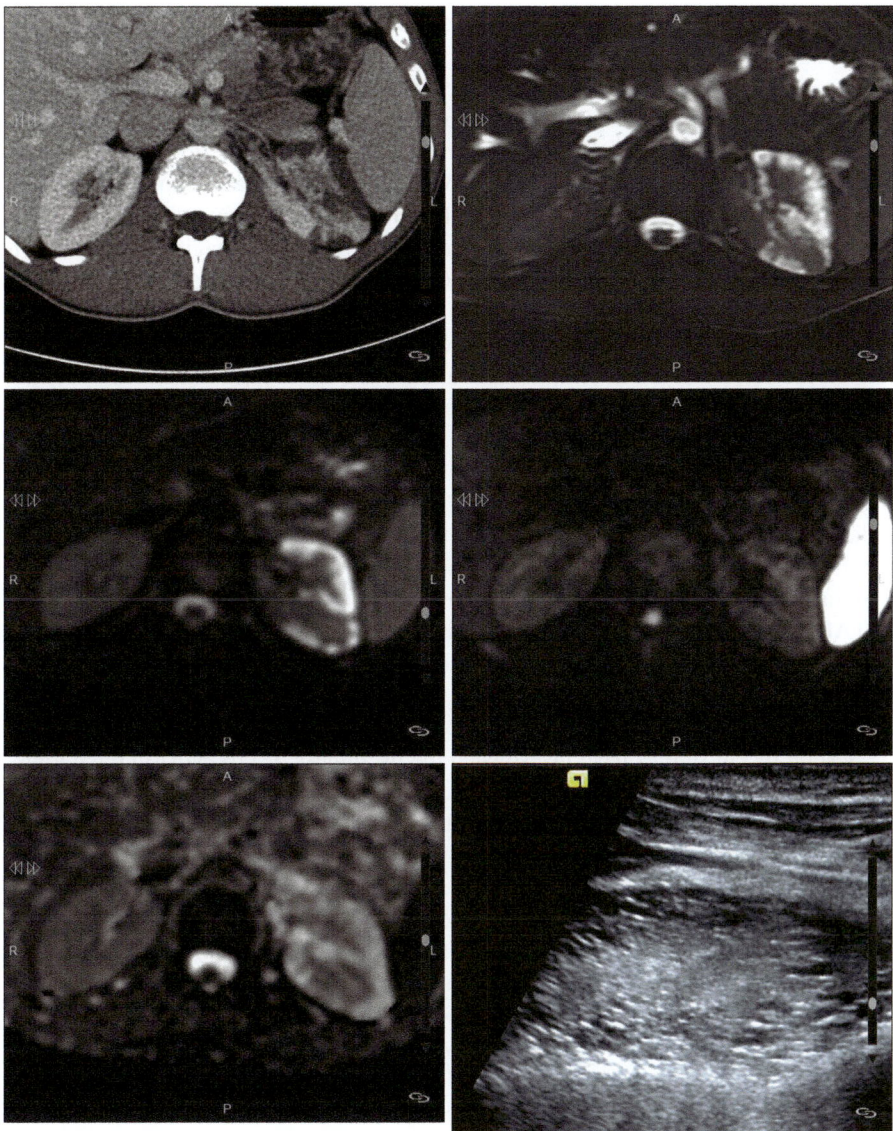

Fig. 2.5 Recurrent pyelonephritis in a 27-year-old man. (1) CT scan showed multifocal wedge-shaped hypoattenuating and non-enhancing areas that extend to the periphery of the kidney. (2) After treatment, a follow-up MR study was performed to avoid radiation exposure. T2 image showed hyperintensity of the peripheral changes seen on previous CT without significant changes in size. (3) DWI with low *b* value = 0, (4) high *b* value = 1000 and (5) ADC map showed fluid component in the peripheral parenchyma without diffusion restriction. No lesions suspicious of abscesses are identified. (6) Follow-up US confirmed the transformation of the peripheral parenchyma into multiple microcysts

2.5   Evaluation of Kidney Transplantation

Kidney transplantation has emerged as the treatment of choice in patients with end-stage renal disease, showing excellent graft survival rates mainly due to improved surgical techniques and rejection management. Allograft dysfunction can be secondary to urinary obstruction and vascular or medical complications including acute tubular necrosis (ATN), acute rejection (AR), drug-related toxicity and delayed graft function, with each requiring different treatment modalities. Imaging is essential in the management of the postoperative care of the kidney recipient, and Doppler US is the first imaging modality used for the immediate stage after transplantation. US is very useful to diagnose urological and vascular complications, but it has a low accuracy in the diagnosis of medical complications. The most common finding of renal dysfunction is an increase of the RI. However, this is a nonspecific finding and does not allow differentiating between ATN, acute or chronic rejection and drug-related toxicity. CT and MRI are usually reserved for further evaluation of US-specific findings or to resolve inconclusive US findings. MRI has the advantage of the absence of radiation and the possibility to obtain functional information. Renal biopsy with histopathological assessment is the gold standard in clinical practice for diagnosing allograft medical dysfunction since the main differential diagnosis lies between ATN and AR. However, renal biopsy is an invasive procedure with the risk of serious complications. Therefore, in recent years, there is increasing investigation regarding functional MRI tools including DW-MRI to identify the aetiology underlying graft dysfunction and to find noninvasive markers to monitor renal function.

Several recent studies have investigated the usefulness of DW-MRI in renal transplantation and have demonstrated that this technique is a promising tool for noninvasive assessment of renal function. Thoeny et al. found no differences in the ADC values in the cortex and medulla in transplanted kidneys with stable function [78], but they did observe lower ADC values in kidneys with renal allograft dysfunction (including ATN and acute or chronic rejection) than in kidneys with adequate renal function [33]. Park et al. also found lower ADC values in patients with allograft dysfunction than in those with normal function ($P < 0.05$) [79]. These results have been corroborated by other studies [80–82]. The role of DW-MRI in the differentiation between AR and ATN has also been investigated, and in the study by Park et al., no significant difference was found in ADC values between AR and ATN ($P > 0.05$) [79]. Neither have several other studies found significant differences [83]. In contrast, Eisenberg et al. reported lower ADC values in kidneys with AR than in those with ATN [84]. In addition, in the study by Abou-El-Ghar et al. performed in 21 patients with acute graft impairment, the ADC map showed a characteristic heterogeneous appearance with a mosaic pattern resembling tiger skin in cases of ATN. These authors speculated that this finding may be due to filling of the tubules with debris and a consequent lack of fluid inside the tubules that appears as sites of signal-void areas [82]. Steiger et al. also described that the combination of qualitative and quantitative DW-MRI parameters correlates with the severity of histopathologic findings in kidney allograft biopsies [85]. In that study, allografts appearing heterogeneous on ADC were associated with severe histopathologic findings, while the morphologic T1- and T2-weighted sequences did not show differences between the group with severe histopathologic changes and that with normal or mild histopathologic changes (Fig. 2.6).

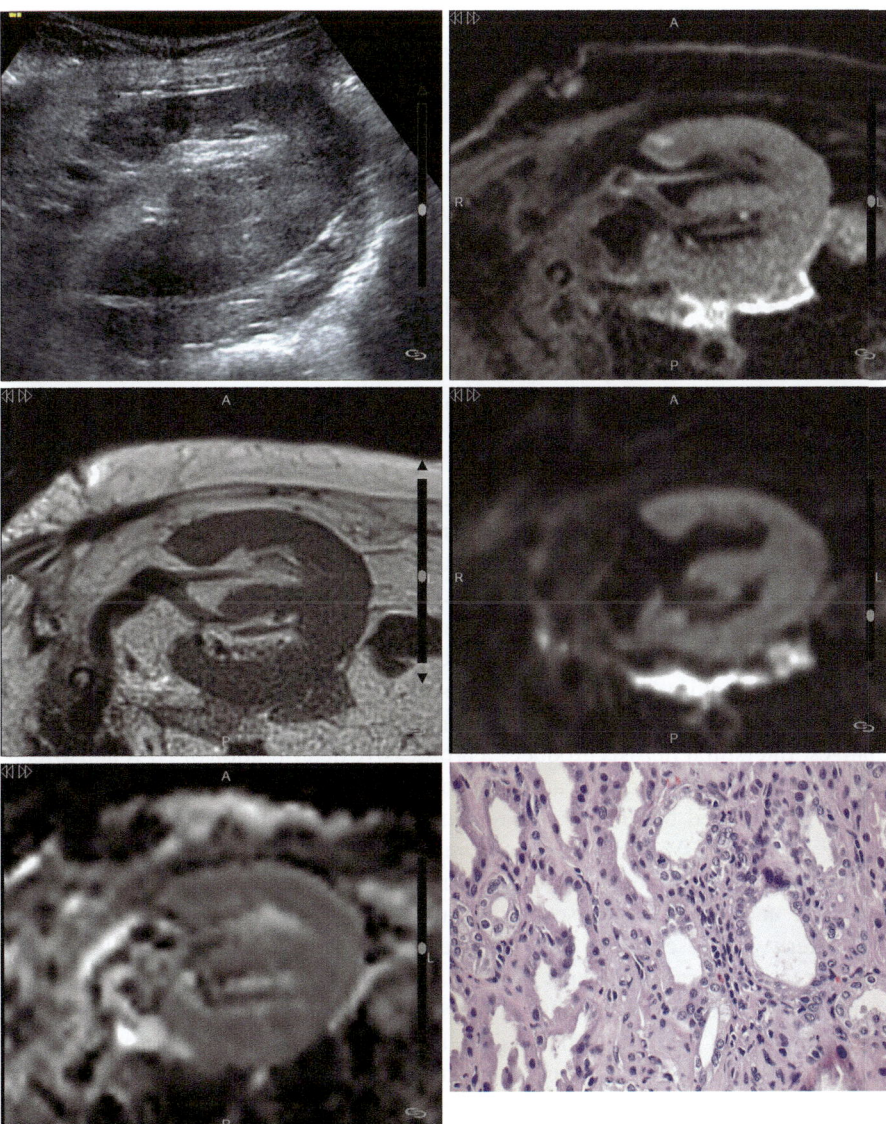

Fig. 2.6 Impaired function of a cadaveric kidney allograft in the early posttransplantation period (day 7) in a 61-year-old man. (1) US showed small perirenal collection without parenchymal changes and RIs of intraparenchymal arteries between 0.75 and 0.8. (2) T1, (3) T2, (4) DWI, with high *b* value = 1000, and (5) ADC map showed homogeneous signal intensity. The perirenal collection was well-depicted in all the sequences. (6) Biopsy was diagnostic of NTA and mild focal inflammatory infiltrate. The renal function improved after treatment

Taking into account that DW-MRI provides information on both diffusion and perfusion simultaneously, some researchers have tried to evaluate the effect of these two components independently. In this way, DTI has demonstrated to be more sensitive than DW-MRI in the detection of pathologic changes in the renal microstructure. Lanzman et al. correlated the ADC and FA values of the cortex and medulla with allograft function determined by eGFR in a group of 40 renal transplant patients [86]. In that study, the mean fractional anisotropy (FA) and ADC of the renal medulla and cortex were significantly higher in patients with good or moderate allograft function (eGFR >30 mL/min/1.73 m^2) than in patients with impaired function (eGFR ≤30 mL/min/1.73 m^2). Even more interestingly, in the group of patients with impaired function, the mean medullary FA correlated with the outcome of renal function, separating patients with recovered or stable renal function and those with renal allograft failure at 6 months following the MRI examination [86]. Recent studies have also reported a high sensitivity of FA obtained using DTI to detect renal disease. DTI tractography revealed impaired medullary microstructure in transplanted kidneys with dysfunction in contrast to healthy kidneys [29]. With respect to the differentiation between AR and ATN, the combination of perfusion and oxygenation techniques (DCE-RM, IVIM PF, ASL and BOLD) has demonstrated to be helpful, with a marked reduction of the perfusion and oxygenation parameters in AR which were not found in ATN [87].

DW imaging can also be useful in the evaluation of chronic nephropathy of kidney allografts that is secondary to progressive scarring of the allograft characterised by interstitial fibrosis and tubular atrophy, with glomerulosclerosis and vascular changes. Interstitial fibrosis produces a progressive deterioration of GFR and affects long-term renal graft function and survival. Nowadays, the diagnosis of interstitial fibrosis is obtained by histological results, and patients are submitted to multiple biopsy protocols. DW-MRI has been postulated as a noninvasive biomarker to evaluate deterioration in graft function and to monitor the response to specific treatment (Figs. 2.7 and 2.8). In the absence of graft dysfunction, DW imaging and BOLD parameters were described to be stable over 3 years in well-functioning allografts in human renal allograft recipients [88]. In addition, several studies have reported a correlation between ADC values and fibrosis or renal function with a progressive reduction of ADC values, medullary FA and tract density with the progression of fibrosis with also changes in renal microstructure using DTI tractography [89–91]. Therefore, DW-MRI can be used for the monitoring of chronic dysfunction [40].

Finally, other clinical situations such as pyelonephritis, ischaemic disease (Fig. 2.9) or the investigation of a dilated collecting system can be explored using DW-MRI similar to what has been described in native kidneys, with the advantage of the absence of not requiring the administration of contrast agents [71].

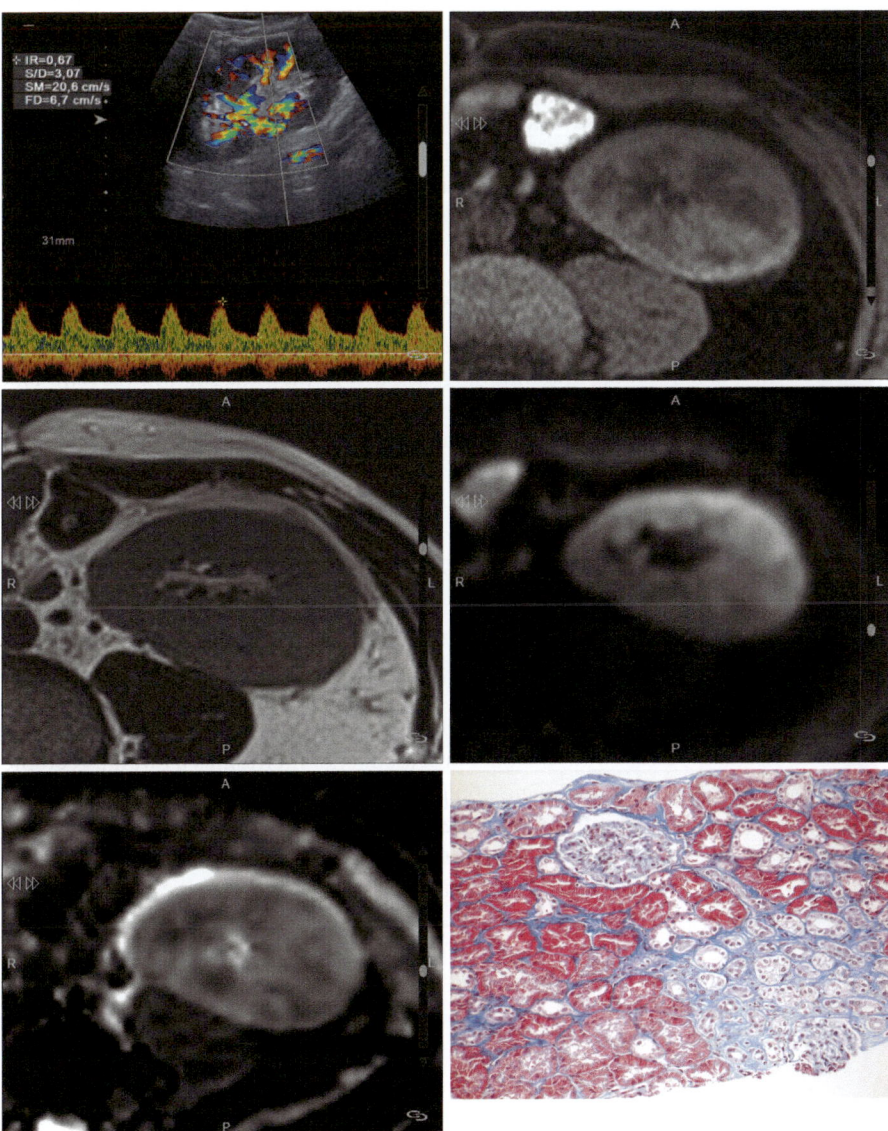

Fig. 2.7 Second kidney transplantation at the left iliac fossa in a 61-year-old man. A protocol biopsy was performed 1 year after transplantation. (1) Doppler ultrasound showed no alterations. (2) T1 and (3) T2 MR images showed homogeneous signal intensity, (4) DWI with high *b* value = 1000, and (5) especially the ADC map showed mild heterogeneity of the signal intensity of the renal parenchyma. (6) Biopsy showed mild histopathologic changes with focal areas of interstitial fibrosis with grade 1 tubular atrophy involving <20% of the renal parenchyma

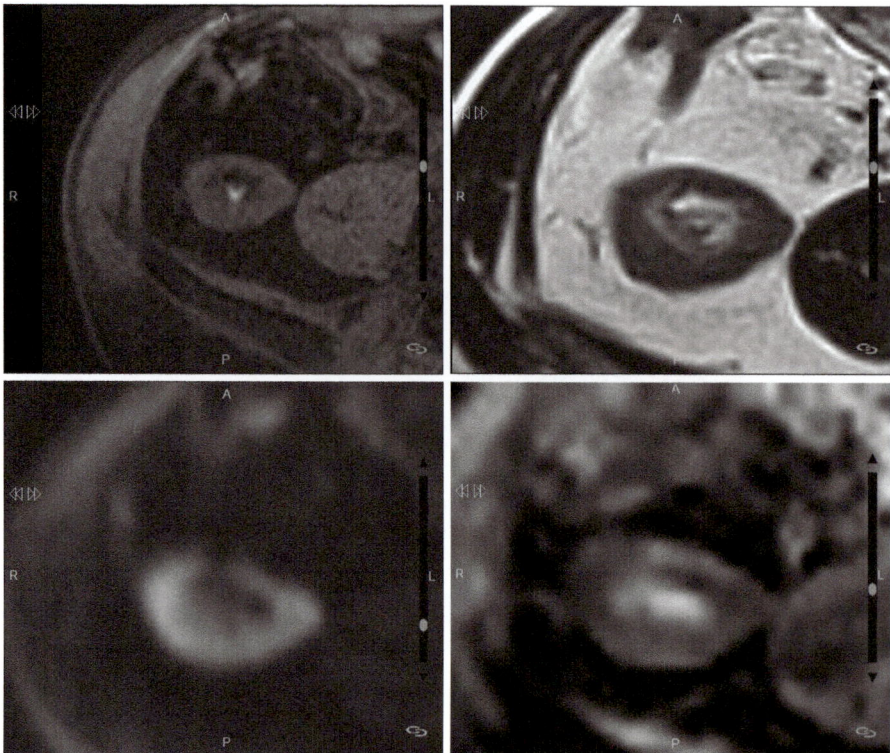

Fig. 2.8 Chronic impaired function of a second transplanted kidney in a 59-year-old man. (1) T1, (2) T2, (3) DWI with high *b* value = 1000 and (4) ADC map showed thinning of the cortex with homogeneous signal intensity of the kidney parenchyma that is diffusely low on the ADC map

Fig. 2.9 Impaired renal function of a cadaveric allograft in the early posttransplantation period in a 71-year-old man that requires haemodialysis. (1) Renal biopsy at the lower pole showed cortical necrosis. (2) Axial enhanced—T1, (3) DWI with high *b* value = 1000 and (4) ADC map of the upper pole showed homogeneous enhancement and signal intensity. (5) Axial enhanced—T1 of the lower pole showed absence of enhancement of the peripheral cortex, (6) DWI with high *b* value = 1000 and (7) ADC map estimated at the same level showed tiny areas of heterogeneity without being able to differentiate between non-necrotic and necrotic parenchyma. (8) Sagittal contrast-enhanced US confirmed the absence of cortical enhancement of the periphery of the lower pole and the deep portion of the middle pole. Contrast agent administration was necessary for a correct diagnosis by MRI and US

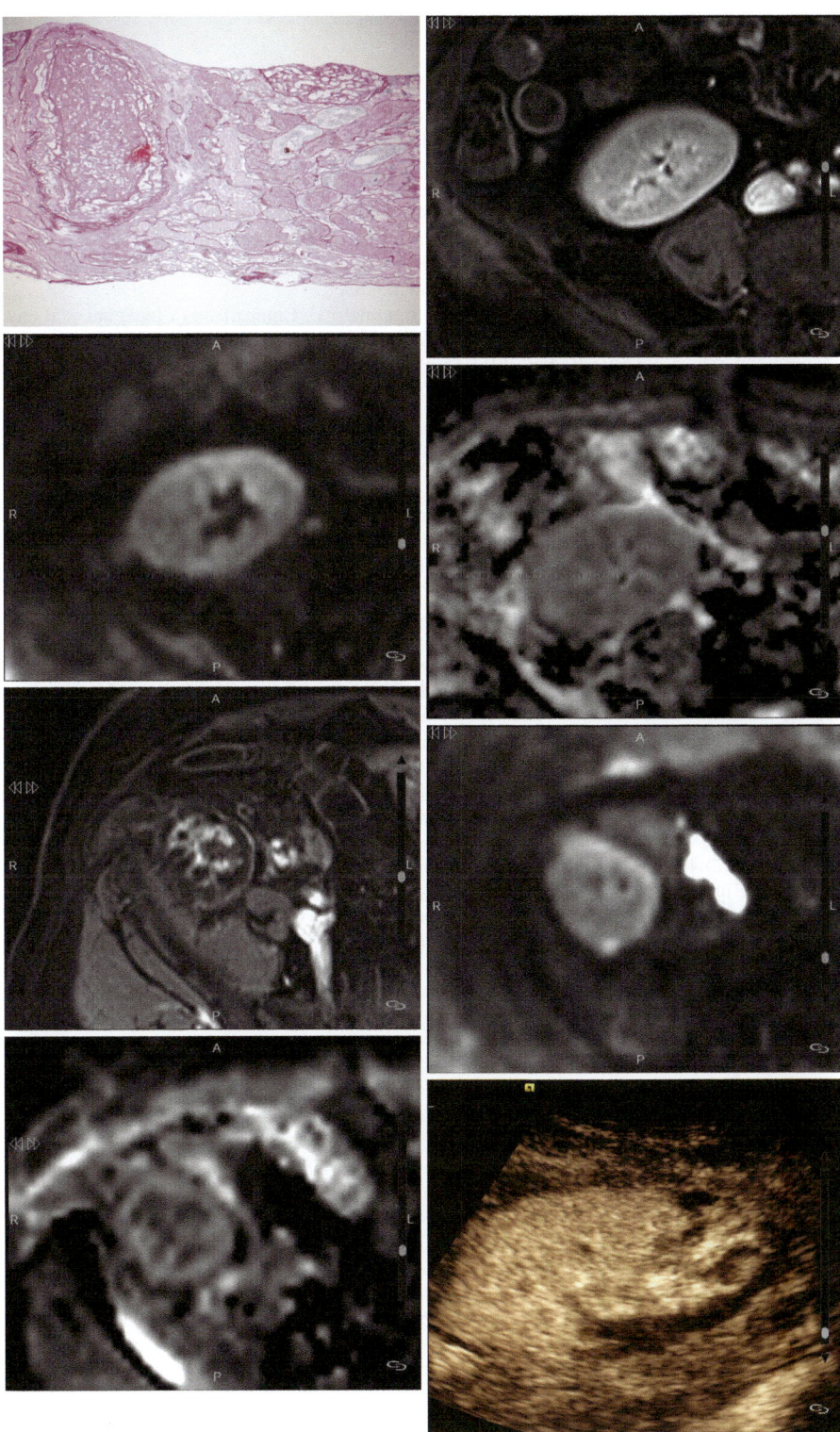

References

1. Padhani AR, Liu G, Koh DM, Chenevert TL, Thoeny HC, Takahara T, et al. Diffusion-weighted magnetic resonance imaging as a cancer biomarker: consensus and recommendations. Neoplasia. 2009;11(2):102–25. http://www.ncbi.nlm.nih.gov/pubmed/19186405.
2. Luna A, Pahwa S, Bonini C, Alcalá-Mata L, Wright KL, Gulani V. Multiparametric MR imaging in abdominal malignancies. Magn Reson Imaging Clin N Am. 2016;24(1):157–86. http://linkinghub.elsevier.com/retrieve/pii/S1064968915001038.
3. Huang Y, Chen X, Zhang Z, Yan L, Pan D, Liang C, et al. MRI quantification of non-Gaussian water diffusion in normal human kidney: a diffusional kurtosis imaging study. NMR Biomed. 2015;28(2):154–61. https://doi.org/10.1002/nbm.3235.
4. Chandarana H, Lee VS, Hecht E, Taouli B, Sigmund EE. Comparison of biexponential and monoexponential model of diffusion weighted imaging in evaluation of renal lesions: preliminary experience. Investig Radiol. 2011;46(5):285–91. http://content.wkhealth.com/linkback/openurl?sid=WKPTLP:landingpage&an=00004424-900000000-99782.
5. Diaz de Leon A, Costa D, Pedrosa I. Role of multiparametric MR imaging in malignancies of the urogenital tract. Magn Reson Imaging Clin N Am. 2016;24(1):187–204. http://www.ncbi.nlm.nih.gov/pubmed/26613881.
6. Taouli B, Beer AJ, Chenevert T, Collins D, Lehman C, Matos C, et al. Diffusion-weighted imaging outside the brain: consensus statement from an ISMRM-sponsored workshop. J Magn Reson Imaging. 2016;44(3):521–40. https://doi.org/10.1002/jmri.25196.
7. Koh D-M, Lee J-M, Bittencourt LK, Blackledge M, Collins DJ, Body Diffusion-weighted MR. Imaging in Oncology: Imaging at 3 T. Magn Reson Imaging Clin N Am. 2016;24(1):31–44. http://linkinghub.elsevier.com/retrieve/pii/S1064968915001051.
8. Rosenkrantz AB, Padhani AR, Chenevert TL, Koh D-M, De Keyzer F, Taouli B, et al. Body diffusion kurtosis imaging: basic principles, applications, and considerations for clinical practice. J Magn Reson Imaging. 2015;42(5):1190–202. https://doi.org/10.1002/jmri.24985.
9. Merkle EM, Dale BM, Paulson EK. Abdominal MR Imaging at 3T. Magn Reson Imaging Clin N Am. 2006;14(1):17–26. http://www.ncbi.nlm.nih.gov/pubmed/16530632.
10. Qayyum A. Diffusion-weighted imaging in the abdomen and pelvis: concepts and applications. Radiographics. 2009;29(6):1797–810. https://doi.org/10.1148/rg.296095521.
11. Le Bihan D, Breton E, Lallemand D, Aubin ML, Vignaud J, Laval-Jeantet M. Separation of diffusion and perfusion in intravoxel incoherent motion MR imaging. Radiology. 1988;168(2):497–505. http://www.ncbi.nlm.nih.gov/pubmed/3393671.
12. Pang Y, Turkbey B, Bernardo M, Kruecker J, Kadoury S, Merino MJ, et al. Intravoxel incoherent motion MR imaging for prostate cancer: an evaluation of perfusion fraction and diffusion coefficient derived from different b-value combinations. Magn Reson Med. 2013;69(2):553–62. https://doi.org/10.1002/mrm.24277.
13. Rheinheimer S, Schneider F, Stieltjes B, Morath C, Zeier M, Kauczor HUU, et al. IVIM-DWI of transplanted kidneys: reduced diffusion and perfusion dependent on cold ischemia time. Eur J Radiol. 2012;81(9):e951–6. http://www.ncbi.nlm.nih.gov/pubmed/22785337.
14. Hennedige T, Koh TS, Hartono S, Yan YY, Song IC, Zheng L, et al. Intravoxel incoherent imaging of renal fibrosis induced in a murine model of unilateral ureteral obstruction. Magn Reson Imaging. 2015;33(10):1324–8. http://linkinghub.elsevier.com/retrieve/pii/S0730725X15001885.
15. Schneider MJ, Dietrich O, Ingrisch M, Helck A, Winter KS, Reiser MF, et al. Intravoxel incoherent motion magnetic resonance imaging in partially nephrectomized kidneys. Investig Radiol. 2016;51(5):323–30. http://content.wkhealth.com/linkback/openurl?sid=WKPTLP:landingpage&an=00004424-900000000-99237.
16. Pentang G, Lanzman RS, Heusch P, Müller-Lutz A, Blondin D, Antoch G, et al. Diffusion kurtosis imaging of the human kidney: a feasibility study. Magn Reson Imaging. 2014;32(5):413–20. http://www.ncbi.nlm.nih.gov/pubmed/24582288.

17. Li H, Liang L, Li A, Hu Y, Hu D, Li Z, et al. Monoexponential, biexponential, and stretched exponential diffusion-weighted imaging models: quantitative biomarkers for differentiating renal clear cell carcinoma and minimal fat angiomyolipoma. J Magn Reson Imaging. 2016. https://doi.org/10.1002/jmri.25524.
18. Hales PW, Olsen ØE, Sebire NJ, Pritchard-Jones K, Clark CA. A multi-Gaussian model for apparent diffusion coefficient histogram analysis of Wilms' tumour subtype and response to chemotherapy. NMR Biomed. 2015;28(8):948–57. https://doi.org/10.1002/nbm.3337.
19. Zhang Y-D, C-J W, Wang Q, Zhang J, Wang X-N, Liu X-S, et al. Comparison of utility of histogram apparent diffusion coefficient and R2* for differentiation of low-grade from high-grade clear cell renal cell carcinoma. Am J Roentgenol. 2015;205(2):W193–201. http://www.ncbi.nlm.nih.gov/pubmed/26204307.
20. Chenevert TL, Brunberg JA, Pipe JG. Anisotropic diffusion in human white matter: demonstration with MR techniques in vivo. Radiology. 1990;177(2):401–5. https://doi.org/10.1148/radiology.177.2.2217776.
21. Pierpaoli C, Jezzard P, Basser PJ, Barnett A, Di Chiro G. Diffusion tensor MR imaging of the human brain. Radiology. 1996;201(3):637–48. http://www.ncbi.nlm.nih.gov/pubmed/8939209.
22. Jaimes C, Darge K, Khrichenko D, Carson RH, Berman JI. Diffusion tensor imaging and tractography of the kidney in children: feasibility and preliminary experience. Pediatr Radiol. 2014;44(1):30–41. http://link.springer.com/10.1007/s00247-013-2774-2.
23. Gürses B, Kiliçkesmez O, Taşdelen N, Firat Z, Gürmen N. Diffusion tensor imaging of the kidney at 3 Tesla MRI: normative values and repeatability of measurements in healthy volunteers. Diagn Interv Radiol. 2011;17(4):317–22. http://www.dirjournal.org/sayilar/37/buyuk/pdf_DIR_379.pdf.
24. Kido A, Kataoka M, Yamamoto A, Nakamoto Y, Umeoka S, Koyama T, et al. Diffusion tensor MRI of the kidney at 3.0 and 1.5 Tesla. Acta Radiol. 2010;51(9):1059–63. https://doi.org/10.3109/02841851.2010.504741.
25. Wang W, Pui MH, Guo Y, Hu X, Wang H, Yang D. MR diffusion tensor imaging of normal kidneys. J Magn Reson Imaging. 2014;40(5):1099–102. http://www.ncbi.nlm.nih.gov/pubmed/24925441.
26. Thoeny HC, De Keyzer F, Oyen RH, Peeters RR. Diffusion-weighted MR imaging of kidneys in healthy volunteers and patients with parenchymal diseases: initial experience. Radiology. 2005;235(3):911–7. http://www.ncbi.nlm.nih.gov/pubmed/15845792.
27. Ries M, Jones RA, Basseau F, Moonen CT, Grenier N. Diffusion tensor MRI of the human kidney. J Magn Reson Imaging. 2001;14(1):42–9. http://www.ncbi.nlm.nih.gov/pubmed/11436213.
28. Bane O, Wagner M, Zhang JL, Dyvorne HA, Orton M, Rusinek H, et al. Assessment of renal function using intravoxel incoherent motion diffusion-weighted imaging and dynamic contrast-enhanced MRI. J Magn Reson Imaging. 2016;44(2):317–26. http://www.ncbi.nlm.nih.gov/pubmed/26855407.
29. Xu Y, Wang X, Jiang X. Relationship between the renal apparent diffusion coefficient and glomerular filtration rate: preliminary experience. J Magn Reson Imaging. 2007;26(3):678–81. http://www.ncbi.nlm.nih.gov/pubmed/17729335.
30. Brezis M, Rosen S. Hypoxia of the renal medulla—its implications for disease. N Engl J Med. 1995;332(10):647–55. http://www.ncbi.nlm.nih.gov/pubmed/7845430.
31. Sigmund EE, Vivier P-H, Sui D, Lamparello NA, Tantillo K, Mikheev A, et al. Intravoxel incoherent motion and diffusion-tensor imaging in renal tissue under hydration and furosemide flow challenges. Radiology. 2012;263(3):758–69. https://doi.org/10.1148/radiol.12111327.
32. Müller MF, Prasad PV, Bimmler D, Kaiser A, Edelman RR. Functional imaging of the kidney by means of measurement of the apparent diffusion coefficient. Radiology. 1994;193(3):711–5. http://www.ncbi.nlm.nih.gov/pubmed/7972811.
33. Thoeny HC, De Keyzer F. Diffusion-weighted MR imaging of native and transplanted kidneys. Radiology. 2011;259(1):25–38. http://www.ncbi.nlm.nih.gov/pubmed/21436095.

34. Gurses B, Kilickesmez O, Tasdelen N, Firat Z, Gurmen N. Diffusion tensor imaging of the kidney at 3 tesla: normative values and repeatability of measurements in healthy volunteers. Diagn Interv Radiol. 2010;17(4):317–22. http://www.ncbi.nlm.nih.gov/pubmed/21108183.

35. Notohamiprodjo M, Dietrich O, Horger W, Horng A, Helck AD, Herrmann KA, et al. Diffusion tensor imaging (DTI) of the kidney at 3 Tesla–feasibility, protocol evaluation and comparison to 1.5 Tesla. Investig Radiol. 2010;45(5):245–54. http://www.ncbi.nlm.nih.gov/pubmed/20375845.

36. Webster AC, Nagler EV, Morton RL, Masson P. Chronic kidney disease. Lancet. 2017;389(10075):1238–52. http://www.ncbi.nlm.nih.gov/pubmed/27887750.

37. Leung G, Kirpalani A, Szeto SG, Deeb M, Foltz W, Simmons CA, et al. Could MRI be used to image kidney fibrosis? A review of recent advances and remaining barriers. Clin J Am Soc Nephrol. 2017:CJN.07900716. http://www.ncbi.nlm.nih.gov/pubmed/28298435.

38. Kettritz U, Semelka RC, Brown ED, Sharp TJ, Lawing WL, Colindres RE. MR findings in diffuse renal parenchymal disease. J Magn Reson Imaging. 1996;6(1):136–44. http://www.ncbi.nlm.nih.gov/pubmed/8851418.

39. Togao O, Doi S, Kuro-o M, Masaki T, Yorioka N, Takahashi M. Assessment of renal fibrosis with diffusion-weighted MR imaging: study with murine model of unilateral ureteral obstruction. Radiology. 2010;255(3):772–80. https://doi.org/10.1148/radiol.10091735.

40. Thoeny HC, Grenier N. Science to practice: can diffusion-weighted MR imaging findings be used as biomarkers to monitor the progression of renal fibrosis? Radiology. 2010;255(3):667–8. http://www.ncbi.nlm.nih.gov/pubmed/20501704.

41. Xu X, Fang W, Ling H, Chai W, Chen K. Diffusion-weighted MR imaging of kidneys in patients with chronic kidney disease: initial study. Eur Radiol. 2010;20(4):978–83. http://www.ncbi.nlm.nih.gov/pubmed/19789876.

42. Zhao J, Wang ZJJ, Liu M, Zhu J, Zhang X, Zhang T, et al. Assessment of renal fibrosis in chronic kidney disease using diffusion-weighted MRI. Clin Radiol. 2014;69(11):1117–22. http://www.ncbi.nlm.nih.gov/pubmed/25062924.

43. Liu Z, Xu Y, Zhang J, Zhen J, Wang R, Cai S, et al. Chronic kidney disease: pathological and functional assessment with diffusion tensor imaging at 3T MR. Eur Radiol. 2014;25(3):652–60. http://www.ncbi.nlm.nih.gov/pubmed/25304821.

44. Wang W, Pui MH, Guo Y, Wang L, Wang H, Liu M. 3T magnetic resonance diffusion tensor imaging in chronic kidney disease. Abdom Imaging. 2014;39(4):770–5. http://www.ncbi.nlm.nih.gov/pubmed/24623033.

45. Lu L, Sedor JR, Gulani V, Schelling JR, O'Brien A, Flask CA, et al. Use of diffusion tensor MRI to identify early changes in diabetic nephropathy. Am J Nephrol. 2011;34(5):476–82. https://doi.org/10.1159/000333044.

46. Chen X, Xiao W, Li X, He J, Huang X, Tan Y. In vivo evaluation of renal function using diffusion weighted imaging and diffusion tensor imaging in type 2 diabetics with normoalbuminuria versus microalbuminuria. Front Med. 2014;8(4):471–6. http://link.springer.com/10.1007/s11684-014-0365-8.

47. Feng Q, Ma Z, Wu J, Fang W. DTI for the assessment of disease stage in patients with glomerulonephritis—correlation with renal histology. Eur Radiol. 2017;25(1):92–8. https://doi.org/10.1007/s00330-014-3336-1.

48. Liu Z, Xu Y, Zhang J, Zhen J, Wang R, Cai S, et al. Chronic kidney disease: pathological and functional assessment with diffusion tensor imaging at 3T MR. Eur Radiol. 2015;25(3):652–60. http://www.ncbi.nlm.nih.gov/pubmed/25304821.

49. Ichikawa S, Motosugi U, Ichikawa T, Sano K, Morisaka H, Araki T. Intravoxel incoherent motion imaging of the kidney: alterations in diffusion and perfusion in patients with renal dysfunction. Magn Reson Imaging. 2013;31(3):414–7. http://www.ncbi.nlm.nih.gov/pubmed/23102943.

50. Preston RA, Epstein M. Ischemic renal disease: an emerging cause of chronic renal failure and end-stage renal disease. J Hypertens. 1997;15(12 Pt 1):1365–77. http://www.ncbi.nlm.nih.gov/pubmed/9431840.

51. Andersson M, Jägervall K, Eriksson P, Persson A, Granerus G, Wang C, et al. How to measure renal artery stenosis—a retrospective comparison of morphological measurement approaches

in relation to hemodynamic significance. BMC Med Imaging. 2015;15(1):42. http://www. ncbi.nlm.nih.gov/pubmed/26459634.

52. Eklöf H, Ahlström H, Magnusson A, Andersson L-G, Andrén B, Hägg A, et al. A prospective comparison of duplex ultrasonography, captopril renography, MRA, and CTA in assessing renal artery stenosis. Acta Radiol. 2006;47(8):764–74. http://www.ncbi.nlm.nih.gov/pubmed/17050355.

53. Vasbinder GB, Nelemans PJ, Kessels AG, Kroon AA, de Leeuw PW, van Engelshoven JM. Diagnostic tests for renal artery stenosis in patients suspected of having renovascular hypertension: a meta-analysis. Ann Intern Med. 2001;135(6):401–11. http://www.ncbi.nlm.nih.gov/pubmed/11560453.

54. Sebastià C, Sotomayor AD, Paño B, Salvador R, Burrel M, Botey A, et al. Accuracy of unenhanced magnetic resonance angiography for the assessment of renal artery stenosis. Eur J Radiol Open. 2016;3:200–6. http://www.ncbi.nlm.nih.gov/pubmed/27536710.

55. Xu X, Lin X, Huang J, Pan Z, Zhu X, Chen K, et al. The capability of inflow inversion recovery magnetic resonance compared to contrast-enhanced magnetic resonance in renal artery angiography. Abdom Radiol. 2017; http://www.ncbi.nlm.nih.gov/pubmed/28470403.

56. Schoenberg SO, Rieger JR, Michaely HJ, Rupprecht H, Samtleben W, Reiser MF. Functional magnetic resonance imaging in renal artery stenosis. Abdom Imaging. 2006;31(2):200–12. http://www.ncbi.nlm.nih.gov/pubmed/16317490.

57. Ikee R, Kobayashi S, Hemmi N, Imakiire T, Kikuchi Y, Moriya H, et al. Correlation between the resistive index by Doppler ultrasound and kidney function and histology. Am J Kidney Dis. 2005;46(4):603–9. http://linkinghub.elsevier.com/retrieve/pii/S0272638605008528.

58. Radermacher J, Chavan A, Bleck J, Vitzthum A, Stoess B, Gebel MJ, et al. Use of doppler ultrasonography to predict the outcome of therapy for renal-artery stenosis. N Engl J Med. 2001;344(6):410–7. http://www.ncbi.nlm.nih.gov/pubmed/11172177.

59. Jiang K, Ferguson CM, Ebrahimi B, Tang H, Kline TL, Burningham TA, et al. Noninvasive assessment of renal fibrosis with magnetization transfer MR imaging: validation and evaluation in murine renal artery stenosis. Radiology. 2017;283(1):77–86. http://www.ncbi.nlm.nih.gov/pubmed/27697008.

60. Yildirim E, Kirbas I, Teksam M, Karadeli E, Gullu H, Ozer I. Diffusion-weighted MR imaging of kidneys in renal artery stenosis. Eur J Radiol. 2008;65(1):148–53. http://www.ncbi.nlm.nih.gov/pubmed/17537606.

61. Ebrahimi B, Rihal N, Woollard JR, Krier JD, Eirin A, Lerman LO. Assessment of renal artery stenosis using intravoxel incoherent motion diffusion-weighted magnetic resonance imaging analysis. Investig Radiol. 2014;49(10):640–6. http://www.ncbi.nlm.nih.gov/pubmed/24743589.

62. Mishima E, Kikuchi K, Ota H, Akiyama Y, Suzuki T, Seiji K, et al. Detection of segmental renal ischemia by diffusion-weighted magnetic resonance imaging: clinical utility for diagnosis of renovascular hypertension. J Clin Hypertens. 2016;18(4):364–5. http://www.ncbi.nlm.nih.gov/pubmed/26360321.

63. Deux J-F, Audard V, Brugières P, Habibi A, Manea E-M, Guillaud-Danis C, et al. Magnetic resonance imaging assessment of kidney oxygenation and perfusion during sickle cell vaso-occlusive crises. Am J Kidney Dis. 2017;69(1):51–9. http://www.ncbi.nlm.nih.gov/pubmed/27663041.

64. Bozgeyik Z, Kocakoc E, Sonmezgoz F. Diffusion-weighted MR imaging findings of kidneys in patients with early phase of obstruction. Eur J Radiol. 2009;70(1):138–41. http://linkinghub.elsevier.com/retrieve/pii/S0720048X08000120.

65. Thoeny HC, Binser T, Roth B, Kessler TM, Vermathen P. Noninvasive assessment of acute ureteral obstruction with diffusion-weighted MR imaging: a prospective study. Radiology. 2009;252(3):721–8. http://www.ncbi.nlm.nih.gov/pubmed/19567650.

66. Chan JH, Tsui EY, Luk SH, Fung SL, Cheung YK, Chan MS, et al. MR diffusion-weighted imaging of kidney: differentiation between hydronephrosis and pyonephrosis. Clin Imaging. 2001;25(2):110–3. http://www.ncbi.nlm.nih.gov/pubmed/11483420.

67. Cova M, Squillaci E, Stacul F, Manenti G, Gava S, Simonetti G, et al. Diffusion-weighted MRI in the evaluation of renal lesions: preliminary results. Br J Radiol. 2004;77(922):851–7. http://www.ncbi.nlm.nih.gov/pubmed/15482997.

68. Gomez H, Ince C, De Backer D, Pickkers P, Payen D, Hotchkiss J, et al. A unified theory of sepsis-induced acute kidney injury: inflammation, microcirculatory dysfunction, bioenergetics, and the tubular cell adaptation to injury. Shock. 2014;41(1):3–11. http://content.wkhealth.com/linkback/openurl?sid=WKPTLP:landingpage&an=00024382-201401000-00003.

69. Imai Y, Parodo J, Kajikawa O, de Perrot M, Fischer S, Edwards V, et al. Injurious mechanical ventilation and end-organ epithelial cell apoptosis and organ dysfunction in an experimental model of acute respiratory distress syndrome. JAMA. 2003;289(16):2104–12. https://doi.org/10.1001/jama.289.16.2104.

70. De Pascale A, Piccoli GB, Priola SM, Rognone D, Consiglio V, Garetto I, et al. Diffusion-weighted magnetic resonance imaging: new perspectives in the diagnostic pathway of non-complicated acute pyelonephritis. Eur Radiol. 2013;23(11):3077–86. http://www.ncbi.nlm.nih.gov/pubmed/23749224.

71. Faletti R, Cassinis MC, Gatti M, Giglio J, Guarnaccia C, Messina M, et al. Acute pyelonephritis in transplanted kidneys: can diffusion-weighted magnetic resonance imaging be useful for diagnosis and follow-up? Abdom Radiol. 2016;41(3):531–7. http://www.ncbi.nlm.nih.gov/pubmed/27039324.

72. Vivier P-H, Sallem A, Beurdeley M, Lim RP, Leroux J, Caudron J, et al. MRI and suspected acute pyelonephritis in children: comparison of diffusion-weighted imaging with gadolinium-enhanced T1-weighted imaging. Eur Radiol. 2014;24(1):19–25. http://www.ncbi.nlm.nih.gov/pubmed/23884301.

73. Verswijvel G, Vandecaveye V, Gelin G, Vandevenne J, Grieten M, Horvath M, et al. Diffusion-weighted MR imaging in the evaluation of renal infection: preliminary results. JBR-BTR. 2002;85(2):100–3. http://www.ncbi.nlm.nih.gov/pubmed/12083620.

74. Rathod SB, Kumbhar SS, Nanivadekar A, Aman K. Role of diffusion-weighted MRI in acute pyelonephritis: a prospective study. Acta Radiol. 2015;56(2):244–9. http://www.ncbi.nlm.nih.gov/pubmed/24443116.

75. Faletti R, Cassinis MC, Fonio P, Grasso A, Battisti G, Bergamasco L, et al. Diffusion-weighted imaging and apparent diffusion coefficient values versus contrast-enhanced MR imaging in the identification and characterisation of acute pyelonephritis. Eur Radiol. 2013;23(12):3501–8. http://www.ncbi.nlm.nih.gov/pubmed/23887662.

76. Kim JW, Lee CH, Yoo KH, Je B-K, Kiefer B, Park YS, et al. Intravoxel incoherent motion magnetic resonance imaging to predict vesicoureteral reflux in children with urinary tract infection. Eur Radiol. 2016;26(6):1670–7. http://link.springer.com/10.1007/s00330-015-3986-7.

77. Lee CH, Yoo KH, Je B-K, Kim IS, Kiefer B, Park YS, et al. Using intravoxel incoherent motion MR imaging to evaluate cortical defects in the first episode of upper urinary tract infections: preliminary results. J Magn Reson Imaging. 2014;40(3):545–51. https://doi.org/10.1002/jmri.24384.

78. Thoeny HC, Zumstein D, Simon-Zoula S, Eisenberger U, De Keyzer F, Hofmann L, et al. Functional evaluation of transplanted kidneys with diffusion-weighted and BOLD MR imaging: initial experience. Radiology. 2006;241(3):812–21. http://www.ncbi.nlm.nih.gov/pubmed/17114628.

79. Park SY, Kim CK, Park BK, Kim SJ, Lee S, Huh W. Assessment of early renal allograft dysfunction with blood oxygenation level-dependent MRI and diffusion-weighted imaging. Eur J Radiol. 2014;83(12):2114–21. http://www.ncbi.nlm.nih.gov/pubmed/25452096.

80. Blondin D, Lanzman RS, Klasen J, Scherer A, Miese F, Kröpil P, et al. Diffusion-attenuated MRI signal of renal allografts: comparison of two different statistical models. AJR Am J Roentgenol. 2011;196(6):W701–5. https://doi.org/10.2214/AJR.10.5775.

81. Palmucci S, Mauro LA, Veroux P, Failla G, Milone P, Ettorre GC, et al. Magnetic resonance with diffusion-weighted imaging in the evaluation of transplanted kidneys: preliminary findings. Transplant Proc. 2011;43(4):960–6. http://linkinghub.elsevier.com/retrieve/pii/S0041134511002417.

82. Abou-El-Ghar ME, El-Diasty TA, El-Assmy AM, Refaie HF, Refaie AF, Ghoneim MA. Role of diffusion-weighted MRI in diagnosis of acute renal allograft dysfunction: a prospective preliminary study. Br J Radiol. 2012;85(1014):e206–11. https://doi.org/10.1259/bjr/53260155.
83. Liu G, Han F, Xiao W, Wang Q, Xu Y, Chen J. Detection of renal allograft rejection using blood oxygen level-dependent and diffusion weighted magnetic resonance imaging: a retrospective study. BMC Nephrol. 2014;15(1):158. http://www.ncbi.nlm.nih.gov/pubmed/25270976.
84. Eisenberger U, Thoeny HC, Binser T, Gugger M, Frey FJ, Boesch C, et al. Evaluation of renal allograft function early after transplantation with diffusion-weighted MR imaging. Eur Radiol. 2010;20(6):1374–83. http://www.ncbi.nlm.nih.gov/pubmed/20013274.
85. Steiger P, Barbieri S, Kruse A, Ith M, Thoeny HC. Selection for biopsy of kidney transplant patients by diffusion-weighted MRI. Eur Radiol. 2017; http://www.ncbi.nlm.nih.gov/pubmed/28374076.
86. Lanzman RS, Ljimani A, Pentang G, Zgoura P, Zenginli H, Kröpil P, et al. Kidney transplant: functional assessment with diffusion-tensor MR imaging at 3T. Radiology. 2013;266(1):218–25. https://doi.org/10.1148/radiol.12112522.
87. Notohamiprodjo M, Reiser MF, Sourbron SP. Diffusion and perfusion of the kidney. Eur J Radiol. 2010;76(3):337–47. http://www.ncbi.nlm.nih.gov/pubmed/20580179.
88. Vermathen P, Binser T, Boesch C, Eisenberger U, Thoeny HC. Three-year follow-up of human transplanted kidneys by diffusion-weighted MRI and blood oxygenation level-dependent imaging. J Magn Reson Imaging. 2012;35(5):1133–8. http://www.ncbi.nlm.nih.gov/pubmed/22180302.
89. Fan W, Ren T, Li Q, Zuo P, Long M, Mo C, et al. Assessment of renal allograft function early after transplantation with isotropic resolution diffusion tensor imaging. Eur Radiol. 2016;26(2):567–75. http://link.springer.com/10.1007/s00330-015-3841-x.
90. Palmucci S, Cappello G, Attinà G, Foti PV, Siverino ROA, Roccasalva F, et al. Diffusion weighted imaging and diffusion tensor imaging in the evaluation of transplanted kidneys. Eur J Radiol Open. 2015;2:71–80. http://www.ncbi.nlm.nih.gov/pubmed/26937439.
91. Hueper K, Gutberlet M, Rodt T, Gwinner W, Lehner F, Wacker F, et al. Diffusion tensor imaging and tractography for assessment of renal allograft dysfunction-initial results. Eur Radiol. 2011;21(11):2427–33. http://link.springer.com/10.1007/s00330-011-2189-0.

Renal, Adrenal, and Retroperitoneal Masses

3

Roberto García-Figueiras and Sandra Baleato-González

3.1 Introduction

Structural imaging techniques have showed clear limitations in the evaluation of patients. Apart from the anatomical assessment, functional imaging techniques, such as diffusion-weighted imaging (DWI), are entering in clinical daily practice and appear to be useful tools for providing insights into lesion phenotype. DWI has revolutionized abdominal MRI. A detailed explanation of the basis of DWI is beyond the scope of this manuscript, but it evaluates the Brownian movement of water molecules at microscopic level, which is related to tissue microstructure, cell membrane integrity, and cellularity. In general, clinical use of DWI is mainly based on the assumption of a Gaussian diffusion behavior of water diffusion (the classical mono-exponential model). However, water proton signal attenuation in vivo tissue with diffusion weighting does not follow a mono-exponential decay due to multiple interacting elements that hindered diffusivity. The deviation from mono-exponential behavior is best observed using the non-Gaussian diffusion models, which include intravoxel incoherent motion (IVIM), diffusion kurtosis imaging (DKI), and stretched-exponential model (SEM) [1–3]. Besides, diffusion tensor imaging (DTI) allows the analysis of the anisotropic properties of tissues. This chapter will review recent developments in DWI and the evolving role for this technique in renal, adrenal, and retroperitoneal masses.

R. García-Figueiras, M.D., Ph.D. (✉) • S. Baleato-González, M.D., Ph.D.
Department of Radiology, Hospital Clínico Universitario de Santiago de Compostela, Santiago de Compostela, Spain
e-mail: roberto.garcia.figueiras@sergas.es; baleatorum@hotmail.com

© Springer International Publishing AG 2018
D. Akata, N. Papanikolaou (eds.), *Diffusion Weighted Imaging of the Genitourinary System*, https://doi.org/10.1007/978-3-319-69575-4_3

47

3.2   Renal Masses

DWI is an established tool in the evaluation of abdominal diseases, including renal masses. The potential of DW-MRI in the evaluation of focal renal lesions is of utmost importance in patients with renal insufficiency, in view of the concerns regarding the risk of development of nephrogenic systemic fibrosis or contrast material-induced nephropathy. In this setting, perfusion fraction (f), a parameter derived from the IVIM model analysis, demonstrated a good correlation with percent enhancement and may provide information regarding lesion vascularity without the use of exogenous contrast agents. Both f and true diffusion (D) showed higher accuracy compared with the apparent diffusion coefficient (ADC) in discriminating enhancing from non-enhancing renal lesions [4]. There are three principle applications of DWI for renal imaging. First, low b-value DW images can replace fat-saturation T2-weighted images, decreasing total examination time. Second, the long b-value DW images may improve renal lesion detection. And last, DWI-derived parameters (i.e., ADC values) could potentially characterize renal lesions [5]. In clinical practice, the use of DWI has been mainly focused on discriminating between malignant and benign renal lesions, differentiating among renal cancer subtypes, distinguishing high- from low-grade tumors, and evaluating tumor characteristics in order to predict patients' outcomes.

3.2.1   Tumor Detection

There were considerable promises on the accuracy of DWI in renal lesion detection [6]. In a meta-analysis including four studies, Tang et al. reported that both low (400–500 s/mm^2) and high b-value (800–1000 s/mm^2) DWI demonstrated a limited diagnostic performance in the detection of renal cell carcinoma (RCC) lesions in the kidney [7]. The ability to detect lesions on DW images is highly dependent on tumor histologic type and grade. Clear cell tumors are less conspicuous on DWI compared with other renal cancer histologic subtypes because of the relatively greater water diffusivity in clear cell renal cell carcinomas (ccRCCs) (Fig. 3.1a–c). Furthermore, it has been noted that well-differentiated or low-grade masses are also less well seen, probably because they often have a more normal appearing histologic structure [8]. The combination of different MRI sequences may improve MRI performance. Yoshida et al. showed that the detection rate using T2-weighted imaging plus DWI (93.4%) was the same as for T2-weighted imaging plus dynamic contrast-enhanced (DCE) MRI but that both were marginally higher comparing to T2 sequences alone (91.8%) [9]. On the other hand, the mean ADC value of TTCs was significantly lower than that of the normal renal parenchyma, which may suggest the utility of DWI to detect upper urinary tract transitional cell carcinomas (TTCs) [10].

3.2.2   Characterization of Renal Masses

Preoperative imaging characterization of benign and malignant renal masses is imperfect. DWI may be a reasonable alternative to conventional cross-sectional imaging to characterize focal renal lesions, especially in patients with impaired

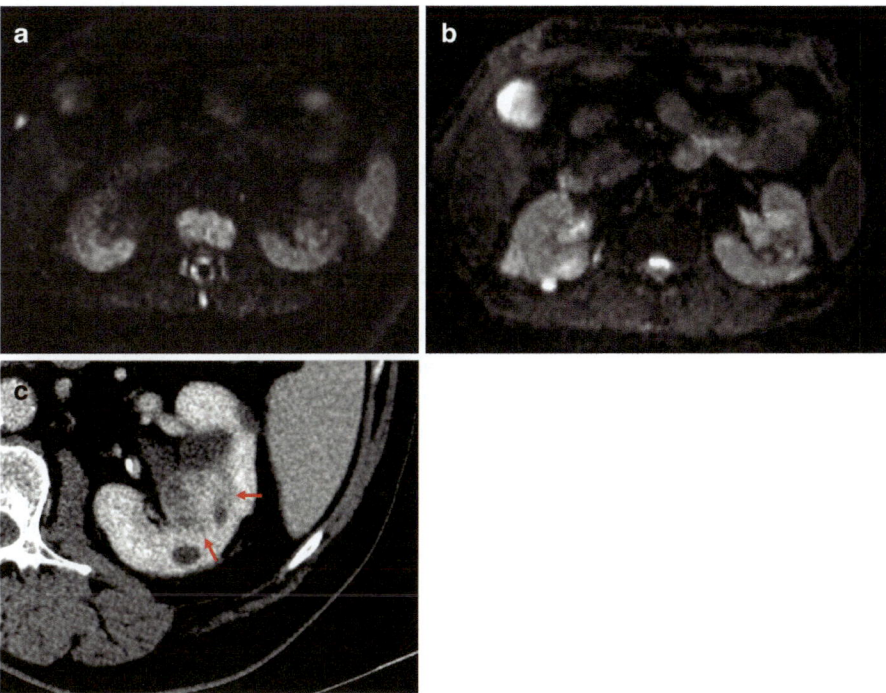

Fig. 3.1 Clear cell renal cell carcinoma. Clear cell tumors are sometimes difficult to detect on DWI compared with other renal cancer histologic subtypes because of the relatively greater water diffusivity in ccRCCs. High b-value ($b = 800$) image (**a**) and the corresponding apparent diffusion coefficient (ADC) map (**b**) did not demonstrate any evident suspicious mass in the kidney. On the contrary, contrast-enhanced CT image in the nephrographic phase (**c**) clearly depicted the tumor in the left kidney (*red arrows*)

renal function [11]. In this group of patients, DWI was able to distinguish pseudo-tumors from RCCs and offered a non-contrast alternative for ruling out malignancy [12]. The ADC values may also be useful for differentiating renal masses and may represent a potential noninvasive biomarker of tumor aggressiveness. A recent meta-analysis has reviewed the role of DWI in the characterization of renal masses. In this paper, Kang et al. found a moderate accuracy (sensitivity and specificity of 86% and 78%, respectively) for differentiating malignant and benign renal masses [13]. On its part, a literature review based on the data of nine publications reported that there were statistically significant differences in ADC values between benign $(2.47 \pm 0.81 \times 10^{-3}$ mm^2/s) and malignant renal lesions $(1.81 \pm 0.41 \times 10^{-3}$ mm^2/s) [14], and Lassel et al. reported also a significant difference between malignant lesions, including clear cell renal cell carcinomas (ccRCCs) and TTCs, and benign lesions $(1.61 \pm 0.08 \times 10^{-3}$ mm^2/s and $1.30 \pm 0.22 \times 10^{-3}$ mm^2/s, respectively, vs. $2.10 \pm 0.09 \times 10^{-3}$ mm^2/s; $P < 0.0001$) [15]. In this latter study, TTCs showed lower ADC values $(1.30 \pm 0.11 \times 10^{-3}$ mm^2/s) than renal cell carcinomas (RCCs). A possible histological explanation for this finding could be that TTCs are usually solid and densely packed hypercellular tumors, while RCCs usually show necrotic and cystic areas and prominent vascularization, which may contribute to their higher

ADC values [16]. There was also a significant difference between ADC values of RCCs and oncocytomas (1.61 ± 0.08 × 10^{-3} mm^2/s vs. 2.00 ± 0.08 × 10^{-3} mm^2/s; $P < 0.0001$) [15]. Besides this, to differentiate the various RCC subtypes is critical for both prognostication and therapy selection in the case of patients with metastatic disease. Patients with chromophobe and papillary RCC (pRCC) have a better prognosis than patients with ccRCC. Some studies have investigated DWI accuracy in this role and evidenced that ADC values usually allowed differentiating between ccRCC and non-ccRCC. A lower ADC has been reported in the papillary subtype of RCC and TCCs compared with other subtypes, whereas cystic RCC and ccRCC showed higher ADC values [17]. However, on the contrary, there was no significant difference in the ADC values between non-ccRCCs (papillary and chromophobe). It is necessary being careful on using ADC values for tumor characterization because there was an overlap of ADC values across the different tumor types and they are based on small sample sizes [14, 15, 18]. The wide confidence intervals that showed the ADC values limit the role of this parameter in clinical practice. Published studies reflect widely variable sensitivities and specificities for DWI with moderate accuracy, mainly because the measurement of ADC value relies on the use of MRI systems, imaging sequences, and other parameters, which restrict its reproducibility. In this setting, some authors recommended the use of a maximum b-value ranging from 800 to 1000 s/mm^2 at 3T in renal evaluation because ADCs obtained with b-values of 0 and 800 s/mm^2 were more effective for distinguishing ccRCC from non-ccRCC (area under the ROC curve, 0.973) comparing to values of 0 and 500 s/ mm^2 [17]. Besides, the ADC values of renal masses are going to depend on perfusion or diffusion characteristics (cellularity, histological composition, etc.) and the type of tumor and grading. Other histological changes also influence DWI measurements. For example, the presence of hemorrhagic changes, which is relatively common in certain tumors, such as pRCC, may potentially alter ADC value measurements due to susceptibility effects. Finally, benign lesions may also exhibit restricted diffusion and may mimic malignancy. AML may show profound diffusion restriction because they contain a combination of varying amounts of vascular, smooth muscle and fat with interstitial stroma, which can explain the reduction in water diffusion. On its part, hemorrhagic cysts may also demonstrate restricted diffusion due to internal viscosity and "T2 blackout" effects. Lastly, renal infections (pyelonephritis or abscesses) commonly exhibit a restricted diffusion. Thus, although different papers have suggested a role of ADC in tumor characterization [19], DWI findings must be always correlated with imaging characteristics on morphological MR sequences, clinical history, and laboratory analysis [5, 20, 21].

More advanced models such as IVIM, DKI, or SEM have shown promise in small studies for the characterization of renal masses. IVIM is a diffusion model that allows to separately quantify tissue diffusivity and tissue capillary perfusion. Diffusion at low b-values (<200 s/mm^2) is significantly affected by perfusion within the normal capillary network (Fig. 3.2), although a correlation between IVIM-related parameters and DCE parameters remains controversial. The DKI model provides more information on tissue structure, reflecting the complexity and heterogeneity of the tissue (Fig. 3.3). And SEM may provide an approximation to the intravoxel diffusion heterogeneity. Concerning the use of these models in the

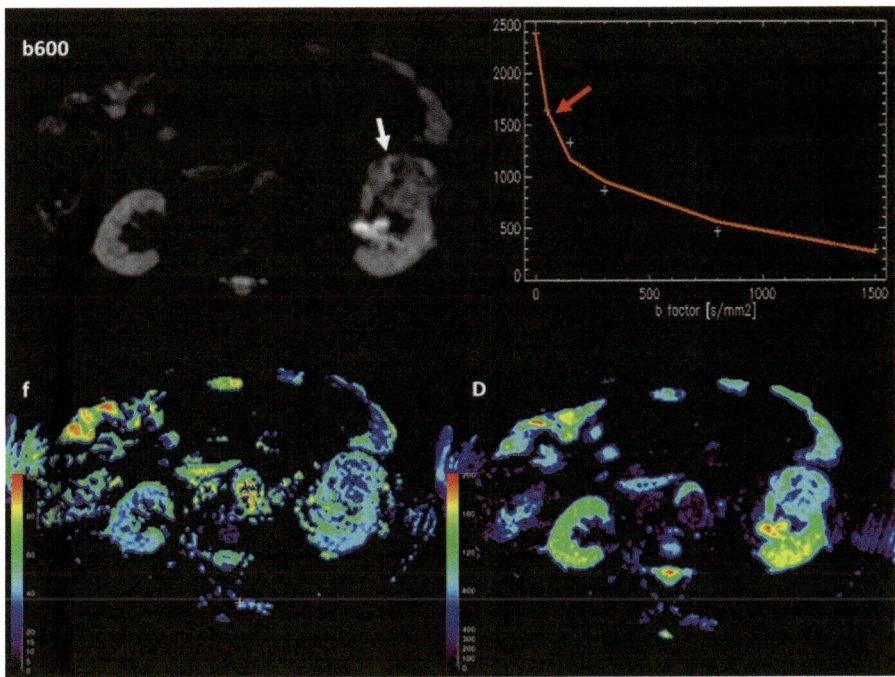

Fig. 3.2 Intravoxel incoherent motion (IVIM) model in renal tumors. IVIM is a diffusion model that allows to separately quantify tissue diffusivity and tissue capillary perfusion. IVIM images in an 86-year-old man patient with clear cell renal cell carcinoma (*white arrow*), including a diffusion-weighted image at $b = 600$, perfusion fraction (f) and true diffusion (D) parametric maps, and diffusion signal intensity attenuation curve (*right-bottom*). Diffusion at low b-values (<200 s/mm²) is significantly affected by perfusion within the normal capillary network causing an intense signal drop with increased b-values (*red arrow*). Tumor mass also showed a high perfusion fraction value in the periphery ($f = 24\%$), which suggested an increased tumor perfusion. Mean D value of the mass was 1.23×10^{-3} mm²/s

evaluation of renal masses, Chandarana et al. reported that perfusion fraction (f) showed a good correlation with model-free parameter initial area under the curve (AUC) of gadolinium concentration at 60 s and could assess the degree of tumor vascularity without the use of exogenous contrast agent. These authors stated that the perfusion-free diffusion (D) seems to provide more accurate information than the ADC for distinguishing different lesion types [22]. However, published data show disparity and Rheinheime et al. found a high correlation of ADC and D [23].

IVIM model can provide certain reliable value in evaluating pathological subtype and differentiation degree of renal cell carcinomas [24]. In the study of Chandarana et al., the combination of f and D diagnosed pRCC and cystic RCC with 100% accuracy and ccRCC and chromophobe RCC with 86.5%. IVIM-derived parameter f had the highest accuracy for the diagnosis of ccRCC (Fig. 3.2) (AUC 0.74). Using a cutoff for f greater than 0.16, the clear cell subtype could be diagnosed with a sensitivity of 100%, specificity of 62.5%, and accuracy of 82.7% (Fig. 3.2) [22]. Besides this, IVIM parameters with inclusion of voxel-based histogram analysis of their

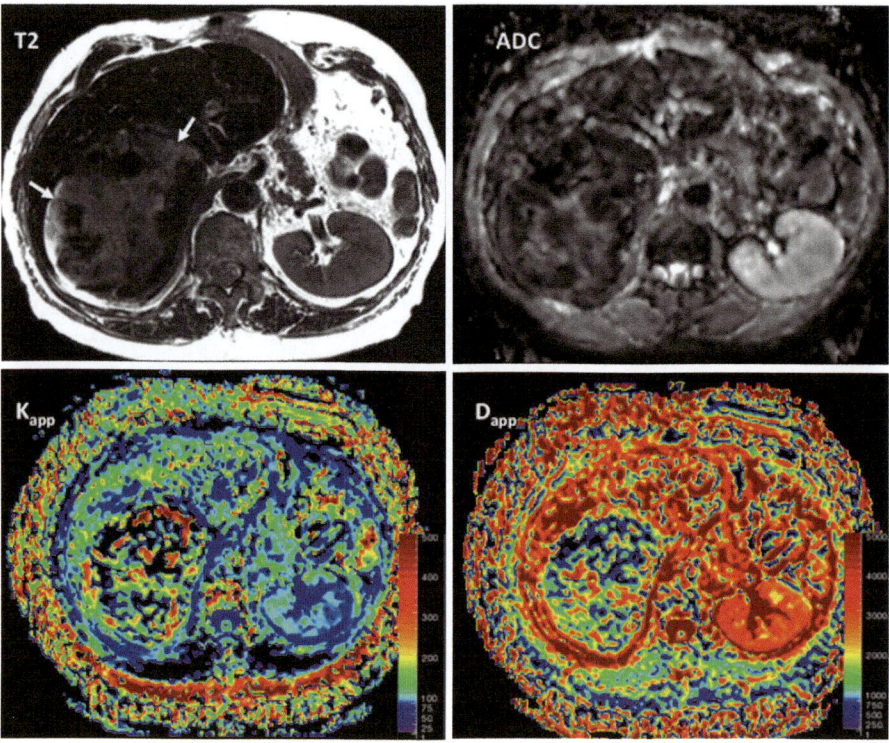

Fig. 3.3 Diffusion kurtosis imaging (DKI) model in renal tumors. DKI potentially provides more information on tissue structure and heterogeneity. MR exam in a 75-year-old man with a high-grade (Fuhrman IV) clear cell carcinoma. Axial T2-weighted MR image (T2) showed a heterogeneous mass in the upper pole of the right kidney with extensive areas of central necrosis (*white arrows*). Diffusion signal intensity attenuation curve (*right-top*) evidenced an intense signal drop with increased *b*-values (*red arrow*). Tumor kurtosis (K_{app}) (*left-bottom*) was increased, and diffusional kurtosis (D_{app}) (*right-bottom*) was reduced when comparing to the normal left kidney (*Courtesy of A. Luna, MD, PhD. Case Western Reserve University, Cleveland, OH (USA), and Grupo Health Time, Jaén (Spain)*)

heterogeneity may help to differentiate malignant from benign lesions as well as various subtypes of renal cancers [25]. Nevertheless, published data are sometimes in contradiction. In a different study, Ding et al. reported no advantage of IVIM parameters comparing to ADC in distinguishing between ccRCCs and fat-poor AMLs [26]. Besides this, it must be considered that some of the IVIM-derived parameters have shown a limited reproducibility in clinical practice.

Other non-Gaussian models analysis might improve the differentiation between fat-poor AML and ccRCC compared with conventional ADC. Li et al. demonstrated that both IVIM-related parameter D and diffusion heterogeneity index (α) derived from SEM could improve the differentiation between fat-poor AML and ccRCC compared with conventional ADC. The area under the curve (AUC) values for both α and D were 0.953 and 0.964, respectively, while it was 0.860 for ADC [27].

Furthermore, other diffusion techniques, such as diffusion tensor imaging (DTI), allow the analysis of the anisotropic properties of tissues, which may be useful in the characterization of renal masses. In a recent study, the differences in fractional anisotropy (FA) values between fat-poor AMLs and ccRCCs were significant. FA values of fat-poor AMLs were higher than that of ccRCCs as a consequence of the presence of the smooth muscle fibers and thick-walled blood vessels in the fat-poor AMLs, which results in an increased anisotropy [28].

Multiparametric MRI may also be a promising tool for the evaluation of renal masses. So, Cornelis et al. proposed to perform a global evaluation of signal intensity on T1-weighted, T2-weighted, fat-saturation, and chemical shift MR images; wash-in and washout analysis of DCE-MRI; and DW images (Fig. 3.4)

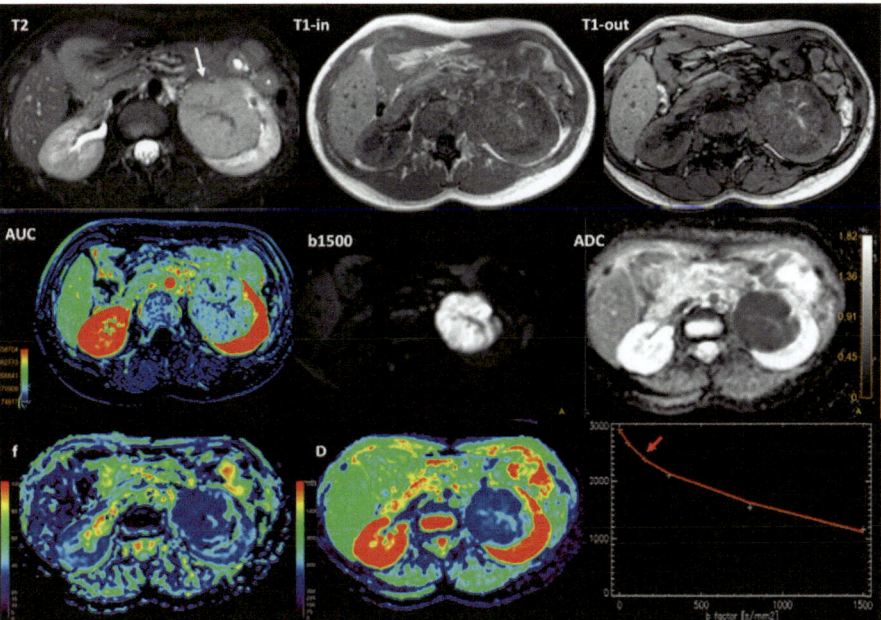

Fig. 3.4 Multiparametric imaging in renal tumors. A 42-year-old woman presented an incidental renal mass on ultrasound examination. MRI allows the evaluation of multiple parameters (signal intensity, degree of enhancement, presence of microscopic or macroscopic fat, restricted diffusion, etc.) in a single exam. MR exam demonstrated a big mass in the left kidney (*white arrow*), which showed a homogeneous decreased signal compared to renal parenchyma on T2-weighted images and a possible central scar. This mass did not show microscopic fat (T1-weighted image in-phase, T1-in, and out of phase, T1-out). In the dynamic acquisition following the administration of contrast media, the mass was hypovascular (area under the curve (AUC) parametric map) relating to the normal kidney. Besides this, there was a marked diffusion restriction with hyperintensity on high *b*-value (b1500) and hypointensity on ADC map (mean ADC value was 0.58×10^{-3} mm^2/s). IVIM model analysis (f = perfusion fraction and D = free perfusion diffusion parametric maps) and signal decay of diffusion signal (*left-bottom*) evidenced that signal decay of diffusion signal at low *b*-values was relatively flat (*red arrow*), revealing low influence of perfusion on diffusion. Final pathological diagnosis was oncocytoma. Unfortunately, the differences in tumor cellularity, vascularization, and hemorrhagic/cystic change contribute to a wide spectrum of imaging findings of renal oncocytomas reported in the literature, which may difficult the diagnosis and may substantially overlap those of common subtypes of clear cell and non-clear cell renal cell carcinomas

[29]. Recent data also suggested that the combination of ADC and peak enhancement and downslope derived from a DCE exam further increased diagnostic accuracy to differentiating ccRCC from other renal cortical tumors [30]. In this sense, Galmiche et al. reported the value of multiparametric imaging including ADC for differentiating oncocytomas from chromophobe RCCs. In this paper, oncocytomas presented significantly higher ADC, faster enhancement, but lower signal intensity index (based on tumor signal intensity on in-phase and opposed-phase T1-weighted images) than carcinomas. This combination of parameters provided sensitivity of 92.3%, specificity of 93.8%, and accuracy of 92.9% for the diagnosis of oncocytoma [31]. Other recent studies have also remarked the added value of DWI to increase the accuracy for diagnosing renal masses [5, 32, 33].

3.2.3 Tumor Grading

Fuhrman grading system is based on a subjective quantification of the nuclear size, nuclear shape, and nucleolar prominence. Tumor cellularity can be characterized by two indices: the number of tumor cell nuclei and the nuclear-to-cytoplasm ratio, which may impact diffusion behavior and may reflect microstructural complexity. The nuclear size of tumor cells in RCC increase with tumor grade. It has been reported in different tumor types a significant correlation between ADC and the number of cells, the total nuclear area, and nucleus/cytoplasm ratio. Different studies have evaluated the use of DWI for discriminating high-grade (Fuhrman grades 3 and 4) from low-grade (Fuhrman grades 1 and 2) RCCs. As a general rule, ADC values were significantly lower with increasing tumor grade [11, 19, 34]. Besides, a strong correlation of the ADC to grading was shown by Rosenkrantz et al. in a study including 57 patients [35]. Apart from this, Yu et al. reported that there were statistically significant differences in the ADC values of low- and high-grade ccRCCs [36]. However, on the contrary, Sandrasegaran et al. observed no significant differences on ADC values related to tumor grading [37]. RCC heterogeneity may explain this contradictory data, because these tumors present areas of different grades, which are often found within the same tumor, and nuclear grading was based on the highest-grade area identified within the tumor independently on its extent. In this setting, ADC map may help to adequately target regions within the renal tumor that indicate greater aggressiveness by selecting regions with low ADC values. Texture or histogram analysis of ADC values may be useful for improving the differentiation between low- and high-stage ccRCCs [38, 39].

   IVIM-derived parameters (D, and pseudodiffusion coefficient, D*) may distinguish well-differentiated renal cancers, which showed significantly higher D values and lower D* measures than moderately and poorly differentiated tumors [24]. Shen et al. reported that pseudodiffusion (also named "fast" ADC) is more accurate compared with the ADC value for characterizing Fuhrman grade of ccRCC [40].

   DKI is a model that allows the measurement of diffusional heterogeneity. The principal parameter, the mean diffusional kurtosis, represents an index of tissue microstructural complexity. Dai et al. reported higher mean diffusion coefficients in grade 1–2 tumors compared to grades 3–4 and vice versa for mean diffusion kurtosis [41].

DTI parameters (ADC, eigenvector E1, and FA) may allow distinguishing high and low nuclear grade tumors. Significant negative correlations between the FA value and cell density and between ADC, E1, and FA values and ki-67 have been reported [42].

Multiparametric MRI may also be a promising tool for ccRCC tumor grading. The study by Cornelis et al. reported that high tumor grade (≥3) was associated with larger tumor size, lower parenchymal wash-in index, and lower ADC ratio (ADC tumor/mean ADC of ipsilateral kidney × 100) [43]. On its part, in a recent paper, Parada Villavicencio et al. demonstrated that the addition of ADC values to a model based on MRI conventional features (hemorrhagic, necrotic, and cystic changes, perirenal fat invasion, and enhancement homogeneity) improved sensitivity and specificity for the differentiation between high-grade and low-grade ccRCC. High-grade ccRCCs showed significantly lower mean ADC values [44]. Notwithstanding, recent data suggest that contrast-enhanced exam (AUC 0.968) was superior to ADC (AUC 0.797) for the differentiation of ccRCC and non-ccRCC [45].

3.2.4 Tumor Staging

DWI may also be useful for tumor staging. In the case of ccRCCs, high ADC values are not associated to an advanced stage (III or IV) [46]. DWI was also significantly more accurate than T2-weighted imaging alone for the diagnosis of tumors with macroscopic renal parenchyma invasion in upper tract TCCs [47]. Besides, Yoshida et al. evidenced that DWI or contrast-enhanced adds an incremental value to T2-weighted sequences in the preoperative T categorization for a relatively inexperienced reader to a level comparable to that of the experienced reader when assessing renal pelvic carcinoma staging [9].

In the case of N-staging, characterization of lymph nodes (LNs) is always challenging for radiologists. Currently, size (i.e., short axis) and morphologic criteria (contour and signal intensity heterogeneity) are used to evaluate LNs with a variable accuracy, because malignant disease may be present even in very small LNs. DWI has demonstrated a good sensitivity for detecting LNs. However, DWI has shown a limited sensitivity and specificity in identifying malignant LNs.

Finally, there is a scarce experience with the use of whole-body DWI in staging renal cancer (Fig. 3.5a, b) [48]. Clear cell carcinomas, which usually have an intrinsically greater water diffusivity and high ADC values, and their metastases can show relative signal suppression on high b-value whole-body DW images and therefore appearing less conspicuous compared with other tumor types on DWI [8, 49]. Besides, it is well known that MR techniques have clear limitations in the detection of lung lesions. Although MR cannot be considered a replacement for CT in the detection of pulmonary metastases from ccRCC, DWI in combination with T1-weighted images may improve the detection of lung metastases ≥0.7 cm [48].

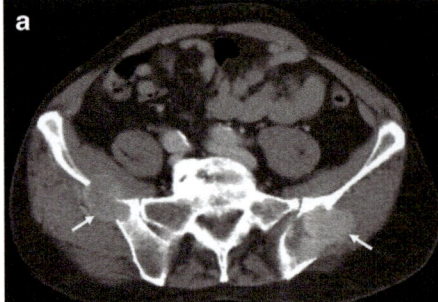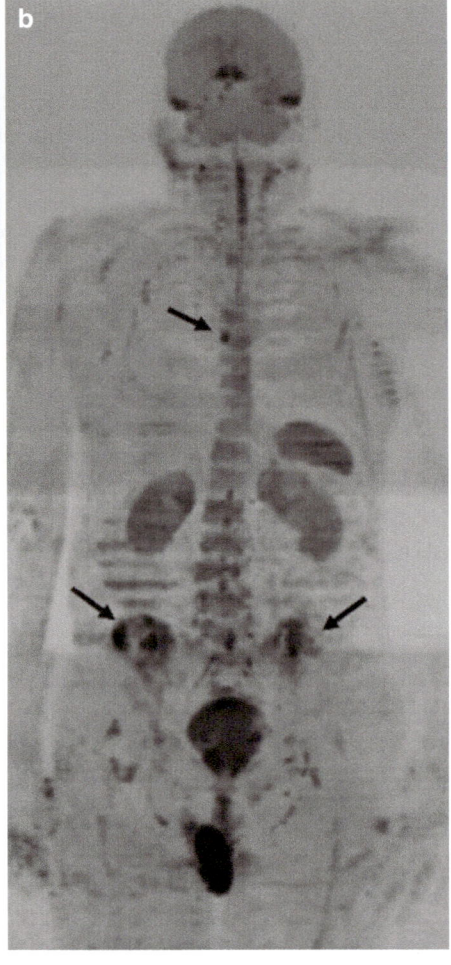

Fig. 3.5 Whole-body diffusion-weighted MRI (WB-DW-MRI). A 53-year-old man with a metastatic renal cell carcinoma. Pelvic contrast-enhanced CT image (**a**) evidenced two lytic metastatic deposits in both iliac bones with soft tissue compound (*white arrows*). Coronal-reformatted WB-DW-MRI with inverted gray scale ($b = 800$ s/mm^2) (**b**) also demonstrated these two metastases and one vertebral lesion (*black arrows*)

3.2.5 Tumor Prognosis

Different studies suggest that ADC may be a prognosis feature in renal tumors. So, the minimum ADC of a tumor was found to be an independent factor for recurrence after nephrectomy in patients with localized RCC [50]. Yoshida et al. demonstrated a statistically significant difference in the ADC between T1a RCC (size ≤4 cm) with or without LNs or distant metastases [51]. Based on these data, perhaps, ccRCCs with low ADC values should be examined extensively for the possibility of distant metastatic lesions.

3.2.6 Treatment Response Evaluation

Functional MR imaging techniques have emerged as important tools in oncology [52, 53]. In this setting, DWI to monitor cancer drug response enables to measure both tumor lesions on axial DWI in the manner as traditional response evaluation is carried out on CT and functional information based on changes in the ADC values. A preliminary study involving only five patients with metastatic renal cancer under antiangiogenic treatment showed a good concordance between measurements of metastatic lesions on high b-value DW images or CT and the corresponding response classification according to RECIST 1.1 [54]. DWI may also play a role as a surrogate marker to reliably predict the probable response early in the course of antiangiogenic therapy for metastatic RCC. Desar et al. demonstrated therapy-related changes in mean ADC with an increasing mean ADC at day 3 followed by a decrease of ADC back to baseline values at day 10 [55]. Unfortunately, these authors did not obtain data about changes in ADC after day 10. In the experience based on preclinical models and in a variety of cancer types treated with antiangiogenic therapy, ADC values showed an early reduction secondary to perfusion decrease, cellular swelling, and intralesional hemorrhage, followed by a progressive increase of ADC values over time due to cell necrosis [56]. On its part, Bharwani et al. evaluated the changes in the primary tumor 10 ± 2 days after completion of three cycles of sunitinib therapy and evaluated the whole-tumor volume and performed histogram analysis. In this study, changes in mean ADC were also not predictive of overall survival, while patients with a decrease in the proportion of the tumor with ADC values lying below the 25th percentile point of the ADC histogram had prolonged survival [57].

Non-mono-exponential DWI models (IVIM or SEM) may offer a robust alternative for the evaluation of early and late antiangiogenic therapy-induced changes. Unfortunately, it results challenging to link changes in the SEM or the IVIM parameters with any particular tissue properties, in particular vascular changes [58], although this point needs to be confirmed in future investigations.

3.2.7 Residual or Relapsing Tumor

DWI may also be helpful to identify foci of residual or relapsing tumor following percutaneous ablation procedures. Tumor tissue may demonstrate restricted diffusion, appearing as bright signal relative to normal renal cortex on DWI at high b-values and as dark signal on ADC maps [59].

3.3 Adrenal Tumors

Normal adrenal glands show high signal intensity on high b-value DWI (Fig. 3.6), although their small size makes ADC measurement difficult. ADC values seem to change with age. Teixeira et al. reported that there was a significant difference in the ADC values of normal adrenal glands between the pre- and postpuberal population [60]. Few reports have discussed the relationships between ADC and adrenal tumor types. ADC measurements are not of value in this differential diagnosis because of

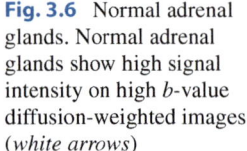

Fig. 3.6 Normal adrenal glands. Normal adrenal glands show high signal intensity on high *b*-value diffusion-weighted images (*white arrows*)

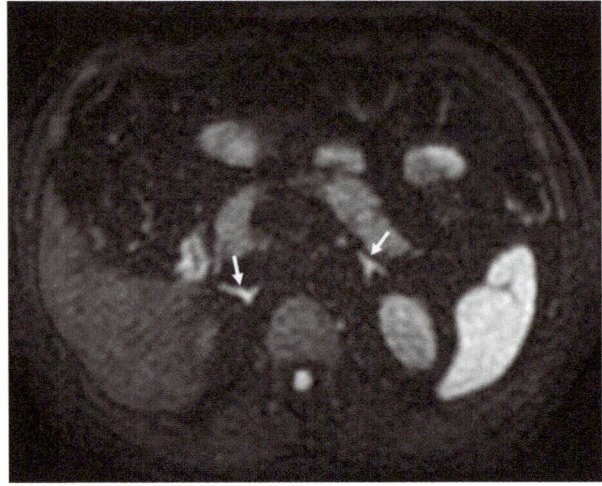

the substantial overlapping of their values between adenomas and metastases [61]. In general, ADC values are not useful in differentiating adrenal masses, but masses that present higher ADC values are more likely to be benign [62, 63].

3.3.1   Characterization of Adrenal Masses

Several studies have compared the ADC values of different adrenal tumors. Most of them were unable to find significant differences in ADC values between benign and malignant adrenal tumors or among the histologic subtypes (Fig. 3.7a–c) [61–69]. There was no difference in ADC values between adenomas and metastatic tumors and pheochromocytomas, although they usually showed higher mean ADC values than those of adenomas or metastatic tumors. It must be stressed that the choice of ROI has a considerable influence on the tumor ADC values. Most of the previous researchers measured mean ADC values by placing the ROI on the solid area of a tumor, avoiding cystic or necrotic areas, which may explain the limited role of mean ADC values in tumor characterization. Apart of this, published data appear to be contradictory. Thus, Tsushima et al. have reported that the mean ADC value of pheochromocytoma was significantly higher than that of adenomas, while Nakajo et al. found that ADC was significantly lower in pheochromocytoma than in lipid-poor adenoma [69, 70]. However, alternative approaches to the analysis of DWI data may improve tumor evaluation. Umanodan et al. retrospectively evaluated 39 adenomas and 13 pheochromocytomas. They found that mean ADC values showed no significant difference between adrenal adenomas and pheochromocytomas. However, ADC histogram analysis was able to differentiate adrenal adenoma from pheochromocytoma. ADC, variance, covariance, and entropy were significantly higher in pheochromocytomas, reflecting a heterogeneous distribution of ADC values related to cystic, hemorrhagic, necrotic, or myxoid changes, which are common in these tumors [71]. As a general rule, ADC measurements used in isolation are not helpful in differentiating benign and malignant lesions. However, in selected populations, DWI may offer

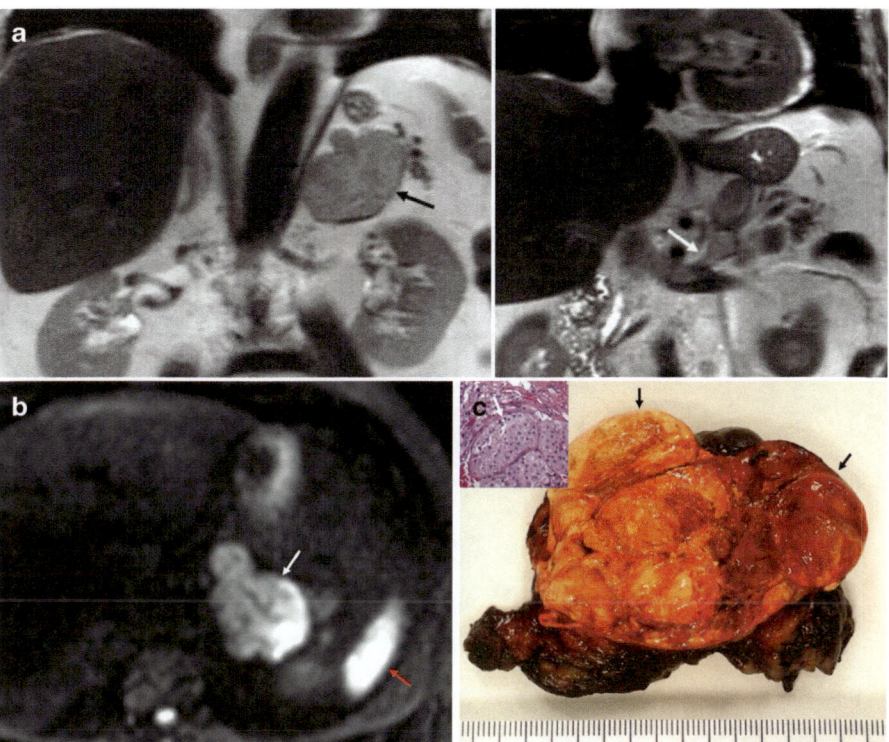

Fig. 3.7 Diffusion-weighted imaging of adrenal mass. A 61-year-old woman with an incidental adrenal mass. Coronal (*left*) and axial (*right*) T2-weighted images (**a**) evidenced a 7.1 cm adrenal mass with irregular shape (*black arrow*) and vascular invasion (*white arrow*). All these imaging findings suggested malignancy. This mass also presented a marked diffusion restriction on the diffusion-weighted images ($b = 1500$ s/mm^2) (**b**). Pathological study (**c**) confirmed an adrenal carcinoma (*black arrows*). The microscopic exam (hematoxylin and eosin staining, 400×) showed high nuclear grade, atypical mitoses, and marked tumor cellularity (*white arrow*), which explained the restriction of water diffusion. In general, diffusion shows clear limitations to distinguish between benign and malignant adrenal tumors or among the histologic subtypes

complementary information in combination with other sequences. Traditionally, chemical shift imaging has been used for characterizing adrenal masses. A decrease of signal intensity more than 20% is considered diagnostic for a lipid-rich adenoma, but signal loss has also been reported in adrenal metastases of tumors that are known to contain intracytoplasmic fat, such as hepatocellular or renal cell carcinomas. In this scenario, several studies have demonstrated that in lesions with less than 16.5% of decrease, low ADC values (1.0×10^{-3} mm^2/s) may help in differentiating benign and malignant lesions. Masses that are indeterminate on chemical shift imaging and that present ADC values of more than 1.5×10^{-3} mm^2/s may be considered benign [62, 66]. Furthermore, advanced methods of DWI as diffusion tensor imaging (DTI) allow the analysis of the anisotropic properties of tissues. Using DTI, Işık et al. demonstrated that the FA values of metastases were significantly lower than those of adenomas [68]. To date, there are not published papers about the use of IVIM or DKI in the characterization of adrenal masses (Fig. 3.8a–d).

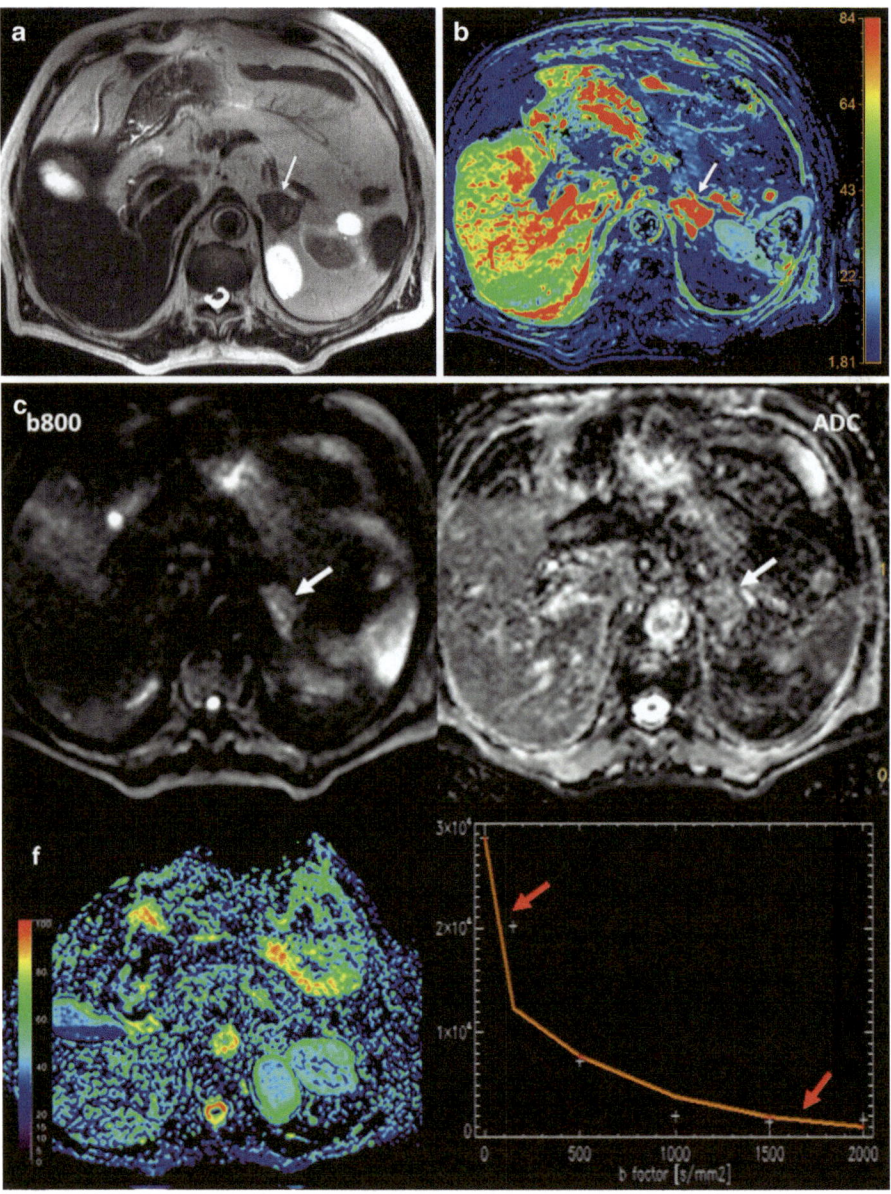

Fig. 3.8 Non-Gaussian diffusion models in the evaluation of adrenal masses. An 83-year-old man with a history of renal cell carcinoma 10 years ago. Axial T2-weighted image (**a**) evidenced a 4 cm adrenal mass (*white arrow*) with heterogeneous signal. Semiquantitative analysis of the dynamic contrast-enhanced MRI acquisition (**b**) showed a hypervascular pattern with a marked wash-in (*white arrow*) within the mass. Mono-exponential and IVIM model analysis of the diffusion (**c**) depicted high ADC values (1.34×10^{-3} mm²/s), an increased perfusion fraction ($f = 21\%$), and an intense signal drop with increased b-values at low b-values (*red arrows*), which also suggested an increased tumor perfusion. Endoscopic ultrasound was performed (**d**) showing a mass that demonstrated a blue pattern with an elastography color score of 5 [range, 1 (soft) to 5 (hard/solid)] (*right*), which suggests malignancy. Biopsy procedure of the mass was performed (*left, arrow*) and confirmed a metastatic deposit of renal cell carcinoma

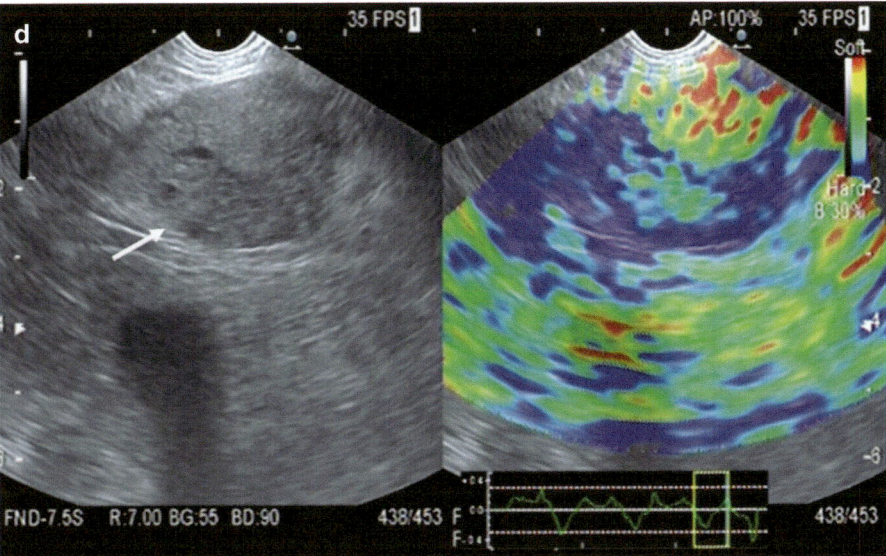

Fig. 3.8 (continued)

3.4 Retroperitoneal Tumors

Retroperitoneal masses include a diverse, and often rare, group of neoplastic and nonneoplastic entities that arise within the retroperitoneal space but outside the major organs in this space. Imaging plays a fundamental role in these entities. The differential diagnosis of retroperitoneal masses can be narrowed down mainly on the basis of their imaging characteristics and patterns of involvement. Imaging evaluation of these tumors is mainly based on determining tumor location and recognizing specific features: patterns of spread and tumor components (fat, myxoid matrix, vascularization, etc.). However, there is still a wide overlapping in their imaging findings [72–77]. Imaging characteristics of retroperitoneal soft tissue masses do not differ from those that show in other parts of the anatomy. Few of them (i.e., lipoma, hemangioma) have specific imaging features that help with characterization. There are a limited number of papers in the literature specifically focused on the use of DWI in the retroperitoneum. DWI may add value to morphologic sequences in the detection, characterization, and post-therapy assessment of retroperitoneal masses [78–80].

3.4.1 Characterization of Retroperitoneal Masses

DWI may add value to morphologic sequences in the characterization of soft tissue malignancies, including those arising in the retroperitoneum [78–80]. A detailed description of the role of DWI in the wide variety of tumor masses that can arise in the retroperitoneum is beyond the scope of this chapter. In general, the lower the

ADC values, the higher the likelihood of malignancy. However, at present no cut-off point of the ADC value has been established in the literature to distinguish benign from malignant soft tissue tumors. ADC values of benign and malignant tumors overlap: not all malignant tumors present more cellularity than the benign, and the benign often have an extracellular matrix similar to the malignant. Besides, cystic, necrotic, myxoid, or cartilaginous masses or portions of a complex mass may exhibit high ADC values regardless of being benign or malignant. Finally, a malignant soft tissue mass may include two or more distinct intermingled components (Fig. 3.9a–c). In consequence, DWI findings must be interpreted alongside

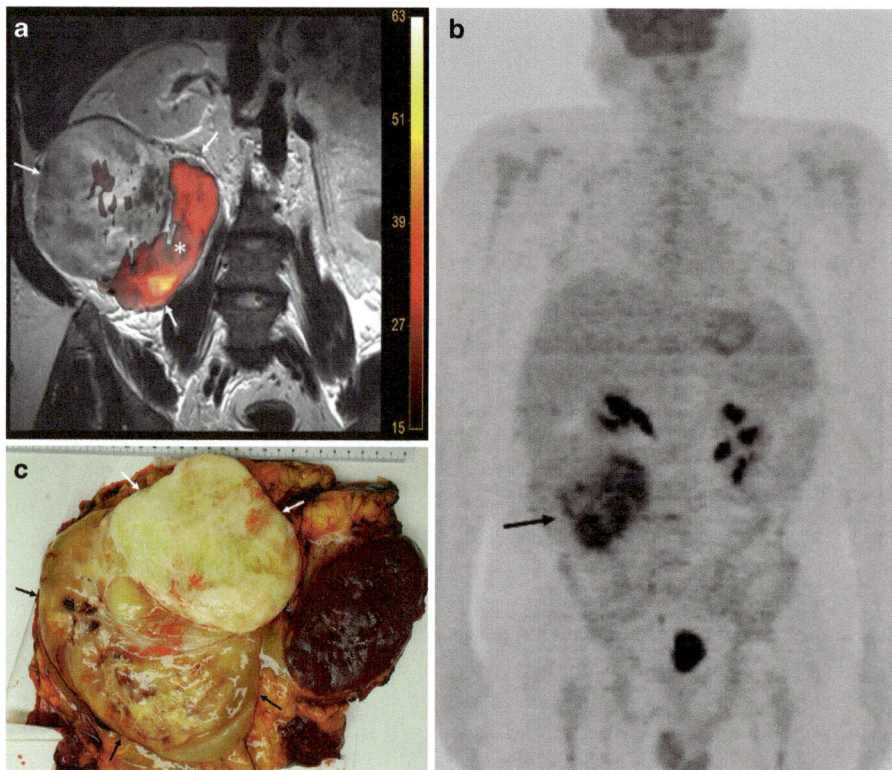

Fig. 3.9 Retroperitoneal mass. A 43-year-old man with a retroperitoneal mass. Fused image superimposing axial T2-weighted MR image and color-coded map derived from high *b*-value diffusion-weighted image (**a**) clearly delineated a 22 cm mass (*white arrows*) containing areas with different behaviors on diffusion-weighted imaging. The cranial part of the tumor did not show restricted diffusion on the fused image, while the caudal part of the tumor (*white asterisk, red areas*) demonstrated marked restriction. PET image (**b**) also evidenced increased metabolic activity on the caudal part of the mass (*black arrow*). Pathologic specimen (**c**) evidenced a big heterogeneous mass, which corresponded to a mixed malignant liposarcoma that presented both myxoid and necrotic areas (*white arrows*, corresponding to the cranial part of the tumor) and solid areas of fibrosarcoma in the caudal part of the mass (*black arrows*). This distribution could explain imaging findings on diffusion and PET scan

its appearance on conventional MR sequences and DCE imaging. Hypercellular masses (i.e., small round cell tumors) or fibrotic tumors usually exhibit low ADC values. Thus, lymphomas, hypercellular lesions composed of small round cells with reduced extracellular space, usually show lower ADC values compared to other malignant or benign retroperitoneal lesions [81, 82]. DWI has also demonstrated a good accuracy in the differentiation of benign masses (i.e., hematomas and retroperitoneal fibrosis [RF]) from malignant lesions [80, 83]. In the case of RF, ADC may allow to differentiate chronic RF (which shows higher ADC values) from active RF or malignant RF and retroperitoneal malignant neoplasms [83]. In the early stages of fibrosis, the high cellular content of the plaque explains the restricted water diffusion (Fig. 3.10a, b). On the contrary, in the chronic stage, the less cellular environment improves the diffusion.

Theoretically, findings on DWI could also be used for biopsy guidance in order to identify the most suspicious areas within the tumor. However, to our knowledge this point has not been reported in the radiological literature in retroperitoneal masses.

Finally, although IVIM-related parameters in soft tissue masses do not have a clear biological explanation [84], preliminary data suggest that IVIM imaging may be helpful for differentiating benign, intermediate, and malignant solid soft tissue tumors [85, 86].

3.4.2 Tumor Staging

Enlarged retroperitoneal LNs are one of the most frequent retroperitoneal masses. Lymphoma and metastatic disease are the main causes of retroperitoneal lymphadenopathy. Most patients with non-Hodgkin's lymphoma have abdominal involvement. Whole-body DWI is gaining increased attention as an alternative to PET/CT in the staging and response evaluation of lymphoma or seminoma as it can assess the entire body, is radiation-free, and does not require use of a contrast agent [87, 88].

3.4.3 Therapy Response

DWI appears to perform well in the assessment of response to therapy of retroperitoneal masses with, in general, an increasing ADC from baseline in the case of good responders. Most studies have shown that successful treatment of lymphoma is reflected by increases in tumor ADC values. Besides, whole-body DWI is a feasible technique in follow-up of patients with testicular cancer. In these patients, DWI may offer an added value data to conventional MRI sequences regarding the activity of residual masses (Fig. 3.11a, b). DWI may also be a useful method for the evaluation of response of RF to treatment without contrast agents. After treatment, lesions showed significantly lower signal intensities on high b-value images and higher ADC values compared with pre-therapy exams [89, 90].

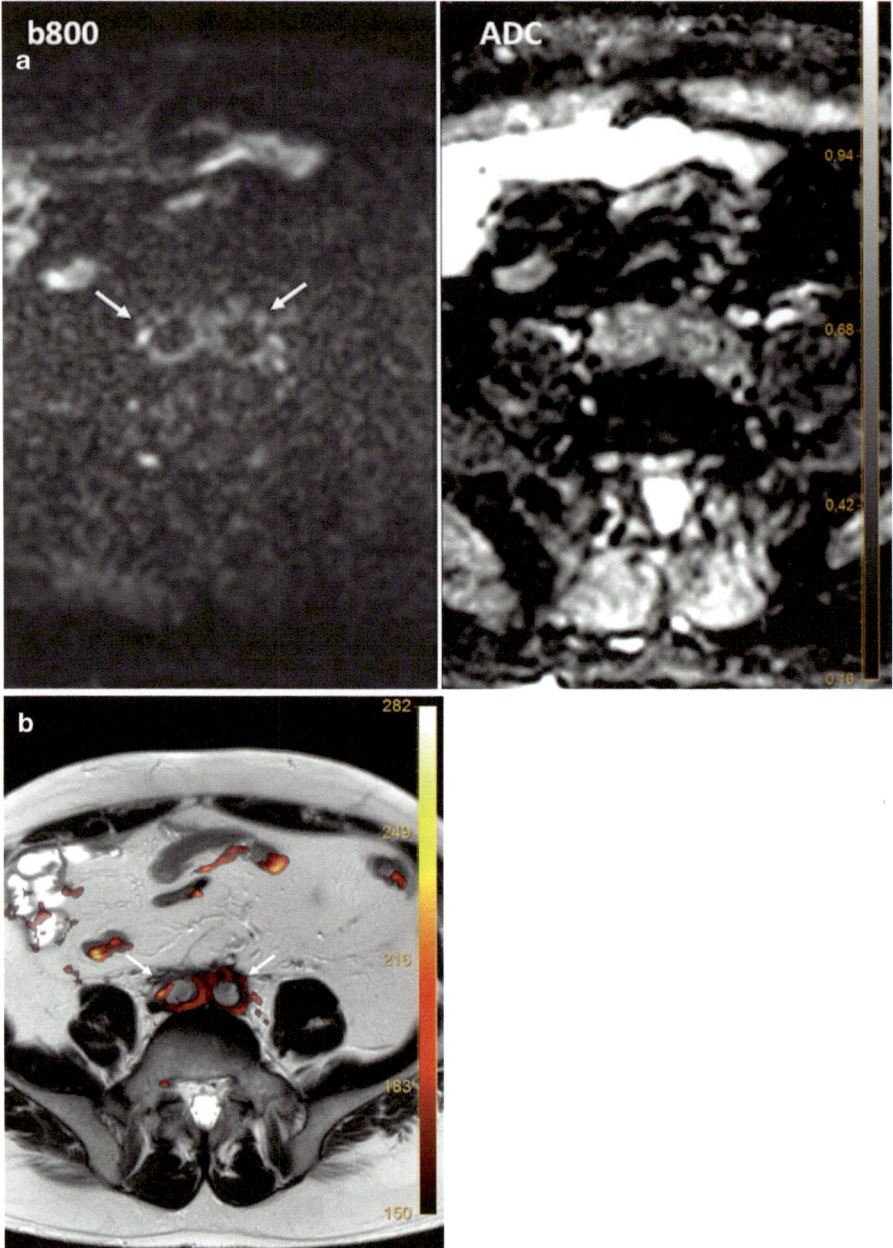

Fig. 3.10 Retroperitoneal fibrosis. Diffusion-weighted image and ADC map (**a**) demonstrated increased signal on diffusion (*white arrows*) around main retroperitoneal vessels (*left*) with patchy areas of decreased ADC values (*right*). Fused image superimposing axial T2-weighted MR image and color-coded map derived from high *b*-value diffusion-weighted image (**b**) clearly delineated areas with restricted diffusion (*white arrows*)

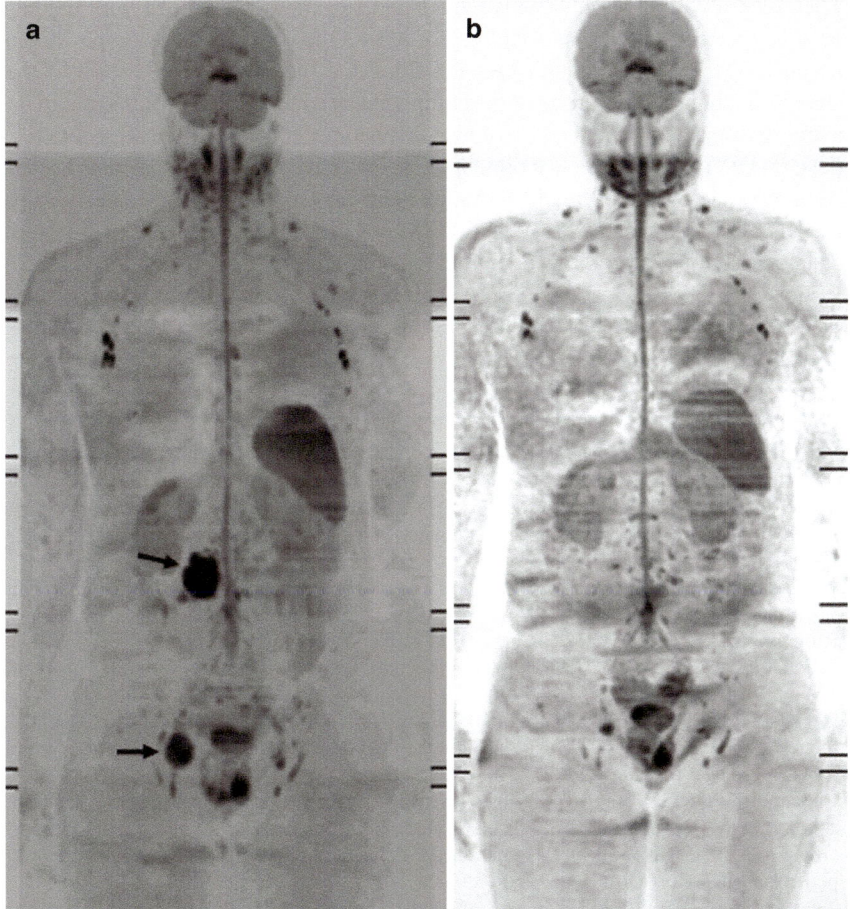

Fig. 3.11 Therapeutic monitoring. A 34-year-old man with seminoma. Whole-body diffusion-weighted MRI (WB-DW-MRI) with inverted gray scale ($b = 800$ s/mm^2) pre-therapy (**a**) demonstrated two metastatic adenopathic conglomerates in the pelvis (iliac chains) and retroperitoneum (*black arrows*). Post-chemotherapy, WB-DW-MRI confirmed the disappearance of these metastatic deposits (**b**)

Conclusions

DWI is being established as a pivotal aspect of MR imaging in the evaluation of tumors, augmenting the morphologic information provided by conventional MR imaging. DWI offers many opportunities in the field of oncologic imaging and can aid in detection, characterization, grading, and staging of tumors and in the prediction and assessment of response to therapy. However, the role of DWI in the evaluation of renal, adrenal, and retroperitoneal masses is limited and depends on the tumor type. To date, published studies have not provided a reliable estimation of DWI performance in the evaluation of renal, adrenal, and retroperitoneal masses.

They reflect widely variable sensitivities and specificities for DWI with moderate accuracy and an overlap of ADC values across the different tumor types, mainly because of the measurement of ADC values and the small sample sizes of these studies. Technical differences of the equipment or conduct of the trials seem to have a major impact on the values of the diffusion-related parameters reported. To develop DWI as a noninvasive biomarker, prospective studies with standardized test parameters are needed. Finally, although there are only preliminary data, advanced models of diffusion analysis, such as IVIM or DKI, may improve the diagnosis and characterization of pathological entities in these areas with diffusion.

Acknowledgments Javier Sánchez González, PhD, and Paula Montesinos Suárez de la Vega, PhD. Clinical Scientist at Philips Spain.

References

1. Taouli B, Beer AJ, Chenevert T, Collins D, Lehman C, Matos C, et al. Diffusion-weighted imaging outside the brain: consensus statement from an ISMRM-sponsored workshop. J Magn Reson Imaging. 2016;44:521–4.
2. Koh DM, Collins DJ, Orton MR. Intravoxel incoherent motion in body diffusion-weighted MRI: reality and challenges. AJR Am J Roentgenol. 2011;196:1351–61.
3. Rosenkrantz AB, Padhani AR, Chenevert TL, Koh DM, De Keyzer F, Taouli B, et al. Body diffusion kurtosis imaging: basic principles, applications, and considerations for clinical practice. J Magn Reson Imaging. 2015;42:1190–202.
4. Chandarana H, Lee VS, Hecht E, Taouli B, Sigmund EE. Comparison of biexponential and monoexponential model of diffusion weighted imaging in evaluation of renal lesions: preliminary experience. Investig Radiol. 2011;46:285–91.
5. Ramamurthy NK, Moosavi B, McInnes MD, Flood TA, Schieda N. Multiparametric MRI of solid renal masses: pearls and pitfalls. Clin Radiol. 2015;70:304–16.
6. Gilet AG, Kang SK, Kim D, Chandarana H. Advanced renal mass imaging: diffusion and perfusion MRI. Curr Urol Rep. 2012;13:93–8.
7. Tang Y, Zhou Y, Du W, Liu N, Zhang C, Ouyang T, et al. Standard b-value versus low b-value diffusion-weighted MRI in renal cell carcinoma: a systematic review and meta-analysis. BMC Cancer. 2014;14:843.
8. Padhani AR, Koh DM, Collins DJ. Whole-body diffusion-weighted MR imaging in cancer: current status and research directions. Radiology. 2011;261:700–18.
9. Yoshida R, Yoshizako T, Maruyama M, Mori H, Ishikawa N, Tamaki Y, et al. The value of adding diffusion-weighted images for tumor detection and preoperative staging in renal pelvic carcinoma for the reader's experience. Abdom Radiol (NY). 2017. https://doi.org/10.1007/s00261-017-1116-5. [Epub ahead of print].
10. Sufana Iancu A, Colin P, Puech P, Villers A, Ouzzane A, Fantoni JC, et al. Significance of ADC value for detection and characterization of urothelial carcinoma of upper urinary tract using diffusion-weighted MRI. World J Urol. 2013;31:13–9.
11. Taouli B, Thakur RK, Mannelli L, Babb JS, Kim S, Hecht EM, et al. Renal lesions: characterization with diffusion-weighted imaging versus contrast-enhanced MR imaging. Radiology. 2009;251:398–407.
12. Goyal A, Sharma R, Bhalla AS, Gamanagatti S, Seth A. Pseudotumours in chronic kidney disease: can diffusion-weighted MRI rule out malignancy. Eur J Radiol. 2013;82:1870–6.
13. Kang SK, Zhang A, Pandharipande PV, Chandarana H, Braithwaite RS, Littenberg B. DWI for renal mass characterization: systematic review and meta-analysis of diagnostic test performance. AJR Am J Roentgenol. 2015;205:317–24.

14. Zhang H, Gan Q, Wu Y, Liu R, Liu X, Huang Z, et al. Diagnostic performance of diffusion-weighted magnetic resonance imaging in differentiating human renal lesions (benignity or malignancy): a meta-analysis. Abdom Radiol (NY). 2016;41:1997–2010.
15. Lassel EA, Rao R, Schwenke C, Schoenberg SO, Michaely HJ. Diffusion-weighted imaging of focal renal lesions: a meta-analysis. Eur Radiol. 2014;24:241–9.
16. Paudyal B, Paudyal P, Tsushima Y, Oriuchi N, Amanuma M, Miyazaki M, et al. The role of the ADC value in the characterisation of renal carcinoma by diffusion-weighted MRI. Br J Radiol. 2010;83:336–43.
17. Wang H, Cheng L, Zhang X, Wang D, Guo A, Gao Y, Ye H. Renal cell carcinoma: diffusion-weighted MR imaging for subtype differentiation at 3.0 T. Radiology. 2010;257:135–43.
18. Sevcenco S, Heinz-Peer G, Ponhold L, Javor D, Kuehhas FE, Klingler HC, et al. Utility and limitations of 3-Tesla diffusion-weighted magnetic resonance imaging for differentiation of renal tumors. Eur J Radiol. 2014;83:909–13.
19. Mytsyk Y, Dutka I, Borys Y, Komnatska I, Shatynska-Mytsyk I, Farooqi AA, et al. Renal cell carcinoma: applicability of the apparent coefficient of the diffusion-weighted estimated by MRI for improving their differential diagnosis, histologic subtyping, and differentiation grade. Int Urol Nephrol. 2017;49:215–24.
20. Agnello F, Roy C, Bazille G, Galia M, Midiri M, Charles T, et al. Small solid renal masses: characterization by diffusion-weighted MRI at 3 T. Clin Radiol. 2013;68:e301–8.
21. Goyal A, Sharma R, Bhalla AS, Gamanagatti S, Seth A. Diffusion-weighted MRI in inflammatory renal lesions: all that glitters is not RCC! Eur Radiol. 2013;23:272–9.
22. Chandarana H, Kang SK, Wong S, Rusinek H, Zhang JL, Arizono S, et al. Diffusion-weighted intravoxel incoherent motion imaging of renal tumors with histopathologic correlation. Investig Radiol. 2012;47:688–96.
23. Rheinheimer S, Stieltjes B, Schneider F, Simon D, Pahernik S, Kauczor HU, et al. Investigation of renal lesions by diffusion-weighted magnetic resonance imaging applying intravoxel incoherent motion-derived parameters—initial experience. Eur J Radiol. 2012;81:e310–6.
24. Cong XY, Chen Y, Zhang J, XD Y, Ye F, WJ Y, et al. Application of diffusion-weighted intravoxel incoherent motion imaging in diagnosis of renal cell carcinoma subtypes. Zhonghua Zhong Liu Za Zhi. 2016;38:434–9.
25. Gaing B, Sigmund EE, Huang WC, Babb JS, Parikh NS, Stoffel D, et al. Subtype differentiation of renal tumors using voxel-based histogram analysis of intravoxel incoherent motion parameters. Investig Radiol. 2015;50:144–52.
26. Ding Y, Zeng M, Rao S, Chen C, Fu C, Zhou J. Comparison of biexponential and monoexponential model of diffusion-weighted imaging for distinguishing between common renal cell carcinoma and fat poor angiomyolipoma. Korean J Radiol. 2016;17:853–63.
27. Li H, Liang L, Li A, Hu Y, Hu D, Li Z, Kamel IR. Monoexponential, biexponential, and stretched exponential diffusion-weighted imaging models: quantitative biomarkers for differentiating renal clear cell carcinoma and minimal fat angiomyolipoma. J Magn Reson Imaging. 2016. https://doi.org/10.1002/jmri.25524. [Epub ahead of print].
28. Feng Q, Ma Z, Zhang S, Wu J. Usefulness of diffusion tensor imaging for the differentiation between low-fat angiomyolipoma and clear cell carcinoma of the kidney. Spring. 2016;5:12.
29. Cornelis F, Grenier N. Multiparametric magnetic resonance imaging of solid renal tumors: a practical algorithm. Semin Ultrasound CT MR. 2017;38:47–58.
30. Hötker AM, Mazaheri Y, Wibmer A, Karlo CA, Zheng J, Moskowitz CS, et al. Differentiation of clear cell renal cell carcinoma from other renal cortical tumors by use of a quantitative multiparametric MRI approach. AJR Am J Roentgenol. 2017;208:W85–91.
31. Galmiche C, Bernhard JC, Yacoub M, Ravaud A, Grenier N, Cornelis F. Is multiparametric MRI useful for differentiating oncocytomas from chromophobe renal cell carcinomas? AJR Am J Roentgenol. 2017;208:343–50.
32. Zhang HM, YH W, Gan Q, Lyu X, Zhu XL, Kuang M, et al. Diagnostic utility of diffusion-weighted magnetic resonance imaging in differentiating small solid renal tumors ($\leq$4 cm) at 3.0T magnetic resonance imaging. Chin Med J. 2015;128:1444–9.

33. Choi YA, Kim CK, Park SY, Cho SW, Park BK. Subtype differentiation of renal cell carcinoma using diffusion-weighted and blood oxygenation level-dependent MRI. AJR Am J Roentgenol. 2014;203:W78–84.
34. Goyal A, Sharma R, Bhalla AS, Gamanagatti S, Seth A. Diffusion-weighted MRI in renal cell carcinoma: a surrogate marker for predicting nuclear grade and histological subtype. Acta Radiol. 2012;53:349–58.
35. Rosenkrantz AB, Niver BE, Fitzgerald EF, Babb JS, Chandarana H, Melamed J. Utility of the apparent diffusion coefficient for distinguishing clear cell renal cell carcinoma of low and high nuclear grade. AJR Am J Roentgenol. 2010;195:W344–51.
36. Yu X, Lin M, Ouyang H, Zhou C, Zhang H. Application of ADC measurement in characterization of renal cell carcinomas with different pathological types and grades by 3.0T diffusion-weighted MRI. Eur J Radiol. 2012;81:3061–6.
37. Sandrasegaran K, Sundaram CP, Ramaswamy R, Akisik FM, Rydberg MP, Lin C, et al. Usefulness of diffusion-weighted imaging in the evaluation of renal masses. AJR Am J Roentgenol. 2010;194:438–45.
38. Kierans AS, Rusinek H, Lee A, Shaikh MB, Triolo M, Huang WC, et al. Textural differences in apparent diffusion coefficient between low- and high-stage clear cell renal cell carcinoma. AJR Am J Roentgenol. 2014;203:W637–44.
39. Zhang YD, CJ W, Wang Q, Zhang J, Wang XN, Liu XS, et al. Comparison of utility of histogram apparent diffusion coefficient and R2* for differentiation of low-grade from high-grade clear cell renal cell carcinoma. AJR Am J Roentgenol. 2015;205:W193–201.
40. Shen L, Zhou L, Liu X, Yang X. Comparison of biexponential and monoexponential DWI in evaluation of Fuhrman grading of clear cell renal cell carcinoma. Diagn Interv Radiol. 2017;23:100–5.
41. Dai Y, Yao Q, Wu G, Wu D, Wu L, Zhu L, et al. Characterization of clear cell renal cell carcinoma with diffusion kurtosis imaging: correlation between diffusion kurtosis parameters and tumor cellularity. NMR Biomed. 2016;29:873–81.
42. Feng Q, Fang W, Sun XP, Sun SH, Zhang RM, Ma ZJ. Renal clear cell carcinoma: diffusion tensor imaging diagnostic accuracy and correlations with clinical and histopathological factors. Clin Radiol. 2017;72(7):560–4.
43. Cornelis F, Tricaud E, Lasserre AS, Petitpierre F, Bernhard JC, Le Bras Y, et al. Multiparametric magnetic resonance imaging for the differentiation of low and high grade clear cell renal carcinoma. Eur Radiol. 2015;25:24–31.
44. Parada Villavicencio C, Mc Carthy RJ, Miller FH. Can diffusion-weighted magnetic resonance imaging of clear cell renal carcinoma predict low from high nuclear grade tumors. Abdom Radiol (NY). 2017;42:1241–9.
45. Yamamoto A, Tamada T, Ito K, Sone T, Kanki A, Tanimoto D, et al. Differentiation of subtypes of renal cell carcinoma: dynamic contrast-enhanced magnetic resonance imaging versus diffusion-weighted magnetic resonance imaging. Clin Imaging. 2017;41:53–8.
46. Nakamura T, Yoshizako T, Araki H, Maruyama M, Uchida K, Tamaki Y, et al. The relation between apparent diffusion coefficient and clinical stage of clear-cell renal cell carcinoma. Clin Imaging. 2015;39:72–5.
47. Akita H, Jinzaki M, Kikuchi E, Sugiura H, Akita A, Mikami S, et al. Preoperative T categorization and prediction of histopathologic grading of urothelial carcinoma in renal pelvis using diffusion-weighted MRI. AJR Am J Roentgenol. 2011;197:1130–6.
48. Liu J, Yang X, Li F, Wang X, Jiang X. Preliminary study of whole-body diffusion-weighted imaging in detecting pulmonary metastatic lesions from clear cell renal cell carcinoma: comparison with CT. Acta Radiol. 2011;52:954–63.
49. Koh DM, Blackledge M, Padhani AR, Takahara T, Kwee TC, Leach MO, Collins DJ. Whole-body diffusion-weighted MRI: tips, tricks, and pitfalls. AJR Am J Roentgenol. 2012;199:252–62.
50. Nishie A, Kakihara D, Asayama Y, Ishigami K, Ushijima Y, Takayama Y, et al. Apparent diffusion coefficient: an associative factor for recurrence after nephrectomy in localized renal cell carcinoma. J Magn Reson Imaging. 2016;43:166–72.

51. Yoshida R, Yoshizako T, Hisatoshi A, Mori H, Tamaki Y, Ishikawa N, et al. The additional utility of apparent diffusion coefficient values of clear-cell renal cell carcinoma for predicting metastasis during clinical staging. Acta Radiol Open. 2017;6:2058460116687174.
52. Benz MR, Vargas HA, Sala E, Functional MR. Imaging techniques in oncology in the era of personalized medicine. Magn Reson Imaging Clin N Am. 2016;24:1–10.
53. García-Figueiras R, Padhani AR, Baleato-González S. Therapy monitoring with functional and molecular MR imaging. Magn Reson Imaging Clin N Am. 2016;24:261–88.
54. Farnebo J, Suzuki C, Vargas-Paris R, Sandström P, Blomqvist L. Measurements of metastatic renal cell tumours as determined by diffusion weighted imaging or computed tomography are in close agreement, a pilot study. Eur J Radiol Open. 2017;4:45–9.
55. Desar IM, ter Voert EG, Hambrock T, van Asten JJ, van Spronsen DJ, Mulders PF, et al. Functional MRI techniques demonstrate early vascular changes in renal cell cancer patients treated with sunitinib: a pilot study. Cancer Imaging. 2012;11:259–65.
56. Jeon TY, Kim CK, Kim JH, Im GH, Park BK, Lee JH. Assessment of early therapeutic response to sorafenib in renal cell carcinoma xenografts by dynamic contrast enhanced and diffusion-weighted MR imaging. Br J Radiol. 2015;88:20150163.
57. Bharwani N, Miquel ME, Powles T, Dilks P, Shawyer A, Sahdev A, et al. Diffusion-weighted and multiphase contrast-enhanced MRI as surrogate markers of response to neoadjuvant sunitinib in metastatic renal cell carcinoma. Br J Cancer. 2014;110:616–24.
58. Orton MR, Messiou C, Collins D, Morgan VA, Tessier J, Young H, et al. Diffusion-weighted MR imaging of metastatic abdominal and pelvic tumours is sensitive to early changes induced by a VEGF inhibitor using alternative diffusion attenuation models. Eur Radiol. 2016;26:1412–9.
59. Iannuccilli JD, Grand DJ, Dupuy DE, Mayo-Smith WW. Percutaneous ablation for small renal masses-imaging follow-up. Semin Intervent Radiol. 2014;31:50–63.
60. Teixeira SR, Elias PC, Leite AF, de Oliveira TM, Muglia VF, Elias Junior J. Apparent diffusion coefficient of normal adrenal glands. Radiol Bras. 2016;49:363–8.
61. Halefoglu AM, Altun I, Disli C, Ulusay SM, Ozel BD, Basak M. A prospective study on the utility of diffusion-weighted and quantitative chemical-shift magnetic resonance imaging in the distinction of adrenal adenomas and metastases. J Comput Assist Tomogr. 2012;36:367–74.
62. Sandrasegaran K, Patel AA, Ramaswamy R, Samuel VP, Northcutt BG, Frank MS, et al. Characterization of adrenal masses with diffusion-weighted imaging. AJR Am J Roentgenol. 2011;197:132–8.
63. Miller FH, Wang Y, McCarthy RJ, Yaghmai V, Merrick L, Larson A, et al. Utility of diffusion-weighted MRI in characterization of adrenal lesions. AJR Am J Roentgenol. 2010;194:W179–85.
64. Hida T, Nishie A, Asayama Y, Ishigami K, Ushijima Y, Takayam Y, et al. Apparent diffusion coefficient characteristics of various adrenal tumors. Magn Reson Med Sci. 2014;13:183–9.
65. Cicekci M, Onur MR, Aydin AM, Gül Y, Ozkan Y, Akpolat N, et al. The role of apparent diffusion coefficient values in differentiation between adrenal masses. Clin Imaging. 2014;38:148–53.
66. Song J, Zhang C, Liu Q, Yu T, Jiang X, Xia Q, et al. Utility of chemical shift and diffusion-weighted imaging in characterization of hyperattenuating adrenal lesions at 3.0T. Eur J Radiol. 2012;81:2137–43.
67. Dong Y, Liu Q. Differentiation of malignant from benign pheochromocytomas with diffusion-weighted and dynamic contrast-enhanced magnetic resonance at 3.0 T. J Comput Assist Tomogr. 2012;36:361–6.
68. Isik Y, Gurses B, Tasdelen N, Kilickesmez O, Firat Z, Ordu C, et al. Diffusion tensor imaging in the differentiation of adrenal adenomas and metastases. Diagn Interv Radiol. 2012;18:189–94.

69. Tsushima Y, Takahashi-Taketomi A, Endo K. Diagnostic utility of diffusion-weighted MR imaging and apparent diffusion coefficient value for the diagnosis of adrenal tumors. J Magn Reson Imaging. 2009;29:112–7.
70. Nakajo M, Nakajo M, Fukukura Y, Jinjuji M, Shindo T, Nakabeppu Y, et al. Diagnostic performances of FDG-PET/CT and diffusion-weighted imaging indices for differentiating benign pheochromocytoma from other benign adrenal tumors. Abdom Imaging. 2015;40:1655–65.
71. Umanodan T, Fukukura Y, Kumagae Y, Shindo T, Nakajo M, Takumi K, et al. ADC histogram analysis for adrenal tumor histogram analysis of apparent diffusion coefficient in differentiating adrenal adenoma from pheochromocytoma. J Magn Reson Imaging. 2017;45:1195–203.
72. Nishino M, Hayakawa K, Minami M, Yamamoto A, Ueda H, Takasu K. Primary retroperitoneal neoplasms: CT and MR imaging findings with anatomic and pathologic diagnostic clues. Radiographics. 2003;23:45–57.
73. Scali EP, Chandler TM, Heffernan EJ, Coyle J, Harris AC, Chang SD. Primary retroperitoneal masses: what is the differential diagnosis? Abdom Imaging. 2015;40:1887–903.
74. Sangster GP, Migliaro M, Heldmann MG, Bhargava P, Hamidian A, Thomas-Ogunniyi J. The gamut of primary retroperitoneal masses: multimodality evaluation with pathologic correlation. Abdom Radiol (NY). 2016;41:1411–30.
75. Osman S, Lehnert BE, Elojeimy S, Cruite I, Mannelli L, Bhargava P, et al. A comprehensive review of the retroperitoneal anatomy, neoplasms, and pattern of disease spread. Curr Probl Diagn Radiol. 2013;42:191–208.
76. Shanbhogue AK, Fasih N, Macdonald DB, Sheikh AM, Menias CO, Prasad SR. Uncommon primary pelvic retroperitoneal masses in adults: a pattern-based imaging approach. Radiographics. 2012;32:795–817.
77. Rajiah P, Sinha R, Cuevas C, Dubinsky TJ, Bush WH Jr, Kolokythas O. Imaging of uncommon retroperitoneal masses. Radiographics. 2011;31:949–76.
78. Vilanova JC, Baleato-Gonzalez S, Romero MJ, Carrascoso-Arranz J, Luna A. Assessment of musculoskeletal malignancies with functional MR imaging. Magn Reson Imaging Clin N Am. 2016;24:239–59.
79. Subhawong TK, Jacobs MA, Fayad LM. Insights into quantitative diffusion-weighted MRI for musculoskeletal tumor imaging. AJR Am J Roentgenol. 2014;203:560–72.
80. Dallaudière B, Lecouvet F, Vande Berg B, Omoumi P, Perlepe V, Cerny M, et al. Diffusion-weighted MR imaging in musculoskeletal diseases: current concepts. Diagn Interv Imaging. 2015;96:327–40.
81. Nakayama T, Yoshimitsu K, Irie H, Aibe H, Tajima T, Shinozaki K, et al. Usefulness of the calculated apparent diffusion coefficient value in the differential diagnosis of retroperitoneal masses. J Magn Reson Imaging. 2004;20:735–42.
82. Rosenkrantz AB, Spieler B, Seuss CR, Stifelman MD, Kim S. Utility of MRI features for differentiation of retroperitoneal fibrosis and lymphoma. AJR Am J Roentgenol. 2012;199:118–26.
83. Bakir B, Yilmaz F, Turkay R, Ozel S, Bilgiç B, Velioglu A, et al. Role of diffusion-weighted MR imaging in the differentiation of benign retroperitoneal fibrosis from malignant neoplasm: preliminary study. Radiology. 2014;272:438–45.
84. Marzi S, Stefanetti L, Sperati F, Anelli V. Relationship between diffusion parameters derived from intravoxel incoherent motion MRI and perfusion measured by dynamic contrast-enhanced MRI of soft tissue tumors. NMR Biomed. 2016;29:6–14.
85. Wu H, Zhang S, Liang C, Liu H, Liu Y, Mei Y, et al. Intravoxel incoherent motion MRI for the differentiation of benign, intermediate, and malignant solid soft-tissue tumors. J Magn Reson Imaging. 2017. https://doi.org/10.1002/jmri.25733. [Epub ahead of print].
86. Du J, Li K, Zhang W, Wang S, Song Q, Liu A, et al. Intravoxel incoherent motion MR imaging: comparison of diffusion and perfusion characteristics for differential diagnosis of soft tissue tumors. Medicine (Baltimore). 2015;94:e1028.

87. Lin C, Luciani A, Itti E, Haioun C, Violaine S, Meignan M, et al. Whole-body diffusion magnetic resonance imaging in the assessment of lymphoma. Cancer Imaging. 2012;12:403–8.
88. Mosavi F, Laurell A, Ahlström H. Whole body MRI, including diffusion-weighted imaging in follow-up of patients with testicular cancer. Acta Oncol. 2015;54:1763–9.
89. Kamper L, Haage P, Brandt AS, Piroth W, Abanador-Kamper N, Roth S, et al. Diffusion-weighted MRI in the follow-up of chronic periaortitis. Br J Radiol. 2015;88:20150145.
90. Kamper L, Brandt AS, Ekamp H, Abanador-Kamper N, Piroth W, Roth S, et al. Diffusion-weighted MRI findings of treated and untreated retroperitoneal fibrosis. Diagn Interv Radiol. 2014;20:459–63.

Bladder and Upper Urinary Tract Urothelial Cancer

4

Mohamed E. Abou El-Ghar, Mohammed A. Badawy, and Tarek A. El-Diasty

Abbreviations

ADC	Apparent diffusion coefficient
BCa	Bladder cancer
CRT	Complete response therapy
CSF	Cerebrospinal fluid
CT	Computed tomography
DCE	Dynamic contrast-enhanced
DTI	Diffusion tensor imaging
DWI	Diffusion-weighted imaging
DW-MRI	Diffusion-weighted magnetic resonance imaging
FA	Fractional anisotropy
FT	Fractional tractography
G1	Grade 1
G2	Grade 2
G3	Grade 3
G4	Grade 4
MDCT	Multidetector computed tomography
MIBC	Muscle-invasive bladder cancer
mpMRI	Multiparametric magnetic resonance imaging
MRI	Magnetic resonance imaging
NMIBC	Non-muscle-invasive bladder cancer
NPV	Negative predictive value
PPV	Positive predictive value

M.E. Abou El-Ghar (✉) • M.A. Badawy • T.A. El-Diasty
Radiology Department, Urology and Nephrology Center, Mansoura University, Dakahlia Governorate, Mansoura, Egypt
e-mail: maboelghar@yahoo.com

© Springer International Publishing AG 2018
D. Akata, N. Papanikolaou (eds.), *Diffusion Weighted Imaging of the Genitourinary System*, https://doi.org/10.1007/978-3-319-69575-4_4

73

RCC	Renal cell carcinoma
ROI	Region of interest
SCC	Squamous cell carcinoma
SI	Signal intensity
SNR	Signal-to-noise ratio
TCC	Transitional cell carcinoma
TE	Time of echo
Tis	Tumor in situ
TURBT	Transurethral resection of bladder tumor
UC	Urothelial carcinoma
UTUC	Upper tract urothelial carcinoma
UUT	Upper urinary tract

Key Points
- Diffusion-weighted MR imaging is a noninvasive fast MRI technique that provides qualitative and quantitative information of tissue cellularity with early detection of early microstructural abnormalities.
- DWI-MRI is a problem solving for many abnormalities detected at conventional MRI sequences specially if there is contraindication for gadolinium contrast administration.
- DWI-MRI improves the preoperative diagnostic accuracy in different urothelial tumors specially bladder carcinoma.
- DWI-MRI provides accurate morphological and functional assessment of tumor response to chemoradiotherapy.

Urothelial tumors originate from kidney collecting systems, ureters, bladder, and urethra. Adequate imaging and diagnosis are crucial as treatment approaches are quite different from those of renal parenchymal tumors [1–3].

Cancer of the urothelium is a multifocal process. Patients with cancer of the upper urinary tract have a 30–50% chance of developing cancer of the bladder at some point in their lives. On the other hand, patients with bladder cancer have only a 2–3% chance of developing cancer of the upper urinary tract. The incidence of renal pelvis tumors is decreasing [4].

Urothelial cancers occur more commonly in men than in women (3:1), with a peak incidence in the seventh decade of life [4].

Transitional cell carcinoma (TCC) constitutes 95% of malignant urothelial tumors (3–6). More than 90% of all bladder cancers are TCC, 5–10% are squamous cell carcinoma (SCC), and the remaining 2–3% are adenocarcinoma [1, 5, 6]. SCC is associated with chronic inflammation, whereas adenocarcinoma is associated with persistent urachal remnants [1–7].

Five percent of urothelial tumors occur from the ureter and renal pelvis or calyces, accounting for approximately 10% of upper urinary tract neoplasms [8]. Upper urinary tract urothelial cancer is one of the most difficult lesions to be shown by imaging studies. Moreover, it is difficult to depict ureteral or renal pelvic small tumors. Conventionally, invasive clinical urology radiography, such as retrograde pyeloureterography using cystoscopy, has been the imaging modality in detecting urothelial tumors [9].

Renal TCC most frequently arises in the extrarenal part of the pelvis, followed by the infundibulocalyceal region [3]. Renal pelvic lesions are four times more common than ureteral lesions. Twenty-five percent of upper tract tumors occur in the ureter, where 60–75% of cases are found in the lower third, with no side predominance [10]. The distribution is equal between the left and right kidneys, with 2–4% of cases occurring bilaterally. Tumor spread occurs by mucosal extension or local, hematogenous, or lymphatic invasion. The most common sites for metastases are the liver, bone, and lungs. The tumor stage at diagnosis influences the development of local recurrence and metastases and hence overall survival [9, 11].

Urinary bladder cancer is one of the most common urinary tract malignancies, causing notable morbidity and mortality [12–14].

Multicentric TCC is common and is associated with poor survival [11]. Synchronous or metachronous tumor of the ipsilateral or contralateral collecting system is also common, necessitating vigilant urologic and radiologic follow-up [15]. For these reasons, a noninvasive diagnostic technique for depicting upper urinary tract cancer would be desirable [16].

The management and prognosis of bladder cancer are based on T staging, pathologic grading of the tumor, and the presence or absence of metastatic disease. Clinical staging of the primary tumor with bimanual examination, cystoscopy, and transurethral resection of bladder tumor (TURBT) is associated with an inaccuracy rate from 23 to 50% [17–21]. Therefore, obtaining an accurate imaging study is important to facilitate choosing optimal management methods [14].

Imaging of urothelium has been for many years by using iodinated radiocontrast media, such as excretory urography and conventional CT that have low diagnostic yield. After the introduction of MDCT in assessment of upper urinary tract, it has improved the sensitivity of upper urinary tract tumor detection up to 89% [16, 22, 23].

Magnetic resonance imaging (MRI) is a feasible and reasonably accurate technique for the local staging of bladder cancer preferred over computed tomography (CT) [24] not only because MRI provides multiplanar images but also because it offers inherently high soft-tissue contrast independent of excretory function. Furthermore, the application of functional images such as diffusion-weighted imaging (DWI) to the anatomic images improves the accuracy of tumor detection and staging and helps in monitoring post-therapy response and identifying recurrences [25–30].

DWI is a functional imaging technique and provides functional and structural information about biological tissues. It can be obtained rapidly and noninvasively without exposure to ionizing radiation and does not require gadolinium contrast administration. This is beneficial to a substantial group of bladder cancer patients who are allergic to contrast medium or who have renal dysfunction because it allows them to avoid contrast medium-induced nephrotoxicity and nephrogenic systemic fibrosis. DWI has played an important role in the multiparametric MRI and is a useful technique to increase the accuracy in detecting and evaluating the extent of bladder cancer. In addition, it provides qualitative evaluation about tissue characterization using ADC values that reflects the magnitude of diffusion of water molecule in tissues. The impact of ADC values within the tumor on the estimation of grade or depth has been shown recently in some malignancies, including bladder cancer to assess its biological behavior and histopathological grading and reflect the aggressiveness of bladder cancer [31–42].

4.1   Techniques of DWI in Urinary Tract

DW imaging is an MR technique that depicts molecular diffusion, which is the Brownian motion of water protons in biologic tissues [43]; it can be added to any MRI protocol. The scan time necessary is largely determined by whether breathhold, free-breathing, respiratory-triggered, or navigator technique is used [44].

Examination of the molecular diffusion with the use of MR relies on sensitization of an imaging sequence with two equally strong but opposed gradients that will cancel each other out if there is no movement of molecules in the meantime. However, movement occurs in any living tissue, and this will induce a remaining dephasing in the moving tissue, which is visible as signal loss on the resulting image [25].

Most DW images are acquired with 1.5-T systems, but 3.0-T systems have the advantage of higher signal to noise ratio (SNR) at the cost of more susceptibility artifacts [45]. However, DW images at 3.0 T are usually of good quality and can be used in a clinical setting [27]. However, the signal intensity on DWI is influenced by both water diffusion and T2 relaxation time (T2 shine-through effect). By using high b value, the signal intensity of watery material such as urine in the ureter or renal pelvis could be reduced while retaining high signal intensity of the tumors [46].

Choosing the b values for the DW acquisition is not always straightforward [47]. DWI sequences with large b values are more sensitive to diffusion at the expense of the SNR [44]. The largest b value used in the sequence defines the echo time of the sequence, and higher maximal b values (and subsequently longer echo times) yield greatly reduced SNR in the resulting images [25]. This signal loss can be overcome with multiple signal averages and increased scan time. The radiologist should be aware of the choice of b values to correctly interpret the resulting ADC values. It is known that by using mainly low b values (<100 s/mm^2), the ADC that is calculated will be higher and reflect a combination of both perfusion and diffusion effects, whereas by using only higher b values (>100 s/mm^2), the resulting ADC values are much lower and better approximate the true diffusion of the tissue [27]. If more than two b values are desired in the abdomen and pelvis, it is recommended to have at least 1 value of 100 or greater and 1 value of 500 or greater for adequate ADC calculation [48].

If three or more b values are utilized, the contributions of perfusion and diffusion can be separated according to the intravoxel incoherent motion model utilizing a bi-exponential decay function instead of the traditional mono-exponential function as described by Le Bihan et al. [49]. A good b-value choice for separation of these components would be a set of b values: 0, 100, 500, and 1000 s/mm^2; whereas the ADC calculated from the first two values would favor perfusion contributions, the ADC calculated from the latter two values approximates the true diffusion of the tissue [27].

Currently used clinical MR systems in abdomen and pelvis should be capable of obtaining DW images with maximal b values of at least 1000 s/mm^2 and have adequate SNR. A range of intermediate b values can be selected depending on the type of quantitative analysis anticipated. Minimally, only two b values (most often $b = 0$ and 1000 s/mm^2) are required to calculate the apparent diffusion coefficient [50].

The application of DW-MRI, particularly in abdominal organs, is challenging and has a variety of shortcomings because of physiological motion artifacts, such as respiratory movements, pulsation, and bowel motion. As a gradient sequence, DWI is sensitive to susceptibility from metal or air, and to limit susceptibility, TE must be kept as low as possible [44]. However, a single-shot echo planar sequence with parallel imaging techniques, high gradient amplitudes, and multichannel coils allows for reduction of scan time with improved image quality [12]. Ghosting can be mitigated with single breath-hold, breath-gating, or navigator techniques [44]. Thoeny et al. [16] reported that DW-MR images without and with breath holding did not show substantial differences in calculated ADC values or image quality. Also Yoshida et al. stated that DW-MRI without breath holding could provide enough MR sections to evaluate UUT neoplasm even with small tumor burden; at the breath-holding technique, only a few MR sections could be obtained [50].

Takahara et al. [51] reported a procedure for body DW-MRI under free-breathing conditions. Such approaches enable longer scan times and more thin-slice images with multiple signal averaging and provide a high-quality multiplanar display. These technological improvements have allowed DW-MRI to be increasingly applied in abdominal and pelvic examinations, and it was quickly introduced as an important diagnostic imaging tool for detecting various types of tumors, including UTUC and bladder cancer [52].

Optimal bladder distension is important in bladder cancer assessment at MRI. With a lack of bladder distention, small tumors will obscured by detrusor muscle thickening. On the other hand, motion artifacts due to discomfort with over-distension and the thinness of the bladder wall can decrease sensitivity for small lesions [53].

4.2   Qualitative and Quantitative Analysis of DW Images

Image analysis is performed qualitatively by means of visual assessment and quantitatively by means of ADC measurements. First-line image interpretation is usually performed with visual assessment of the SI on images acquired at high b values and their corresponding ADC maps. Typical malignant lesions display high signal intensity (SI) on images acquired at high b values of $\geq 800-1000$ s/mm^2 and corresponding low ADC values on the ADC maps, due to diffusion restriction caused by hypercellularity of the lesion [50]. Quantitative measurement can be done after the generation of ADC maps. ADC could be calculated by applying a circular region of interest (ROI) manually placed on the ADC maps that was maximally covering but not extending beyond the boundaries of the masses [54]. The placement and size of the ROI are important for accurate ADC calculation. In heterogeneous lesions, the ROIs should always be placed on the solid parts of the lesions, excluding the necrosis as possible to avoid false high ADC values and thereby misclassifying the lesion as benign. These solid components of the lesions can be separated from cystic and necrotic components, which display intermediate or low SI on images acquired at high b values but yield high ADC values on the corresponding ADC maps. Edema or inflammation may be sometimes mistaken for tumor tissue and display high SI on high b-value images due to the T2 shine-through effect; the distinction between tumor and inflammation or edema is only possible based on assessment of the ADC map, where a high ADC is present in both edema and inflammation but not in tumors [50].

4.3 Role of DWI in Imaging in the Bladder and Upper Urinary Tract Urothelial Cancer

4.3.1 Upper Urinary Tract

The clinical presentation of UUT cancer and other diseases of the UUT are non-specific; thus, the majority of urinary tract lesions require evaluation with imaging modalities [55]. Upper urinary tract (calyces, renal pelvis and ureter) urothelial cancer is one of the most difficult lesions to be shown by imaging studies. Moreover, it is difficult to depict ureteral or renal pelvic small tumors. The accurate diagnosis of UUT disease is important, as it may significantly affect the choice of therapeutic approach in many cases [56]. MRI has been used by a number of retrospective studies to assess already diagnosed cases of upper urinary tract urothelial cancer using the DWI technique [9, 16, 57]. The diagnostic ability of DWI with anatomic information from T1- and T2-weighted imaging for detecting upper urinary tract cancer in a non-invasive manner was excellent (Fig. 4.1). The addition of DWI to T1- and T2-weighted imaging significantly improves the accuracy and sensitivity for upper urinary tract cancer detection, although this did not improve the specificity because the specificity of T1- and T2-weighted imaging for upper urinary tract cancer was already sufficiently high. Wu et al. also demonstrated a significantly higher accuracy of DW-MRI with different b values in the diagnosis of UUT cancer compared with conventional MRI alone [58]. DWI shows the tumor as high signal intensity, and ADC values are related to the proportion of extracellular and intracellular components. Since a

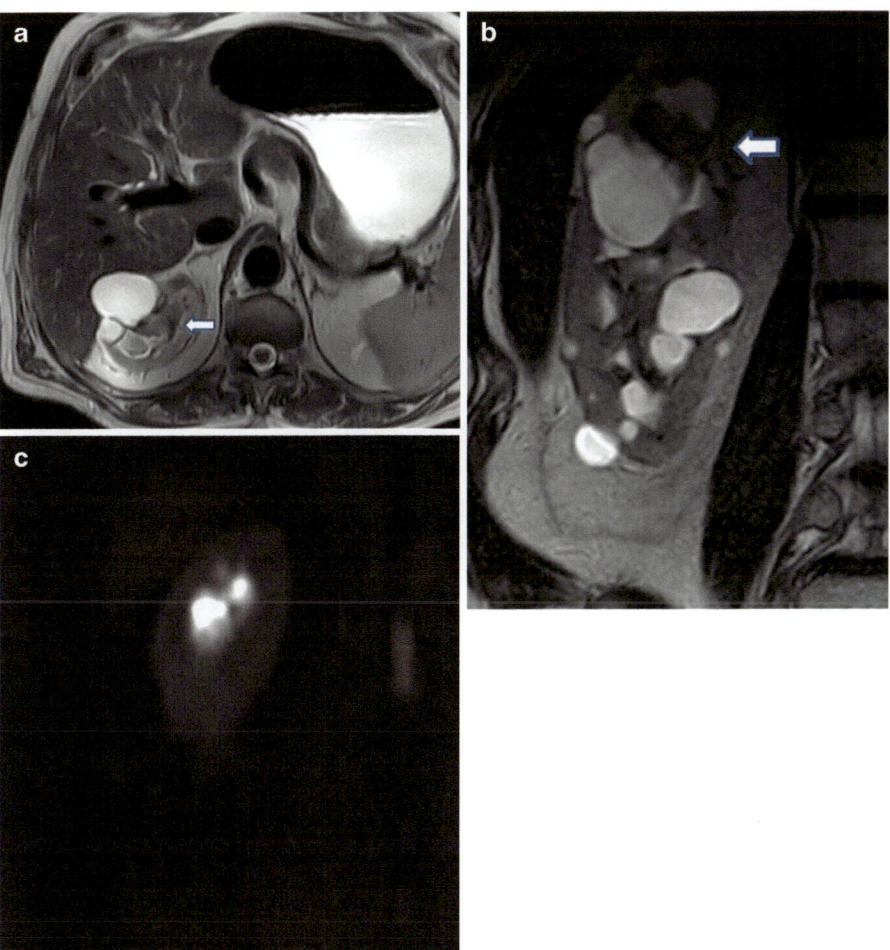

Fig. 4.1 Right pelvicalyceal low-grade urothelial carcinoma invading the subepithelial layer. A 69-year-old male patient presented with hematuria. 3 Tesla MRI: (**a**, **b**) Axial and coronal T2w images of the right kidney show hypointense calyceal lesion (*arrows*) with irregular dilated calyces. (**c**) Coronal DW image of the kidney using *b* value of 800 s/mm² shows diffusion restriction at the lesion and no parenchymal infiltration

malignant tumor often has a larger cell diameter and cellularly denser than normal tissue, the ADC values of tumors may decrease as well (Fig. 4.2) [9].

Several studies investigated DWI for UUT cancer detection [9, 16, 48, 57]. One study reported that combining DWI with standard MRI can improve the accuracy of UUT cancer diagnosis because malignant tissue has higher signal intensity than

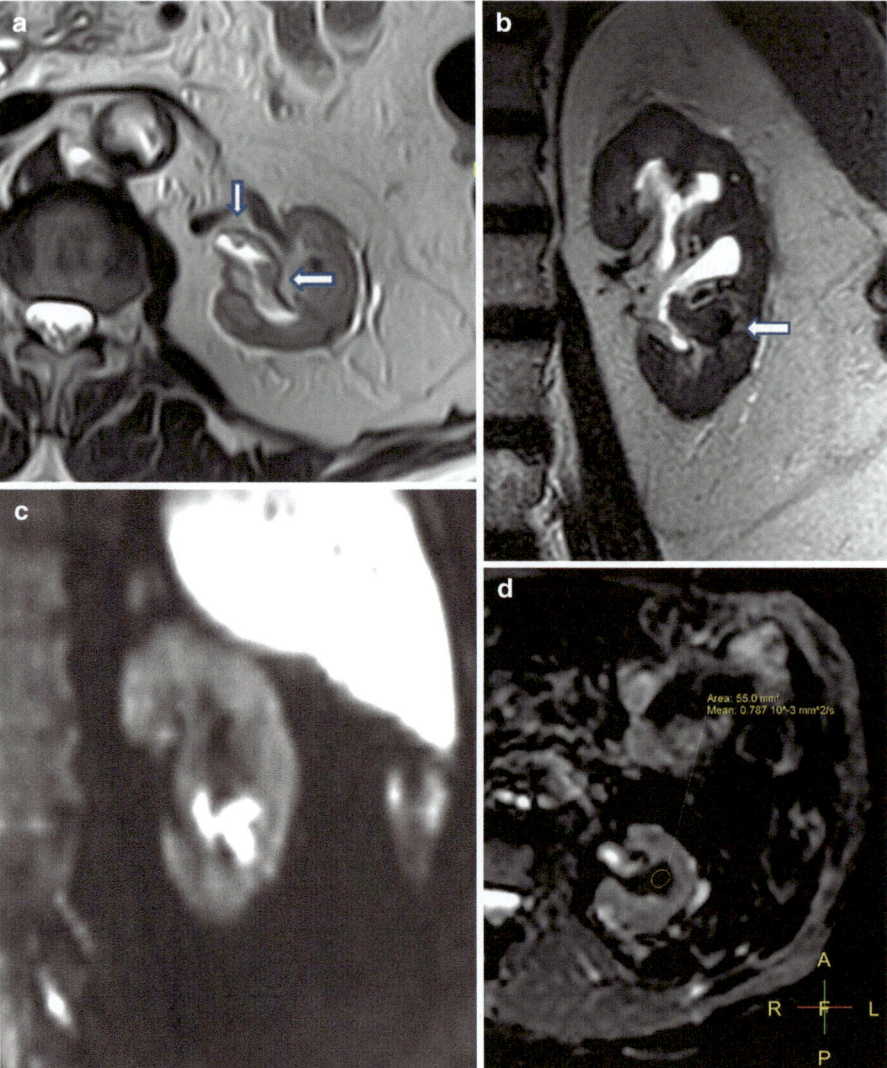

Fig. 4.2 Left lower calyceal urothelial cancer. A 73-year-old male patient presented with hematuria. 3 Tesla MRI: (**a, b**) Axial and coronal T2w images of the left kidney shows ill-defined lower calyceal lesion of low SI associated with nodular thickening of the renal pelvis (*arrows*). (**c, d**) DWI and ADC map of the left kidney *b* value = 800 s/mm² show diffusion restriction of lower calyceal cancer at the left lower calyces with no diffusion restriction of the chronic inflammatory changes at the renal pelvis. ADC of the mass displays 6.78×10.3 mm/s with renal parenchyma 1.78×10^{-3} mm²/s

normal tissue (Figs. 4.3 and 4.4) [14]. DWI provides good contrast between the tumor and surrounding tissues even if the tumor is not visible by MR imaging; thus, it improves the sensitivity in UUT cancer diagnosis [14, 59, 60]. Shebel et al. reported that the mean ADC values of all lesions in their study whether malignant or inflammatory were significantly lower than that of the renal parenchyma. A cutoff value of ADC 1.5 is of high sensitivity and specificity 79% and 82%, respectively, in differentiating inflammatory lesions from urothelial cancer, and ADC more than 1.5 is

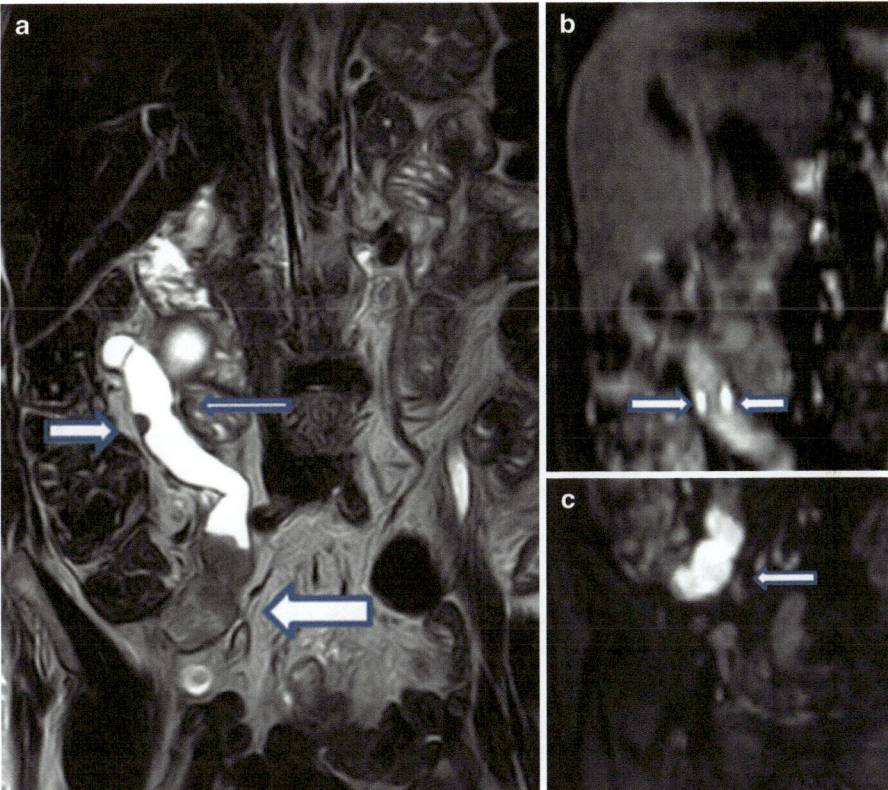

Fig. 4.3 A case of right multicentric ureteric tumor. A 66-year-old male patient presented with hematuria. There is a history of radical cystectomy 3 years ago. 3 Tesla MRI: (**a**) Coronal T2w image of the abdomen and pelvis shows multiple right ureteric soft tissue nodules at the lumbar and iliac portions of the ureter (*arrows*), (**b**, **c**) Coronal DWI of the abdomen and pelvis, *b* value = 800 s/mm². There is diffusion restriction at the nodules with no periureteric extension

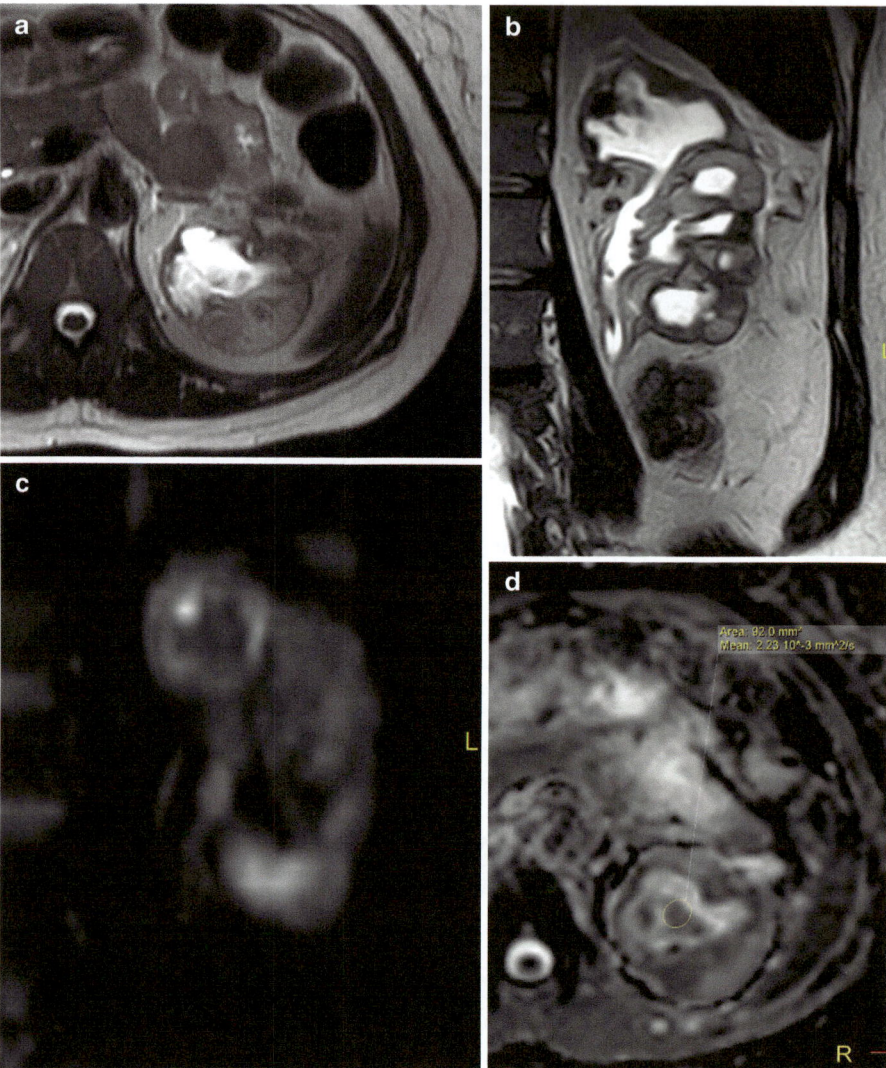

Fig. 4.4 Chronic pyelonephritis of the left kidney with impaired renal function. A 37-year-old female presented with chronic urinary tract infection. 3 Tesla MRI: (**a, b**) Axial and coronal T2w images of the left kidney show chronic pyelonephritic changes with irregular mucosal thickening and irregular dilated PCS. (**c, d**) DWI and ADC map show intracalyceal areas of restricted diffusion with high ADC values (2.32×10^{-3} mm^2/s)

more likely to be benign (Fig. 4.5). However, in some cases with acute renal infection, there may be a decrease in the ADC values of the lesions, and mistaken with tumors, the clinical data and negative urine cytology help in differentiation (Fig. 4.6). DWI can differentiate benign urothelial thickening associated with chronic pyelonephritis with no diffusion restriction from malignant one with diffusion restriction (Fig. 4.7). Yoshida et al. [16] demonstrated significantly lower ADC values of the renal pelvic and ureteral tumors than of the surrounding tissues (Fig. 4.8) [23]. In another study by Nishizawa et al., they detected all upper UUT urothelial carcinomas with DWI except carcinoma in situ regardless of the tumor grade. The mean ADC value of the urothelial tumor was significantly lower than those of the renal tissue. The mean ADC value of the tumor was 1.125×10^{-3} mm^2/s, while the values of the renal parenchyma were 1.984×10^{-3} mm^2/s [9].

Both PPV for all upper urinary tract cancer and NPV for upper urinary tract cancer with negative urinary cytology of DWI were more than 90%. This indicates that a positive DWI is virtually indicative of upper urinary tract cancer and a negative DWI nearly excludes upper urinary tract cancer in cases with negative urinary cytology [58].

Yoshida et al. reported that they were able to obtain high signal intensity of small renal pelvic tumors (5 and 7 mm in diameter) on DWI, despite unclear conventional morphological MRI, while the smallest tumor depicted by Nishizawa et al. was approximately 8 mm in diameter [9].

The value of ADC measurements within the tumor on the prediction of tumor grade or depth has been shown in some malignancies, including bladder cancer [61–67]. Some studies showed that high-grade upper urinary tract cancers likely had lower ADC values, whereas the ADC values did not allow the readers to discriminate the extra-muscular extension. DWI could be a useful adjunct to preoperative evaluation of histologic grade of upper urinary tract cancer [58]. In a series of 40 pelvicalyceal urothelial cancers (UCs), Akita et al. [57] have showed that the mean ADC of high-grade was significantly lower than that of low-grade tumors ($p < 0.01$). Nishizawa et al. [9] were not able to demonstrate a significant difference in ADC values between grades of 17 upper urinary tract urothelial cancers (UTUCs). Sufana Iancu et al. also failed to demonstrate a significant correlation between the ADC value and grade of the UTUCs at their study [68].

DWI in addition to conventional sequences could be a helpful tool to obtain a better preoperative staging. Akita et al. [57] reported a higher accuracy for the detection of locally advanced T3b pelvicalyceal UCs using DWI in addition to T2-weighted sequence MRI compared with T2-weighted sequence alone. While the T factor was determined according to the 2010 American Joint Committee on Cancer categories. Subsequently, tumors that had directly invaded the renal parenchyma were subdivided

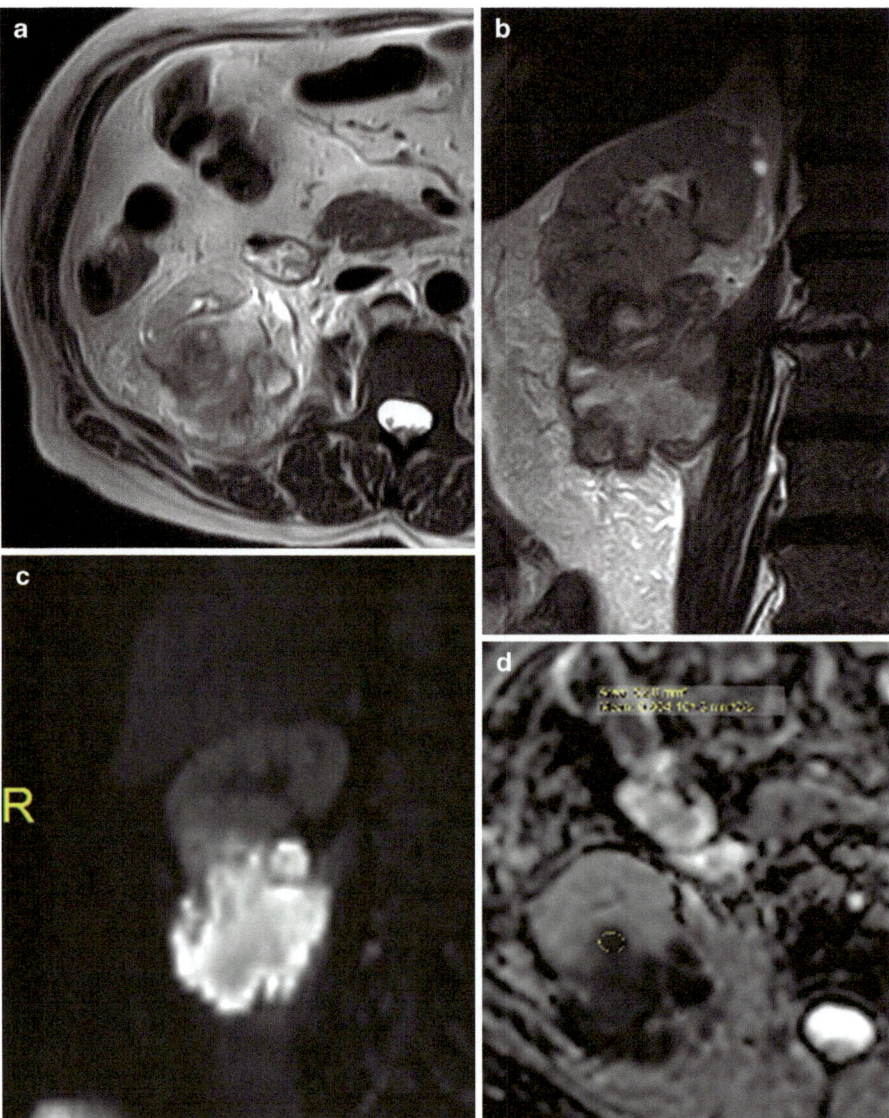

Fig. 4.5 Right renal and perirenal abscess. A 73-year-old male patient presented with fever and right loin pain. 3 Tesla MRI: (**a, b**) Axial and coronal T2w images of the right kidney show renal and perirenal inflammatory lesion encroaching upon the lower calyces. (**c**) Coronal DWI of the right kidney b value = 800 s/mm^2 shows diffusion restriction with low ADC value at ADC map (0.654×10^{-3} mm^2/s)

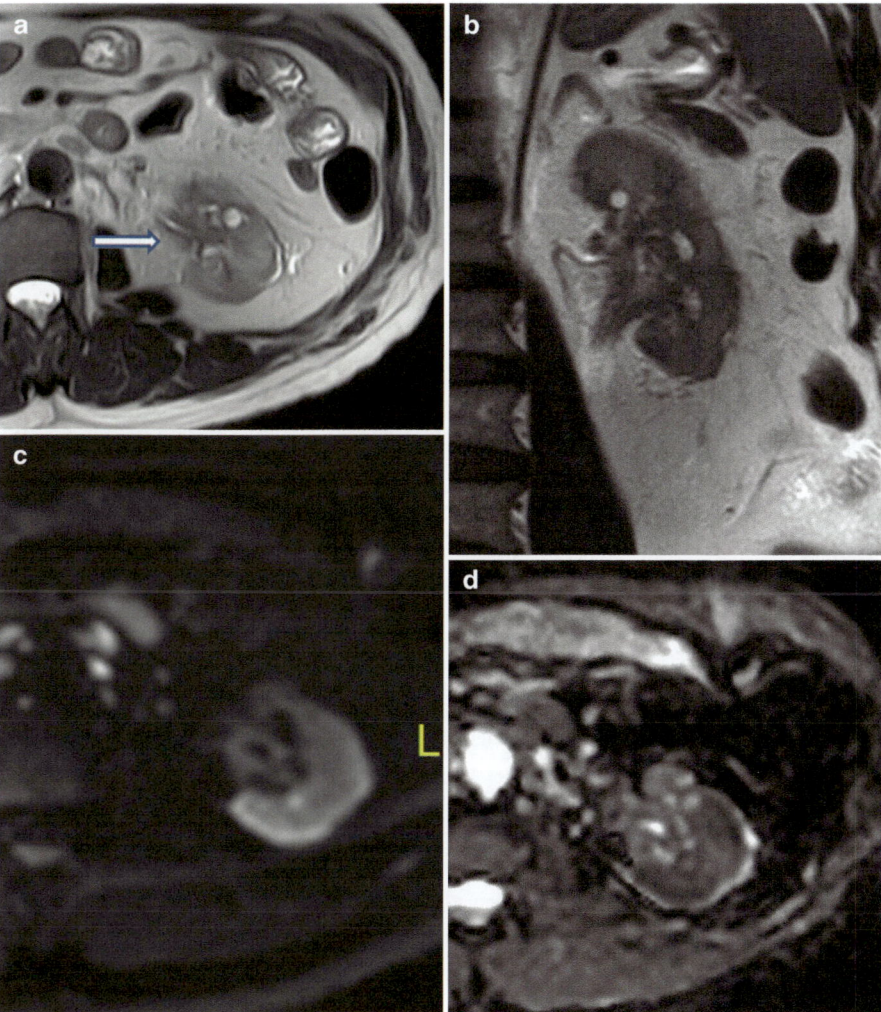

Fig. 4.6 Chronic pyelonephritis of the left kidney. A 60-year-old male patient. 3 Tesla MRI: (**a**, **b**) Axial and coronal T2w MR images of the left kidney show diffuse thickening of the left renal pelvis (*arrow*) with no diffusion restriction at DWI and ADC (**c**, **d**) and negative cytology

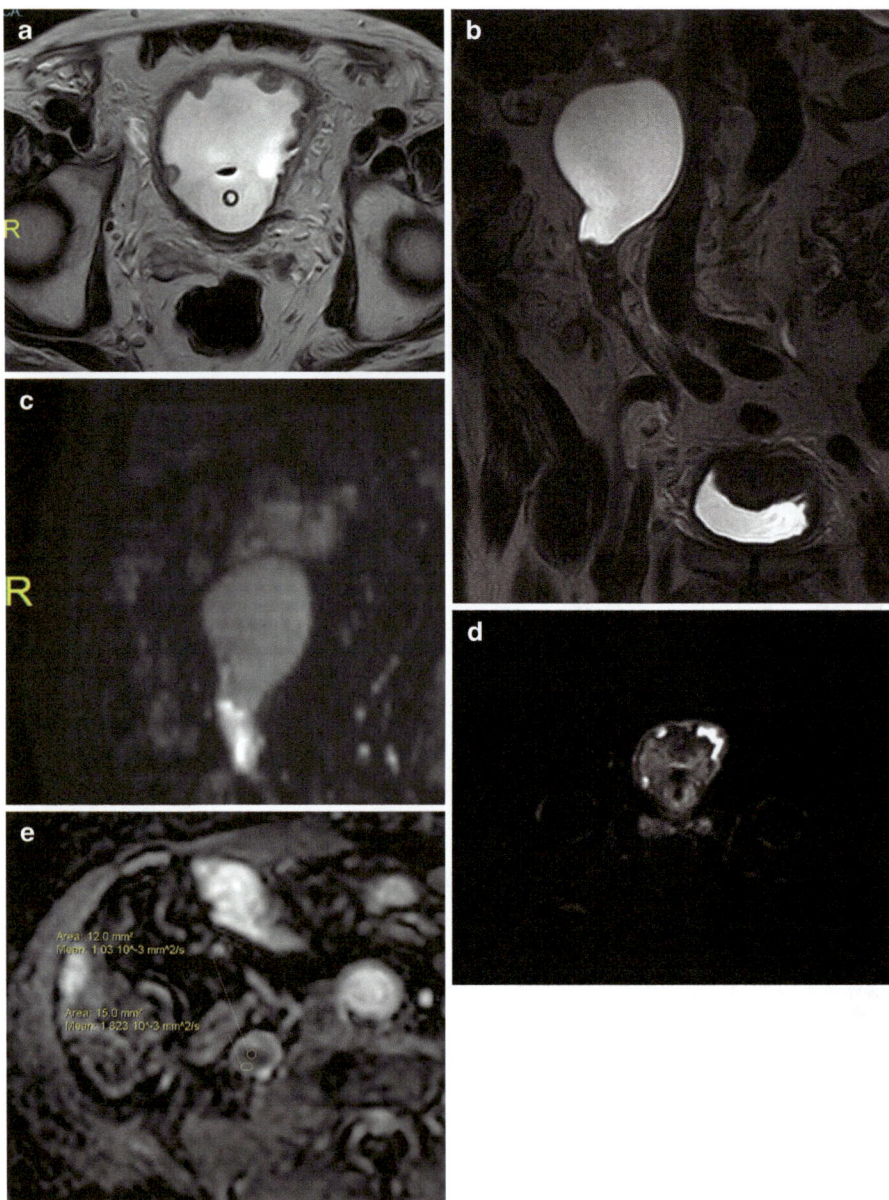

Fig. 4.7 High-grade multicentric urothelial cancer of the bladder and right ureter. An 83-year-old male patient presented with recurrent attacks of hematuria. 3T MRI: (**a, b**) Axial and coronal T2w images of the abdomen and pelvis show multiple lesions at the lumbar ureter and bladder dome of low T2w SI. (**c, d**) DWI *b* value = 800 s/mm^2 shows restricted diffusion at the lesions. (**e**) ADC map, the nodule measures 1.03×10^{-3} mm^2/s and the ureteric wall 1.823×10^{-3} mm^2/s

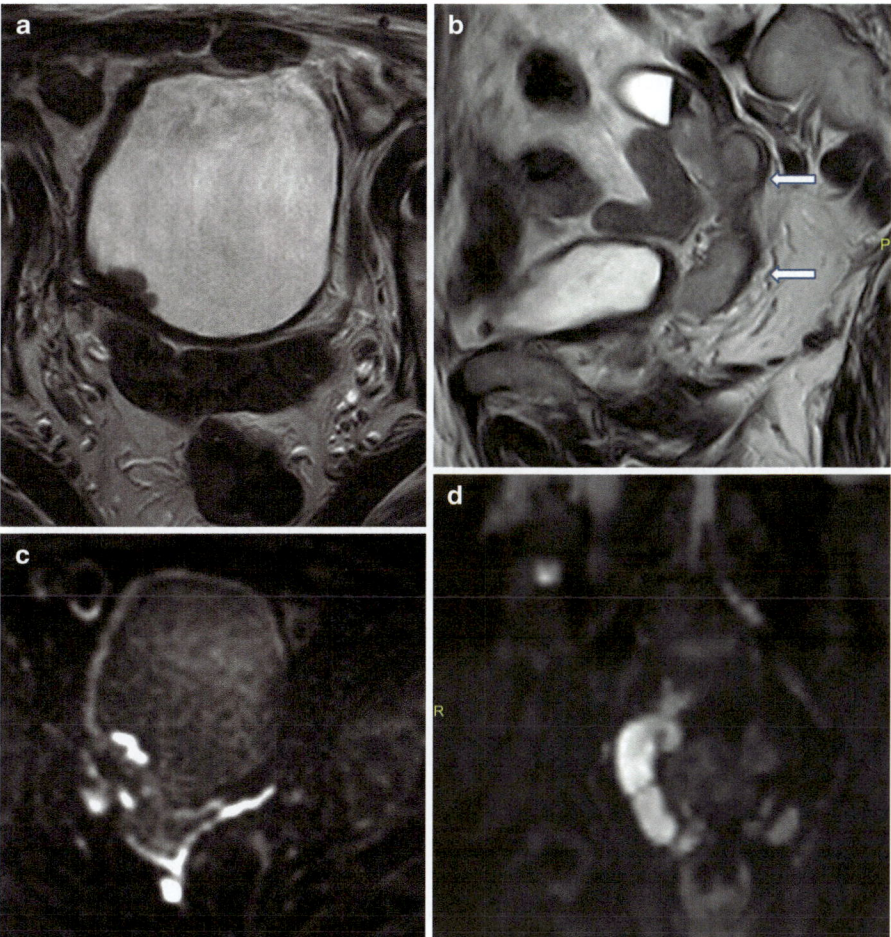

Fig. 4.8 Multicentric T1 bladder mass and right ureteric urothelial cancer. A 75-year-old male patient presented with hematuria and history of right simple nephrectomy. 3 Tesla MRI: (**a**) Axial T2w MR image of the bladder shows irregular thickening of the bladder wall with a nodular growth at the right side of posterior bladder wall. (**b**) Sagittal T2w MR image of the right ureteric stump shows a large lesion along the pelvic ureter (*arrow*). (**c**) Axial DWI, *b* value = 800 s/mm^2, the bladder shows a superficial bladder mass limited to the lamina propria. (**d**) Coronal DWI *b* value = 800 s/mm^2 of the right ureteric stump shows the mass with diffuse restriction and wall invasion (*arrows*)

into microscopic invasion (within 5 mm in depth, defined as pT3a) and macroscopic invasion (more than 5 mm in depth, defined as pT3b). Kobayashi et al. have demonstrated the inverse correlation of ADC value with pT stage for bladder UCs. Sufana Iancu et al., in contrary to these previous reports, failed to demonstrate a significant association between muscle-invasive or locally advanced disease and ADC value [69].

Distinguishing between centrally infiltrative urothelial carcinoma of the kidney and central RCC can be a diagnostic challenge on imaging. Urine cytology is an inexpensive noninvasive screening test with an accuracy of up to 98% for high-grade urothelial carcinoma; sensitivities and specificities as low as 8.5% and 50%, respectively, have been reported for low-grade papillary urothelial carcinoma [69]. Low SI of the lesion with diffusion restriction and positive urine cytology has a high positive predictive value in diagnosis of urothelial carcinoma.

Wehrli et al. [71] investigated the utility of ADC for distinguishing renal pelvic urothelial carcinoma from central RCC. The utility of standard ADC values and ADC values normalized to CSF, a technique motivated to help offset variability between examinations relating to differences in scanners and sequence parameters, as well as possible biologic effects contributing to variability [70, 71]. Although ADC was not significantly different between the two groups, normalized ADC was significantly lower in urothelial carcinoma compared with RCC ($p = 0.008$), and optimal threshold of normalized ADC value was 0.451. This threshold was associated with 83% sensitivity and 71% specificity in distinguishing renal pelvic urothelial carcinoma and central RCC [71].

4.3.2 Urinary Bladder

The feasibility of using DW-MR imaging for the detection of a urinary bladder carcinoma has been reported by Matsuki et al. [72]. Their study included 15 patients with bladder carcinomas; all lesions had high SI relative to the surrounding structures. The sensitivity and PPV of DW imaging in that study were both 100% for detection of carcinomas. There were several limitations at this study. First, it was a retrospective study of a small number of patients. In addition, MR examinations of all patients were performed after biopsy, which may have affected the results. Furthermore, all patients included in the study were known to have bladder tumors; thus, there was case selection bias in the report. The same findings were also reported by El-Assmy et al. [73]. However, all included cases were known to have bladder tumors; thus, there was a selection bias [38].

In another study by Abou El-Ghar et al., DW-MR images showed excellent agreement with those at conventional cystoscopy. Reviewers could identify almost all bladder lesions and missed only two lesions that were less than 4 mm in diameter. The sensitivity and PPV for the diagnosis of bladder tumors were 98.1% and 100%, respectively [38]. Matsuki et al. [74] reported the same results for identification of the cause of hematuria; the sensitivity and PPV of DW MR imaging were 98.3% and 100%, respectively [38].

Bladder cancers generally had higher SI than surrounding tissues on high b-value DWI [74, 75]. The reported sensitivity, specificity, and accuracy for identifying bladder cancers are 90–98%, 85–93%, and 89–97%, respectively (Fig. 4.8) [26, 38, 75, 76, 89]. Nevertheless, because of poor spatial resolution of DW images, small tumors less than 1 cm may be missed on DWI due to insufficiency of tissue contrast between small tumors and normal bladder wall [26, 38, 70, 78]. However, with advancement of DWI sequences especially at 3 Tesla machines, small lesions of few millimeters in diameter can be detected at DWI (Fig. 4.9).

The urinary epithelial cancers in the urinary bladder demonstrate low ADC value $(1.1890.19 \times 10^{-3} \text{ mm}^2/\text{s}$ and $1.4090.51 \times 10^{-3} \text{ mm}^2/\text{s}$, respectively). The cause of high intensity in cancerous lesions is not clear, but both decreased ADC of the cancer tissue, due to its denser cellularity compared to normal tissue, and long T2 relaxation time of the tumors may contribute to the signal increase on DWI (Fig. 4.10) [74, 75].

The different T stages include carcinomas in situ (Tis), T1 tumors invade the subepithelial connective tissue, T2 tumors invade the superficial muscle (T2a) and the deep muscle (T2b), T3 tumors invade the microscopic (T3a) or macroscopic (T3b) perivesical tissue, and T4 tumors invade the adjacent prostate, uterus, vagina, or peritoneal reflection (T4a) or the pelvic and/or abdominal wall (T4b). The management and prognosis of bladder cancer are based on T staging, pathologic grading of the tumor, and the presence or absence of metastatic disease. Clinical staging of the primary tumor with bimanual examination, cystoscopy, and transurethral resection of bladder tumor (TURBT) is associated with an inaccuracy rate from 23 to 50% [17–21]. To distinguish between stage T1 and stages T2 or higher is of particular importance, as superficial T1 tumors can be treated with transurethral resection, whereas invasive tumors of stage T2 or higher usually require a radical cystectomy, a radiation therapy or chemotherapy, or their combination [36–38, 77–79]. So, accurate imaging study is important for adequate staging to facilitate choosing optimal management methods (Figs. 4.11 and 4.12).

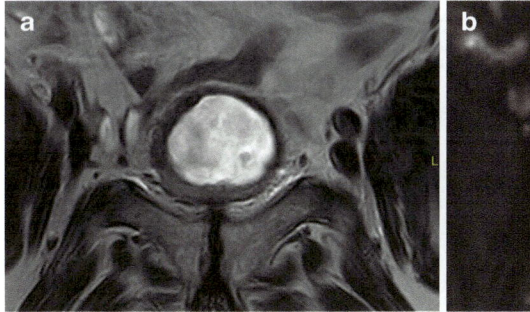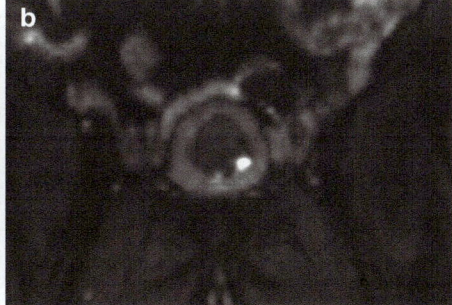

Fig. 4.9 Small superficial bladder carcinoma. A 78-year-old male patient presented with history of multiple previous resections of superficial bladder urothelial cancer. 3 Tesla MRI: (**a**) Coronal T2w image shows irregular thickening of bladder wall with no definite masses. (**b**) Coronal DWI b value = 800 s/mm² shows a small papillary urothelial cancer at the left wall

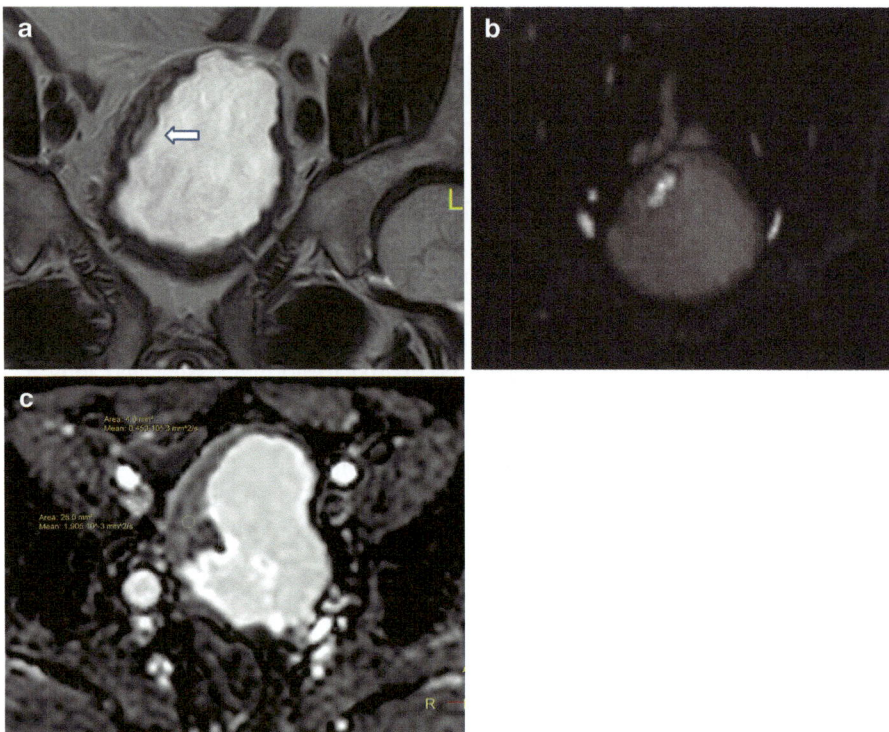

Fig. 4.10 Low-grade T1 papillary urothelial bladder cancer with chronic non-specific cystitis at the bladder. A 60-year-old male patient presented with hematuria post-transurethral resection of bladder urothelial cancer. 3 Tesla MRI: (**a**) Coronal T2w image shows irregular diffuse thickening of the bladder wall with nodular area of intermediate SI at the right wall (*arrow*). (**b**) DWI *b* value = 800 s/mm^2 shows restricted diffusion at the right lateral wall nodule no muscle invasion, ADC value of the bladder wall measures 1.905×10^{-3} mm^2/s and at the nodule 0.453×10^{-3} mm^2/s

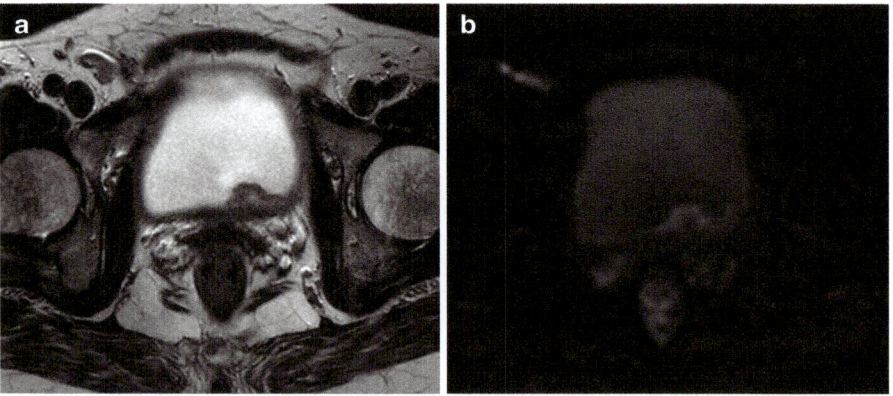

Fig. 4.11 T1 urothelial bladder cancer. A 42-year-old male patient presented with recurrent attacks of hematuria. 3T MRI: (**a**) Axial T2w image of the bladder shows irregular bladder thickening at the posterior wall to the left. (**b, c**) Axial DWI *b* value = 800 s/mm^2 and ADC map show superficial growth at the posterior wall to the left with restricted diffusion and no muscle invasion

Fig. 4.11 (continued)

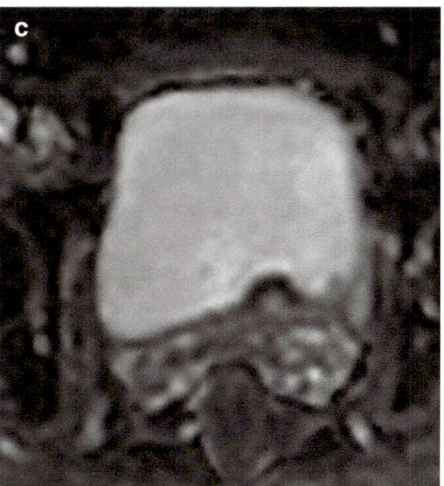

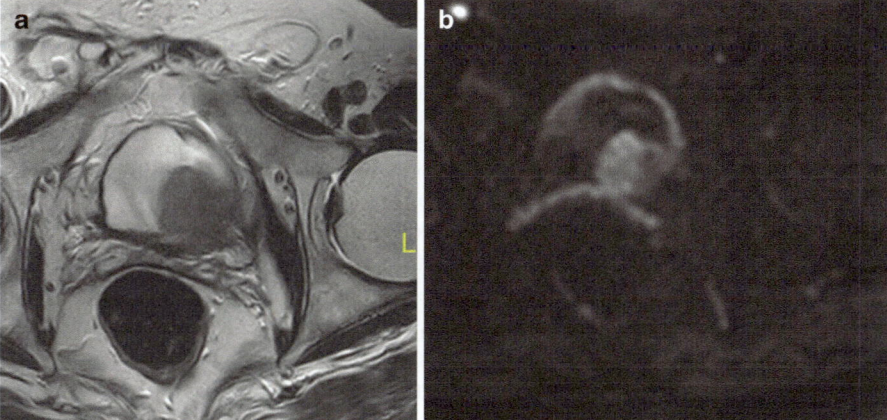

Fig. 4.12 Recurrent T2 papillary bladder tumor. A 65-year-old male patient had history of previous transurethral resection of bladder cancer. 3 Tesla MRI: (**a**) Axial T2w image of the bladder shows a soft tissue mass at the low left bladder wall with distortion of the related perivesical fat. (**b**) Axial DWI of the bladder b value = 800 s/mm^2 restricted diffusion at the mass with invasion of the deep muscle and no extravesical extension

Urine may persistently show mild high SI in patients with bladder cancer especially in patients with hematuria, this will lead to missing of intraluminal tumor. Tumor recognition and differentiation need careful comparison of ADC map, T2WI, and DCE, or the use of an ultrahigh b-value DWI would improve [80–82].

The potential role of DWI in staging bladder cancers was investigated in several studies. It was reported that the accuracy of using DWI alone to discriminate muscle-invasive bladder cancer (MIBC) from non-muscle-invasive bladder cancer (NMIBC) ranges from 63.6 to 92% [27, 28, 70, 83]. Staging of bladder cancer by DWI alone is generally unsatisfactory [30], although accuracy increases with the combination of T2WI [30, 84]. Wu et al. [98] prospectively evaluated 362 bladder cancer patients and showed that combining DWI and T2WI can significantly improve the diagnostic performance in preoperative evaluation of the T category. Accuracy rates for differentiating between T1 and T2 tumors ranged between 92% and 98%, respectively. Watanabe et al. evaluated the performance of DWI in tumor staging of 40 patients with 52 bladder tumors. DW-MRI combined with T2w-MRI was able to differentiate between T1 or lower tumors and T2 or higher tumors with 96% accuracy and between T2 or lower tumors and from T3 to T4 tumors with 92% accuracy based on morphologic findings at high b values, increasing the performance of T2w-MRI alone. Overall T stage accuracy increased from 67% using T2w-MRI alone to 88% when DW-MRI was added [85]. El-Assmy et al. evaluated 106 bladder cancer patients and reported staging accuracy rates of 63.6 and 69.6% in differentiating superficial from invasive tumors and organ-confined from non-organ-confined tumors, respectively, when DW-MRI alone was evaluated, although accuracy for T2w-MRI alone was even worse (6.1% and 15.1%, respectively) [26]. This may be due to low image quality in this early report. A recent study by Ohgiya and colleagues showed that the specificity and accuracy in differentiating T1 tumors from T2 and higher stage tumors were significantly higher when using T2w imaging combined with DW-MR imaging than with T2w imaging alone (specificity, 83.3% vs. 50%, $P = 0.02$ and accuracy, 84.6% vs. 66.7%, $P = 0.02$). A similar result was revealed by Wu and colleagues [86], who found a higher specificity of T2w combined with DWI than with DW-MR imaging alone ($P < 0.05$) when differentiating Tis to T1 tumor stages from T2 to T4 tumor stages [87]. Staging a tumor with a stalk showing imaging of "inchworm sign" which is not only seen in stage Ta or stage T1 tumors but also can be seen in stage T2 tumors (Figs. 4.13 and 4.14) [88, 89].

In differentiating T2 from T3, inflammatory change or fibrosis surrounding the tumor could lead to overestimation of the T staging using T2WI or DCEI, but DWI could differentiate them clearly because these changes cause signal suppression [90]. Differentiating T2b from T3a is quite difficult because of the limited spatial resolution; if the contour of the mass invading the muscle is irregular or has a ridge protruding into the perivesical space, the T stage is thought to be T3 [92]. However, it is not a serious problem because the treatment procedure and prognosis are the same for both these T stages [92]. If the extent of high SI reflecting cancer invasion is seen in adjacent organs on DWI, the stage is T4 (Figs. 4.15, 4.16, 4.17, and 4.18) [92].

Infiltrative scattered tumors may not generate enough high signals on DWI to be discriminated from normal bladder that can be underdetected and lead to understaging [91].

4.4   Bladder Cancer Characterization

Because of the rarity of non-TCC, there is limited literature focus on distinguishing TCC from non-TCC of bladder on DWI. Generally, non-TCC of bladder is reported to be more aggressive and usually extends beyond the bladder wall and is usually larger than TCC of the bladder at the initial time of diagnosis [92].

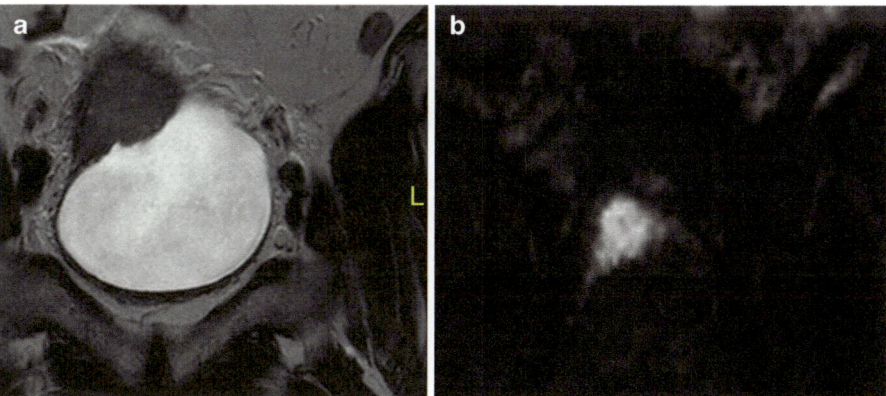

Fig. 4.13 T3b high-grade urothelial carcinoma of the bladder. A 63-year-old male patient presented with recurrent attacks of hematuria. 3 Tesla MRI: (**a**) Sagittal T2w image of the bladder shows large mass of the posterior wall and invading the perivesical fat with thickened-related peritoneal reflection. (**b**) DW image of the bladder with b value = 800 s/mm^2 shows restricted diffusion at the mass with invasion of the perivesical fat but no invasion of the peritoneal reflection (*arrow*)

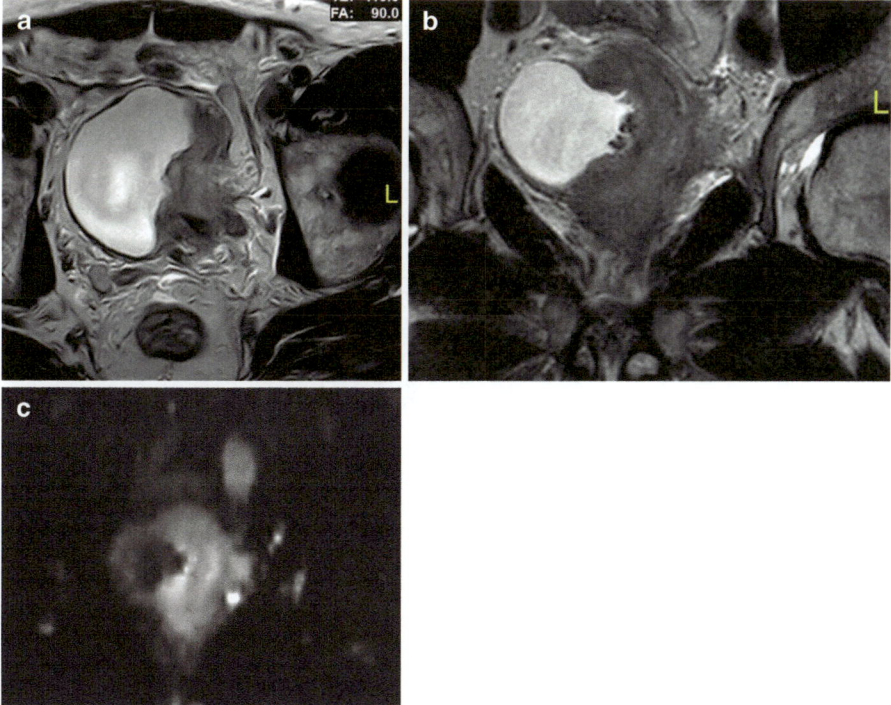

Fig. 4.14 High-grade T3b urothelial carcinoma of the bladder. A 59-year-old male patient presented with hematuria. 3T MRI: (**a**) Coronal T2w image of the bladder shows a large left-sided bladder mass involving the dome and bladder base with perivesical fat infiltration; the mass is nearby the left acetabulum. (**b**) Coronal DWI b value = 800 s/mm^2 shows restricted diffusion of the mass with invasion of the perivesical fat

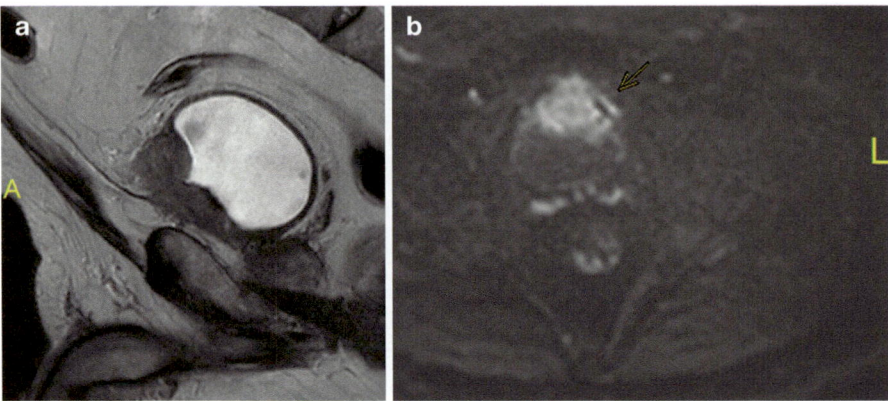

Fig. 4.15 T4a high-grade invasive urothelial carcinoma of the bladder. A 63-year-old male presented with recurrent attacks of hematuria. 3 Tesla MRI: (**a**) Sagittal T2w image of the pelvis shows large exophytic anterior vesical wall mass invading the perivesical fat with close adhesion at the anterior peritoneal reflection. (**b**) Axial DW image of the bladder b value = 800 s/mm^2 shows restricted diffusion at the mass and the infiltrated peritoneal reflection (*arrow*)

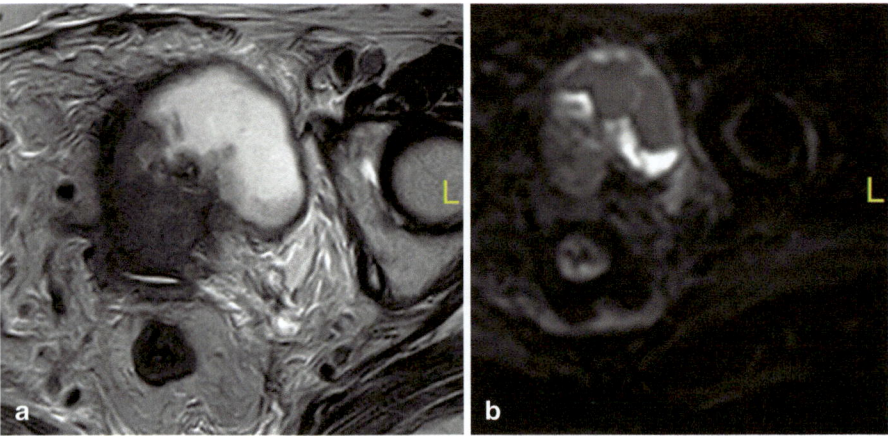

Fig. 4.16 T4a high-grade urothelial carcinoma of the bladder. A 74-year-old female patient presented with total hematuria and clot retention. 3 Tesla MRI: (**a**) Axial T2w image of the pelvis shows large posterior wall mass to the right infiltrating the anterior vaginal wall (*arrow*). (**b**) Axial DW image b value = 800 s/mm^2 shows that the fungating extravesical component has lower diffusion restriction than the intravesical part with infiltration of the anterior vaginal wall

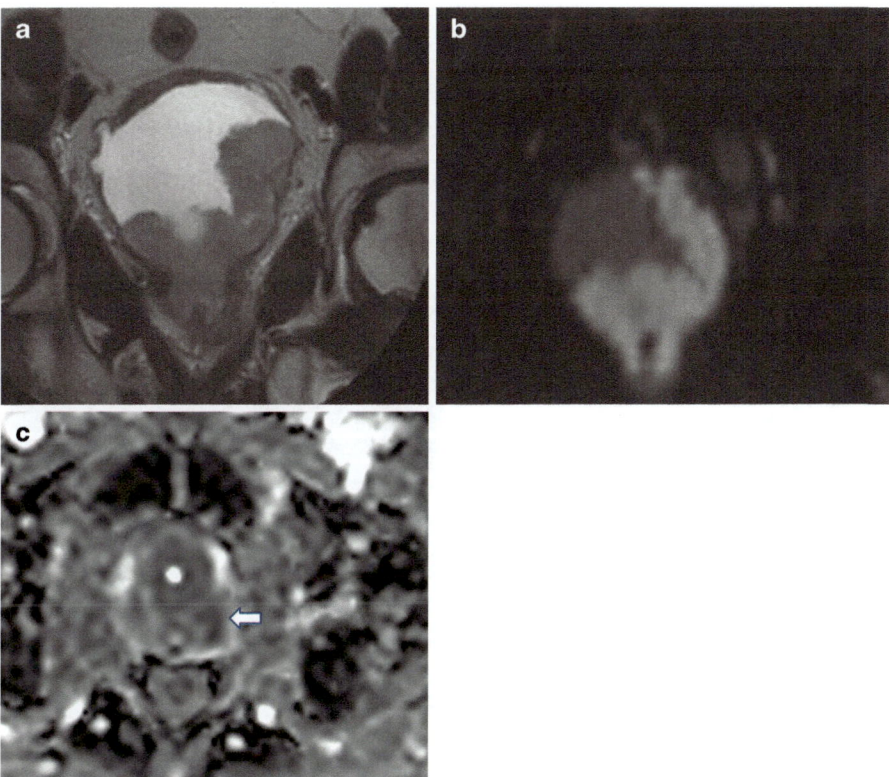

Fig. 4.17 Multicentric high-grade invasive urothelial carcinoma of the bladder and urethra. A 53-year-old male patient presented with hematuria. 3T MRI: (**a**) Coronal T2w image of the pelvis shows large vesical mass extending along the urethra. (**b**) Coronal DWI *b* value = 800 s/mm^2 shows restricted diffusion at the mass. (**c**) ADC map at the prostate shows tumor invasion into the prostate (*arrow*)

Detection of cell type and the histologic grade of bladder carcinoma are fundamental prognostic factors. Daggulli et al. [78] found that the ADC values of transitional cell carcinoma were significantly higher than those of squamous cell carcinoma, but El-Assmy et al. [75] did not. UCCs are categorized as high- or low-grade tumors based on the rate of cellular abnormality at microscopy. ADC values could be a biomarker predicting histopathological grading, aggressiveness, and tumor response to chemoradiation therapy. Some researchers reported that the mean ADC values of high-grade cancers and MIBCs were lower than those of lower grade cancers and NMIBCs [25, 30, 78, 85, 89, 93–95].

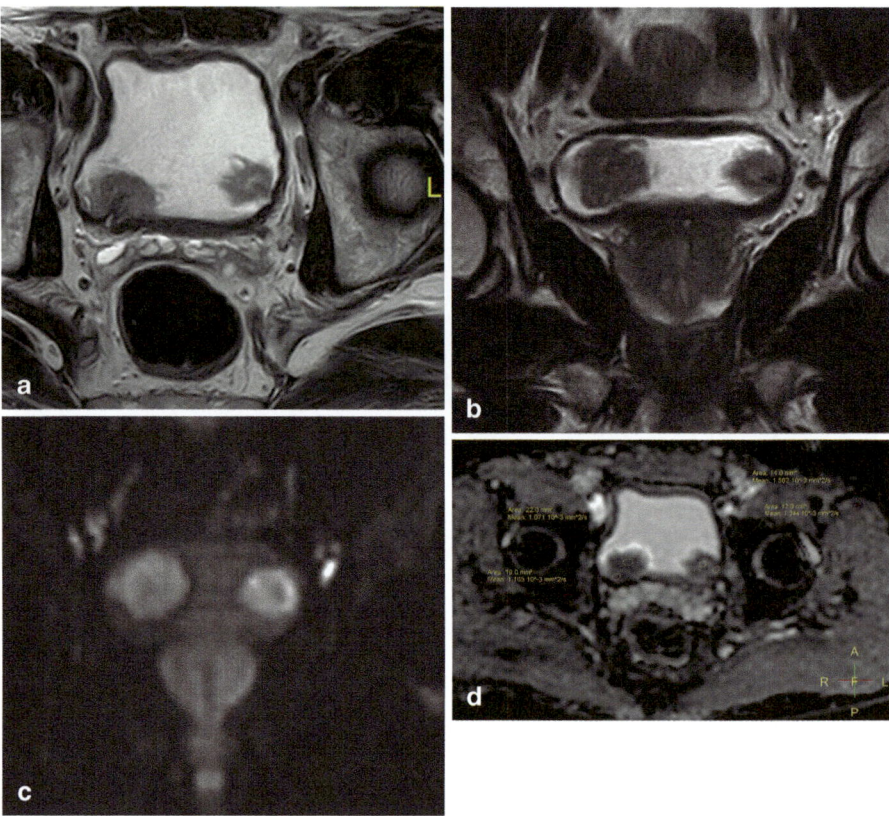

Fig. 4.18 Two papillary low-grade urothelial carcinomas of the bladder. A 64-year-old male patient presented with recurrent attacks of hematuria. 3T MRI: (**a**, **b**) Axial and coronal T2w images show two lesions from both lateral walls with central connective tissue stalk of low SI. (**c**) Coronal DWI b value = 800 s/mm² of the bladder shows restricted diffusion at both lesions with invasion of superficial muscle at the left side, while the right one is seen invading the deep muscle, no perivesical fat. (**d**) ADC map shows low ADC value of the mass ($1071-1.165 \times 10^{-3}$ mm²/s) with relative high value of the stalk (1.562×10^{-3} mm²/s)

One study of 121 patients aimed to investigate whether ADC values provide useful information on the clinical aggressiveness of a tumor, because ADC values have been shown to be significantly lower in high-grade disease (median 0.79×10^{-3} mm²/s) in comparison to low-grade tumors (median 0.99×10^{-3} mm²/s; $P < 0.0001$) [89]. Takeuchi et al. [25], using a tumor classification with three grades, reported that the differences in the ADC values were significant between both G1 and G3 and between G2 and G3 tumors, but not between G1 and G2 tumors [96]. In another study, in 39 patients with 60 bladder tumors, ADC values for muscle-invasive and G3 grade bladder cancers were significantly lower than those of non-muscle-invasive and G1 grade cancers ($P < 0.01$) [97].

Panebianco et al. evaluated 76 patients with suspected or confirmed bladder lesions to determine the ability of multiparametric magnetic resonance imaging (mpMRI) to differentiate muscle-invasive bladder carcinoma (MIBC) from non-muscle-invasive bladder carcinoma (NMIBC); they found only five cases that were misclassified by the MRI examination. Of these, two T2 lesions had early microscopic invasion at histopathology (T2a) and were classified as non-muscle-invasive bladder cancer, while three pT1 lesions showing a very similar signal intensity of tumor and sub-mucosa at DWI were labeled as muscle-invasive bladder cancer [98].

4.5   Monitoring Treatment Response and Tumor Recurrence

Evaluation of response to induction chemotherapy is important in determining if patients will be candidates for cystectomy or in case of incomplete response, additional radiation therapy is recommended [99, 100]. Yoshida and his colleagues had two studies assessing the bladder cancer response to chemotherapy. In the first one [101], they compared different imaging techniques to predict a complete response in 20 patients based on histopathology and found that DW-MR imaging had a significantly higher specificity (92%) and accuracy (80%) than conventional T2w imaging (45% and 44%) or dynamic contrast-enhanced (DCE) MR imaging (18% and 33%). In the second one, their aim was to predict sensitivity to chemoradiotherapy (CRT) in patients with muscle-invasive bladder cancers [102]. They found that tumors with a pathologic complete response to chemoradiotherapy had significantly lower ADC values than patients with tumors that were resistant (median, 0.63×10^{-3} mm^2/s vs. 0.84×10^{-3} mm^2/s; $P < 0.0001$) [89].

DW-MR imaging has been shown to be superior to DCE-MR imaging in differentiating recurrent tumor from chronic inflammation and fibrosis in patients after cystectomy or transurethral resection of bladder cancer. Chronic inflammatory or fibrotic tissues have lower cellular density or larger extracellular space so that the relatively free water movement is reflected as increased diffusion with hypointensity on high b-value DWI (Fig. 4.19) [103].

Both recurrent bladder tumors and postoperative benign changes have similar morphological MRI appearance as nodular, papillary, or flat lesions. Inflammation and fibrosis can enhance with intravenous contrast because of peri-tumoral neovascularization. Wang and colleagues [29] found significantly higher accuracies, sensitivities, specificities, and positive predictive values of DW-MR imaging compared with DCE-MR imaging for detecting recurrent tumors. They found higher sensitivity of 100% (16/16) on DWI than that of DCE MRI (81.3%, 13/16) for detecting recurrent tumor. DWI detected three lesions smaller than 5 mm that were missed at dynamic contrast-enhanced MRI study. Their results were similar to those of El-Assmy et al. [75], they reported high accurate diagnosis of 32/34 recurrent tumors and 21/23 benign lesions after TURBT on DWI without quantitative ADC analysis. Wang et al. were able to correctly diagnose inflammation or fibrosis that appeared slightly hyperintense on both DWI and ADC maps. The recurrent tumors had significantly lower ADC of 0.845 ± 0.166 mm^2/s (range 0.726–0.963 mm^2/s) than ADC of 1.239 ± 0.191 mm^2/s (range 1.092–1.387 mm^2/s) for benign lesions ($P < 0.05$) [29].

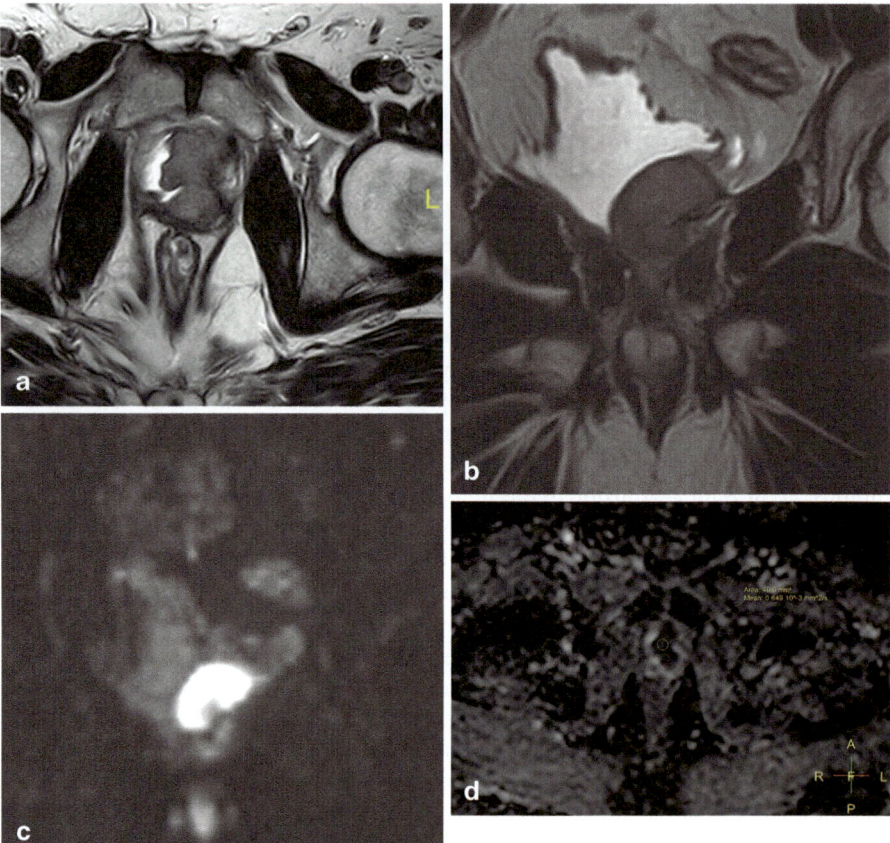

Fig. 4.19 High-grade urethral recurrence after radical cystectomy for bladder urothelial cancer. A 58-year-old male patient presented with recurrent attacks of hematuria. 3T MRI: (**a**, **b**) Axial and coronal T2w images of the pelvis show soft tissue mass at the pouch-urethral anastomosis. (**c**) Coronal DW image shows diffusion at the mass with low ADC (0.649×10^{-3} mm^2/s) at ADC map (**d**)

Conventional cystoscopy and biopsy are still indicated to identify posttreatment recurrence due to limitations of DWI in differentiating small or microscopic viable tumors from post-therapeutic inflammatory changes and fibrosis [29, 104, 107]. There is still also an overlap of ADC values between recurrent tumors and the surrounding bladder wall that may be attributable to the inflammatory reaction from previous TURBT [75].

4.6   Future Developments

DW-MRI could serve as a biomarker for monitoring response in patients to targeted therapies in malignant patients. It can detect early changes in tumor metabolism in response to treatment regardless the change in tumor size [105].

Also, validation of cutoff values for the noninvasive differentiation between benign and malignant tumors and their LN metastases, and eventually for discrimination of various histologic subtypes and grading, might allow individualized patient management. This is requiring standardization of DW-MRI for various organs [106].

Diffusion tensor imaging (DTI), with the fractional anisotropy (FA) methodology and fiber tractography (FT) has been recently evaluated by Panebianco et al. In this study they demonstrated the need to integrate all the sequences information for an optimal bladder evaluation. The diagnostic accuracy of inclusion of DTI into an mpMRI was 94% in differentiating MIBC from NMIBC [100].

They also demonstrated in this study that the diffusion tensor parameters of invasive and noninvasive bladder cancer differ significantly. The FA values were not significantly different in normal muscle tissue and interface between tumor and bladder wall in NMIBC. The FA value was significantly higher at the interface between tumor and bladder wall in MIBC [100].

References

1. Arslan H, Tezcan FM, Alğin O. Urothelial cancers: clinical and imaging evaluation. Turk J Med Sci. 2012;42(Sup.2):1355–64.
2. Gödekmerdan A, Yahşi S, Semerciöz A, İlhan F, Akpolat N, Yekeler H. Determination of nuclear matrix protein 22 levels in cystitis, urothelial dysplasia and urothelial carcinoma. Turk J Med Sci. 2006;36:93–6.
3. Wong-You-Cheong JJ, Woodward PJ, Manning MA, Sesterhenn IA. From the archives of the AFIP: neoplasms of the urinary bladder: radiologic-pathologic correlation. Radiographics. 2006;26:553–80.
4. Hurwitz M, Spiess PE, Garcia JA and Louis L. Pisters LL. Urothelial and kidney cancers. Cancer Management. Published on Cancer Network. http://www.cancernetwork.com. Accessed 1 June 2016.
5. Vikram R, Sandler CM, Ng CS. Imaging and staging of transitional cell carcinoma. Part 2. Upper urinary tract. AJR Am J Roentgenol. 2009;192:1488–93.
6. Akbulut Z, Tuzlalı M, Canda AE, Ercan K, Kandemir O, Balbay MD. Factors affecting adrenal gland involvement in patients who underwent radical nephrectomy for renal cell carcinoma. Turk J Med Sci. 2009;39:215–22.
7. Rafla S. Tumors of the upper urothelium. Am J Roentgenol Radium Therapy, Nucl Med. 1975;123:540–51.
8. Hall MC, Womack S, Sagalowsky AI, Carmody T, Erickstad MD, Roehrborn CG. Prognostic factors, recurrence, and survival in transitional cell carcinoma of the upper urinary tract: a 30-year experience in 252 patients. Urology. 1998;52:594–601.
9. Nishizawa S, Imai S, Okaneya T, Nakayama T, Kamigaito T, Minagawa T. Diffusion weighted imaging in the detection of upper urinary tract urothelial tumors. Int Braz J Urol. 2010;36(1):18–28.
10. Kirkali Z, Tuzel E. Transitional cell carcinoma of the ureter and renal pelvis. Crit Rev Oncol Hematol. 2003;47:155–69.
11. Chan V, Pantanowitz L, Vrachliotis TG, Rabkin DJ. CT demonstration of a rapidly growing transitional cell carcinoma of the ureter and renal pelvis. Abdom Imaging. 2002;27:222–3.
12. Yoshikawa K, Nakata Y, Yamada K, Nakagawa M. Early pathological changes in the parkinsonian brain demonstrated by diffusion tensor MRI. J Neurol Neurosurg Psychiatry. 2004;75:481–4.

13. Eastwood JD, Lev MH, Wintermark M, et al. Correlation of early dynamic CT perfusion imaging with whole-brain MR diffusion and perfusion imaging in acute hemispheric stroke. Am J Neuroradiol. 2003;24:1869–75.
14. Koh DM, Collins DJ. Diffusion-weighted MRI in the body: applications and challenges in oncology. AJR. 2007;188:1622–35.
15. Browne RF, Meehan CP, Colville J, Power R, Torreggiani WC. Transitional cell carcinoma of the upper urinary tract: spectrum of imaging findings. Radiographics. 2005;6:1609–27.
16. Yoshida S, Masuda H, Ishii C, Tanaka H, Fujii Y, Kawakami S, Kihara K. Usefulness of diffusion-weighted MRI in diagnosis of upper urinary tract cancer. AJR Am J Roentgenol. 2011;196(1):110–6.
17. MacVicar AD. Bladder cancer staging. BJU. 2000;86:111–22.
18. Stein JP, Lieskovsky G, Cote R, Groshen S, Feng AC, Boyd S, Skinner E, Bochner B, Thangathurai D, Mikhail M, et al. Radical cystectomy in the treatment of invasive bladder cancer: long-term results in 1,054 patients. J Clin Oncol. 2001;19:666–75.
19. Dutta SC, Smith Jr JA, Shappell SB, Coffey CS, Chang SS, Cookson MS. Clinical under staging of high risk nonmuscle invasive urothelial carcinoma treated with radical cystectomy. J Urol. 2001;166:490–3.
20. Ficarra V, Dalpiaz O, Alrabi N, Novara G, Galfano A, Artibani W. Correlation between clinical and pathological staging in a series of radical cystectomies for bladder carcinoma. BJU Int. 2005;95:786–90.
21. Mehrsai A, Mansoori D, Taheri Mahmoudi M, Sina A, Seraji A, Pourmand GH. A comparison between clinical and pathologic staging in patients with bladder cancer. Urol J. 2004; 1:85–9.
22. Anderson EM, Murphy R, Rennie AT, Cowan NC. Multidetector computed tomography urography (MDCTU) for diagnosing urothelial malignancy. Clin Radiol. 2007;62:324–32.
23. Caoili EM, Cohan RH, Inampudi P, et al. MDCT urography of upper tract urothelial neoplasms. AJR. 2005;184:1873–81.
24. Siegel R, Naishadham D, Jemal A. Cancer statistics. CA Cancer J Clin. 2013;63:11–30.
25. Takeuchi M, Sasaki S, Ito M, Okada S, Takahashi S, Kawai T, Suzuki K, Oshima H, Hara M, Shibamoto Y. Urinary bladder cancer: diffusion—weighted MR imaging—accuracy for diagnosing T stage and estimating histologic grade. Radiology. 2009;251:112–21.
26. El-Assmy A, Abou-El-Ghar ME, Mosbah A, El-Nahas AR, Refaie HF, Hekal IA, El-Diasty T, Ibrahiem el H. Bladder tumour staging: comparison of diffusion- and T2-weighted MR imaging. Eur Radiol. 2009;19:1575–81.
27. Thoeny HC, Forstner R, De Keyzer F. Genitourinary applications of diffusion-weighted MR imaging in the pelvis. Radiology. 2012;263:326–42.
28. Rosenkrantz AB, Mussi TC, Melamed J, Taneja SS, Huang WC. Bladder cancer: utility of MRI in detection of occult muscle-invasive disease. Acta Radiol. 2012;53:695–9.
29. Wang HJ, Pui MH, Guo Y, Yang D, Pan BT, Zhou XH. Diffusion-weighted MRI in bladder carcinoma: the differentiation between tumor recurrence and benign changes after resection. Abdom Imaging. 2014;39:135–41.
30. Avcu S, Koseoglu MN, Ceylan K, Bulut MD, Unal O. The value of diffusion-weighted MRI in the diagnosis of malignant and benign urinary bladder lesions. Br J Radiol. 2011;84:875–82.
31. Bammer R. Basic principles of diffusion-weighted imaging. Eur J Radiol. 2003;45:169–84.
32. Okada Y, Ohtomo K, Kiryu S, Sasaki Y. Breathhold T2-weighted MRI of hepatic tumors: value of echo planar imaging with diffusion-sensitizing gradient. J Comput Assist Tomogr. 1998;22:364–71.
33. Squillaci E, Manenti G, Di Stefano F, Miano R, Strigari L, Simonetti G. Diffusion-weighted MR imaging in the evaluation of renal tumours. J Exp Clin Cancer Res. 2004;23:39–45.
34. Abe Y, Yamashita Y, Tang Y, Namimoto T, Takahashi M. Calculation of T2 relaxation time from ultrafast single shot sequences for differentiation of liver tumors: comparison of echo-planar, HASTE, and spin-echo sequences. Radiat Med. 2000;18:7–14.
35. Yamashita Y, Tang Y, Takahashi M. Ultrafast MR imaging of the abdomen: echo planar imaging and diffusion-weighted imaging. J Magn Reson Imaging. 1998;8:367–74.

36. Ito K, Mitchell DG, Matsunaga N. MR imaging of the liver: techniques and clinical applications. Eur J Radiol. 1999;32:2–14.
37. Park SW, Lee JH, Ehara S, et al. Single shot fast spin echo diffusion-weighted MR imaging of the spine: is it useful in differentiating malignant metastatic tumor infiltration from benign fracture edema? Clin Imaging. 2004;28:102–8.
38. Abou-El-Ghar ME, El-Assmy A, Refaie HF, El-Diasty T. Bladder cancer: diagnosis with diffusion-weighted MR imaging in patients with gross hematuria. Radiology. 2009;251:415–21.
39. Higano S, Yun X, Kumabe T, et al. Malignant astrocytic tumors: clinical importance of apparent diffusion coefficient in prediction of grade and prognosis. Radiology. 2006;241:839–46.
40. Matoba M, Tonami H, Kondou T, et al. Lung carcinoma: diffusion-weighted MR imaging—preliminary evaluation with apparent diffusion coefficient. Radiology. 2007;243:570–7.
41. Watanabe H, Kanematsu M, Kondo H, et al. Preoperative T staging of urinary bladder cancer: does diffusion-weighted MRI have supplementary value? AJR. 2009;192:1361–6.
42. Zelhof B, Pickles M, Liney G, et al. Correlation of diffusion-weighted magnetic resonance data with cellularity in prostate cancer. BJU Int. 2009;103:883–8.
43. Yamanouchi Y, Yamamoto K, Noda K, Tomori K, Kinoshita T. Renal infarction in a patient with spontaneous dissection of segmental arteries: diffusion-weighted magnetic resonance imaging. Am J Kidney Dis. 2008;52:788–91.
44. Dunn DP, Kelsey NR, Lee KS, Smith MP, Mortele KJ. Non-oncologic applications of diffusion-weighted imaging (DWI) in the genitourinary system. Abdom Imaging. 2015;40(6):1645–4.
45. Kataoka M, Kido A, Koyama T, et al. MRI of the female pelvis at 3T compared to 1.5T: evaluation on high-resolution T2- weighted and HASTE images. J Magn Reson Imaging. 2007;25(3):527–34.
46. Takeuchi M, Matsuzaki K, Kubo H, Nishitani H. Diffusion-weighted magnetic resonance imaging of urinary epithelial cancer with upper urinary tract obstruction: preliminary results. Acta Radiol. 2008;49(10):1195–9.
47. Karakas E, Karakas O, Cullu N, et al. Diffusion-weighted MRI of the testes in patients with varicocele: a preliminary study. AJR. 2014;202:324–8.
48. Padhani AR, Liu G, Koh DM, et al. Diffusion-weighted magnetic resonance imaging as a cancer biomarker: consensus and recommendations. Neoplasia. 2009;11:102–25.
49. Le Bihan D, Breton E, Lallemand D, et al. Separation of diffusion and perfusion in intravoxel incoherent motion MR imaging. Radiology. 1988;168:497–505.
50. Thoeny HC, Binser T, Roth B, Kessler TM, Vermathen P. Noninvasive assessment of acute ureteral obstruction with diffusion-weighted MR imaging: a prospective study. Radiology. 2009;252:721–8.
51. Takahara T, Imai Y, Yamashita T, Yasuda S, Nasu S, Van Cauteren M. Diffusion weighted whole body imaging with background body signal suppression (DWIBS): technical improvement using free breathing, STIR and high resolution 3D display. Radiat Med. 2004;22:275–82.
52. Nagel KNA, Schouten MG, Hambrock T, et al. Differentiation of prostatitis and prostate cancer by using diffusion weighted MR imaging and MR-guided biopsy at 3T. Radiology. 2013;267:164–72.
53. Roy C. Tumour pathology of the bladder: the role of MRI. Diagn Interv Imaging. 2012;93:297–309.
54. Mazaheri Y, Hricak H, Fine SW, et al. Prostate tumor volume measurement with combined T2-weighted imaging and diffusion weighted MR: correlation with pathologic tumor volume. Radiology. 2009;252(2):449–57.
55. Wang J, Wang H, Tang G, et al. Transitional cell carcinoma of upper urinary tract vs. benign lesions: distinctive MSCT features. Abdom Imaging. 2009;34:94–106.
56. Fritz GA, Schoellnast H, Deutschmann HA, et al. Multiphasic multidetector-row CT (MDCT) in detection and staging of transitional cell carcinomas of the upper urinary tract. Eur Radiol. 2006;16:1244–52.
57. Akita H, Jinzaki M, Kikuchi E, Sugiura H, Akita A, Mikami S, et al. Preoperative T categorization and prediction of histopathologic grading of urothelial carcinoma in renal pelvis using diffusion-weighted MRI. AJR Am J Roentgenol. 2011;197(5):1130–6.

58. Colagrande S, Carbone SF, Carusi LM, Cova M, Villari N. Magnetic resonance diffusion weighted imaging: extraneurological applications. Radiol Med. 2006;111(3):392–419.
59. Wu GY, Lu Q, Wu LM, Zhang J, Chen XX, Xu JR. Comparison of computed tomographic urography, magnetic resonance urography and the combination of diffusion weighted imaging in diagnosis of upper urinary tract cancer. Eur J Radiol. 2014;83(6):893–9.
60. Shebel H, Elhawary G, Sheir K, Sultan A. Characterization of upper urinary tract urothelial lesions in patients with gross hematuria using diffusion-weighted MRI: a prospective study. Egypt J Radiol Nucl Med. 2014;45:943–8.
61. Namimoto T, Yamashita Y, Sumi S, et al. Focal liver masses: characterization with diffusion-weighted echo-planar MR imaging. Radiology. 1997;204:739–44.
62. Yamada I, Aung W, Himeno Y, et al. Diffusion coefficients in abdominal organs and hepatic lesions: evaluation with intravoxel incoherent motion echo-planar MR imaging. Radiology. 1998;210:617–23.
63. Kim T, Murakami T, Takahashi S, et al. Diffusion-weighted single-shot echo-planar MR imaging for liver disease. AJR Am J Roentgenol. 1999;173:393–8.
64. Bammer R, Keeling SL, Augustin M, et al. Improved diffusion-weighted single-shot echo-planar imaging (EPI) in stroke using sensitivity encoding (SENSE). Magn Reson Med. 2001;46:548–54.
65. Hunsche S, Moseley ME, Stoeter P, et al. Diffusion-tensor MR imaging at 1.5 and 3.0 T: initial observations. Radiology. 2001;221:550–6.
66. Boulanger Y, Amara M, Lepanto L, et al. Diffusion-weighted MR imaging of the liver of hepatitis C patients. NMR Biomed. 2003;16:132–6.
67. Aubé C, Racineux PX, Lebigot J, et al. Diagnosis and quantification of hepatic fibrosis with diffusion weighted MR imaging: preliminary results. J Radiol. 2004;85:301–6.
68. Sufana Iancu A, Colin P, Puech P, Villers A, Ouzzane A, Fantoni JC, Leroy X, Lemaitre L. Significance of ADC value for detection and characterization of urothelial carcinoma of upper urinary tract using diffusion weighted MRI. World J Urol. 2013;31(1):13–9.
69. Wehrli NE, Kim MJ, Matza BW, Melamed J, Taneja SS, Rosenkrantz AB. Utility of MRI features in differentiation of central renal cell carcinoma and renal pelvic urothelial carcinoma. AJR Am J Roentgenol. 2013;201(6):1260–7.
70. Sasaki M, Yamada K, Watanabe Y, et al. Variability in absolute apparent diffusion coefficient values across different platforms may be substantial: a multivendor, multi-institutional comparison study. Radiology. 2008;249:624–30.
71. Rosenkrantz AB, Kopec M, Kong X, et al. Prostate cancer vs. post-biopsy hemorrhage: diagnosis with T2- and diffusion-weighted imaging. J Magn Reson Imaging. 2010;31:1387–94.
72. Matsuki M, Inada Y, Tatsugami F, Tanikake M, Narabayashi I, Katsuoka Y. Diffusion weighted MR imaging for urinary bladder carcinoma: initial results. Eur Radiol. 2007;17(1):201–4.
73. El-Assmy A, Abou-El-Ghar ME, Refaie HF, El-Diasty T. Diffusion-weighted MR imaging in diagnosis of superficial and invasive urinary bladder carcinoma: a preliminary prospective study. ScientificWorldJournal. 2008;8:364–70.
74. Kilickesmez O, Cimilli T, Inci E, Kayhan A, Bayramoglu S, Tasdelen N, Gurmen N. Diffusion-weighted MRI of urinary bladder and prostate cancers. Diagn Interv Radiol. 2009;15:104–10.
75. Halefoglu AM, Sen EY, Tanriverdi O, Yilmaz F. Utility of diffusion-weighted MRI in the diagnosis of bladder carcinoma. Clin Imaging. 2013;37:1077–83.
76. Daggulli M, Onur MR, Firdolas F, Onur R, Kocakoc E, Orhan I. Role of diffusion MRI and apparent diffusion coefficient measurement in the diagnosis, staging and pathological classification of bladder tumors. Urol Int. 2011;87:346–52.
77. Babjuk M, Oosterlinck W, Sylvester R, et al. EAU guidelines on non-muscle-invasive urothelial carcinoma of the bladder, the 2011 update. Eur Urol. 2011;59(6):997–1008.
78. Josephson D, Pasin E, Stein JP. Superficial bladder cancer: part 2. Management. Expert Rev Anticancer Ther. 2007;7(4):567–81.
79. Sherif A, Jonsson MN, Wiklund NP. Treatment of muscle-invasive bladder cancer. Expert Rev Anticancer Ther. 2007;7(9):1279–83.

80. Katahira K, Takahara T, Kwee TC, Oda S, Suzuki Y, Morishita S, Kitani K, Hamada Y, Kitaoka M, Yamashita Y. Ultra-high-b-value diffusion-weighted MR imaging for the detection of prostate cancer: evaluation in 201 cases with histopathological correlation. Eur Radiol. 2011;21:188–96.
81. Kozlowski P, Chang SD, Goldenberg SL. Diffusion-weighted MRI in prostate cancer—comparison between single-shot fast spin echo and echo planar imaging sequences. Magn Reson Imaging. 2008;26:72–6.
82. Hambrock T, Futterer JJ, Huisman HJ, Hulsbergen-vandeKaa C, van Basten JP, van Oort I, Witjes JA, Barentsz JO. Thirty-two-channel coil 3 T magnetic resonance–guided biopsies of prostate tumor suspicious regions identified on multimodality 3 T magnetic resonance imaging: technique and feasibility. Investig Radiol. 2008;43:686–94.
83. Zhou G, Chen X, Zhang J, Zhu J, Zong G, Wang Z. Contrast-enhanced dynamic and diffusion-weighted MR imaging at 3.0 T to assess aggressiveness of bladder cancer. Eur J Radiol. 2014;83:2013–8.
84. Rosenkrantz AB, Obele C, Rusinek H, Balar AV, Huang WC, Deng FM, Ream JM. Whole-lesion diffusion metrics for assessment of bladder cancer aggressiveness. Abdom Imaging. 2015;40:327–32.
85. Dietrich O, Biffar A, Reiser MF, Baur-Melnyk A. Diffusion-weighted imaging of bone marrow. Semin Musculoskelet Radiol. 2009;13:134–44.
86. Kim CK, Park BK, Kim B. High-b-value diffusion-weighted imaging at 3 T to detect prostate cancer: comparisons between b values of 1,000 and 2,000 s/mm^2. AJR Am J Roentgenol. 2010;194:W33–7.
87. Maurer MH, Härmä KH, Thoeny H. Diffusion-weighted genitourinary imaging. Radiol Clin N Am. 2017;55(2):393–411.
88. Ohgiya Y, Suyama J, Sai S, Kawahara M, Takeyama N, Ohike N, Sasamori H, Munechika J, Saiki M, Onoda Y, et al. Preoperative T staging of urinary bladder cancer: efficacy of stalk detection and diagnostic performance of diffusion-weighted imaging at 3T. Magn Reson Med Sci. 2014;13:175–81.
89. Saito W, Amanuma M, Tanaka J, Heshiki A. Histopathological analysis of a bladder cancer stalk observed on MRI. Magn Reson Imaging. 2000;18:411–5.
90. Buxton RB. The diffusion sensitivity of fast steady-state free precession imaging. Magn Reson Med. 1993;29:235–43.
91. Lin WC, Chen JH. Pitfalls and limitations of diffusion-weighted magnetic resonance imaging in the diagnosis of urinary bladder cancer. Transl Oncol. 2015;8(3):217–30.
92. Tekes A, Kamel IR, Chan TY, Schoenberg MP, Bluemke DA. MR imaging features of non-transitional cell carcinoma of the urinary bladder with pathologic correlation. AJR Am J Roentgenol. 2003;180:779–84.
93. Yamada Y, Kobayashi S, Isoshima S, et al. The usefulness of diffusion-weighted magnetic resonance imaging in bladder cancer staging and functional analysis. J Cancer Res Ther. 2014;10:878–82.
94. Sevcenco S, Ponhold L, Heinz-Peer G, et al. Prospective evaluation of diffusion-weighted MRI of the bladder as a biomarker for prediction of bladder cancer aggressiveness. Urol Oncol. 2014;32:1166–71.
95. Wang HJ, Pui MH, Guo Y, et al. Multiparametric 3-T MRI for differentiating low-versus high-grade and category T1 versus T2 bladder urothelial carcinoma. AJR Am J Roentgenol. 2015;204:330–4.
96. Grignon DJ. The current classification of urothelial neoplasms. Mod Pathol. 2009;22:60–9.
97. Wang Y, Li Z, Meng X, et al. Nonmuscle-invasive and muscle-invasive urinary bladder cancer: image quality and clinical value of reduced field-of view versus conventional single-shot echo-planar imaging DWI. Medicine (Baltimore). 2016;95(10):e2951.
98. Panebianco V, De Berardinis E, Barchetti G, Simone G, Leonardo C, Grompone MD, Del Monte M, Carano D, Gallucci M, Catto J, Catalano C. An evaluation of morphological and functional multiparametric MRI sequences in classifying non muscle and muscle invasive bladder cancer. Eur Radiol. 2017;2:4758–3.

99. Chung PW, Bristow RG, Milosevic MF, et al. Long-term outcome of radiation-based conservation therapy for invasive bladder cancer. Urol Oncol. 2007;25(4):303–9.
100. Zapatero A, Martin de Vidales C, Arellano R, Bocardo G, Pérez M, Ros P. Updated results of bladder-sparing trimodality approach for invasive bladder cancer. Urol Oncol. 2010;28(4):368–74.
101. Yoshida S, Koga F, Kawakami S, et al. Initial experience of diffusion-weighted magnetic resonance imaging to assess therapeutic response to induction chemoradiotherapy against muscle-invasive bladder cancer. Urology. 2010;75(2):387–91.
102. Yoshida S, Koga F, Kobayashi S, et al. Role of diffusion-weighted magnetic resonance imaging in predicting sensitivity to chemoradiotherapy in muscle-invasive bladder cancer. Int J Radiat Oncol Biol Phys. 2012;83(1):e21–7.
103. Lim KS, Tan CH. Diffusion-weighted MRI of adult male pelvic cancers. Clin Radiol. 2012;67:899–908.
104. Inoue T, Ogasawara K, Beppu T, Ogawa A, Kabasawa H. Diffusion tensor imaging for preoperative evaluation of tumor grade in gliomas. Clin Neurol Neurosurg. 2005;107:174–80.
105. Thoeny HC, Ross BD. Predicting and monitoring cancer treatment response with diffusion-weighted MRI. J Magn Reson Imaging. 2010;32:2–16.
106. Giannarini G, Petralia G, Thoeny HC. Potential and limitations of diffusion-weighted magnetic resonance imaging in kidney, prostate, and bladder cancer including pelvic lymph node staging: a critical analysis of the literature. Eur Urol. 2012;61(2):326–40.
107. El-Assmy A, Abou-El-Ghar ME, Refaie HF, Mosbah A, El-Diasty T. Diffusion-weighted magnetic resonance imaging in follow-up of superficial urinary bladder carcinoma after transurethral resection: initial experience. BJU Int. 2012;110:e622–27.

MR Imaging of Ovarian Masses

5

Ali Devrim Karaosmanoğlu, Musturay Karcaaltıncaba,
Mustafa N. Özmen, and Deniz Akata

Abbreviations

ADC	Apparent diffusion coefficient
DCE	Dynamic contrast enhanced
DTI	Diffusion tensor imaging
DWI	Diffusion-weighted imaging
EPI	Echo planar imaging
IV	Intravenous
IVIM	Intra-voxel incoherent motion
Kapp	Apparent diffusional kurtosis
LNs	Lymph nodes
MPG	Motion-probing gradients
MRI	Magnetic resonance imaging
OT	Ovarian torsion
TOA	Tubo-ovarian abscesses
US	Ultrasonography

5.1 General Overview

Solid and cystic ovarian lesions are commonly encountered during routine imaging practice. Differentiation of benign lesions from the malignant ones is of paramount importance to guide the proper clinical management. Despite the commonly detected benign ovarian lesions, the borderline and frankly malignant lesions are

A.D. Karaosmanoğlu, M.D. • M. Karcaaltıncaba, M.D. • M.N. Özmen • D. Akata, M.D. (✉)
Department of Radiology, Hacettepe University School of Medicine, Ankara, Turkey
e-mail: dakata@hacettepe.edu.tr

© Springer International Publishing AG 2018
D. Akata, N. Papanikolaou (eds.), *Diffusion Weighted Imaging of the Genitourinary System*, https://doi.org/10.1007/978-3-319-69575-4_5

also not rare and prompt diagnosis, and differentiation of neoplastic lesions is one of the main tasks of the imaging specialists.

Malignant tumors of the ovaries are not rare and may be seen in all age groups. The lifetime risk of a woman in the United States developing ovarian cancer is around 1 in 70 [1]. Epithelial tumors account for most of the cases (90–95%) followed by the germ cell (15–20%) and sex cord-stromal tumors (5–10%). Metastatic ovarian tumors account for 1–5% of the ovarian malignancies and usually arise from breast, colon, endometrial, stomach, and cervical cancers [1]. Ovarian tumors comprise approximately 23% of all gynecologic tumors but are responsible for 47% of all deaths from malignant tumors of the female genital tract. Germ cell tumors of the ovaries are more commonly seen in younger women (<20 years), while epithelial ovarian tumors are more commonly seen in older women in their 50s [1].

Nonneoplastic diseases of the ovaries are also not rare. Infectious diseases of the ovary, including tubo-ovarian abscess, may also closely mimic the neoplastic ovarian diseases.

Imaging plays a crucial role in the diagnosis of neoplastic and nonneoplastic ovarian abnormalities. Ultrasonography (US) has conventionally been the modality of choice for evaluating the ovaries. Morphological evaluation of adnexal lesions is generally accurate for the identification of low- or high-risk lesions [2]. US provides high-quality images with unmatched cost-effectiveness with no associated radiation burden to the patient. Despite the mentioned advantages of US, magnetic resonance imaging (MRI) is gaining ever-increasing acceptance in the evaluation of ovarian abnormalities.

5.2   Technical Considerations of Pelvic MRI

Fasting for 3–4 h before the MRI exam is recommended. The use of antispasmodic drugs to reduce bowel peristalsis is a subject of debate, but in our current practice, we find it useful unless there is any presence of medical reason to not use it. The use of antiperistaltic medication also allows better evaluation of the pelvic peritoneal surfaces.

5.2.1   Conventional Imaging Technique

The conventional sequences include small field-of-view (FOV) high-resolution T2-weighted images without fat suppression in three orthogonal (axial, coronal, and sagittal) planes of the pelvis and large FOV axial T1 of the pelvis extended up to the aortic bifurcation. *These images provide us the panoramic anatomic view of the internal genitalia with high imaging resolution.* Intravenous (IV) contrast injection and dynamic post-contrast gradient echo 3D T1-weighted imaging in the axial plane with fat suppression are mandatory to reveal the enhancement of septa or to identify any solid or papillary projection in a cystic mass. The 3D contrast-enhanced imaging with fat-suppressed pre-contrast series is needed for subtraction when it is necessary.

Table 5.1 Our institutional MRI protocol for evaluating the ovariest

MRI protocol
Axial, coronal, sagittal plane high-resolution non-fat-sat T2W images
Axial plane high-resolution non-fat-sat T1W images
Axial plane T1W and T2W fat saturated images
Axial plane DWI with three different b-values (0, 300, 800 s/mm^2)
Axial plane post-contrast dynamic gradient 3D echo T1W images with fat saturated
Axial plane post-contrast dynamic spin echo 2D echo T1W images with fat saturated

Proper acquisition of these T1- and T2-weighted images is of fundamental importance for evaluating pelvic anatomy and optimal tissue characterization [3–5] (Table 5.1).

5.2.2 Imaging Technique of Diffusion-Weighted MR Imaging

In case of a totally unrestricted environment, water molecules would move randomly, a phenomenon also known as the Brownian motion [6]. Diffusion-weighted MR (DWI-MR) imaging basically exploits the random motion of water molecules in different human tissues. DW-MR imaging measures the length of the path traveled by the water molecules within a certain time period by the application of two diffusion-sensitizing gradients, both of which have opposing polarity, also called as motion-probing gradients (MPG). DW-MR imaging is sensitive to the random displacement of the water molecules within tissues. With the combined use of MPGs and echo planar imaging (EPI), DW-MR images are acquired. The intensity of MPG pulses is represented by the b-value (s/mm^2), a measure of the amplitude and strength of diffusion-sensitizing gradients. With the use of different b-value MPGs, one can effectively map and quantitatively calculate the apparent diffusion coefficient (ADC) [7].

DW-MR imaging can be quickly obtained without any IV contrast use and provides invaluable information regarding the microenvironment of any tissue in the human body. With this unique ability, the use of DWI-MR imaging is gaining popularity in diagnostic imaging outside the central nervous system.

5.3 Use of DWI-MR Imaging in Ovarian Inflammatory Lesions

Tubo-ovarian infections are relatively common, and clinical evaluation may sometimes be insufficient for a diagnosis. Imaging may play a crucial role in the diagnosis of tubo-ovarian abscesses (TOA), and differentiation from ovarian neoplasms may sometimes be extremely difficult. TOA usually appears as a complex cystic mass with variable amount of fluid content. Also associated are intense inflammatory changes in the pelvic fat planes and other neighboring pelvic organs. Hydro- or pyosalpinx may also associate the intense inflammatory changes in the adnexa (Fig. 5.1).

TOAs typically appear as a hypointense lesion in pre-contrast T1-weighted MR images with heterogeneous hyperintense signal on T2-weighted images. The wall of the abscess may appear hyperintense in case of microscopic hemorrhage. It may also reflect the formation of granulation tissue [8].

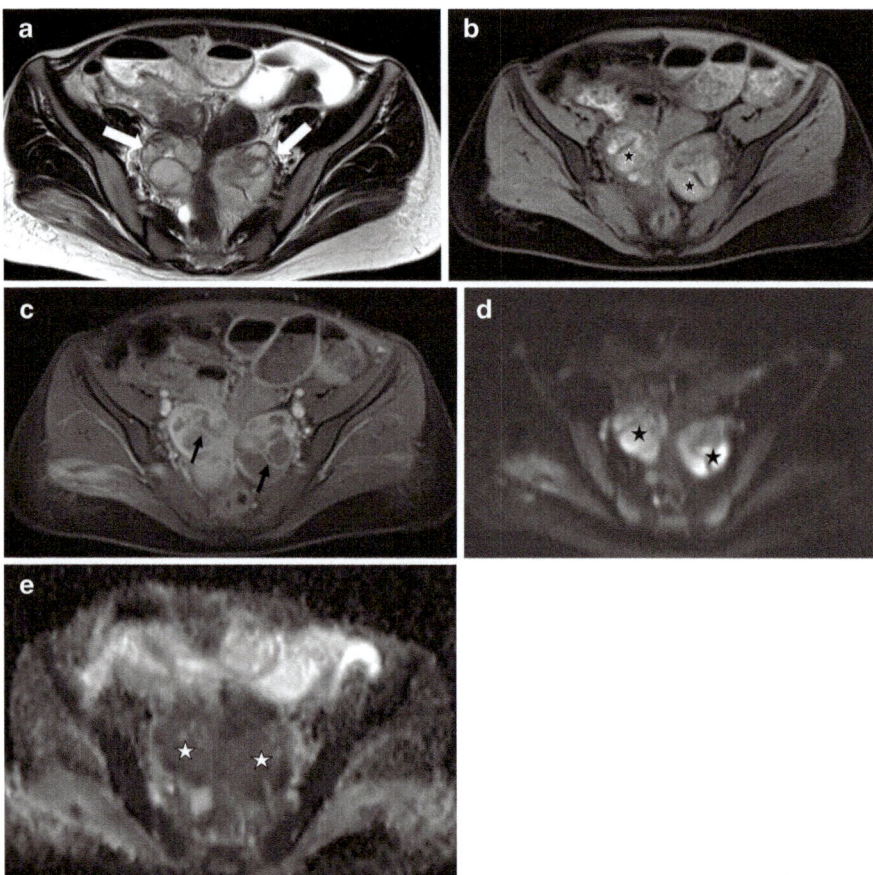

Fig. 5.1 A 33-year-old woman presenting with intense abdominal pain, foul-smelling vaginal discharge, and high fever. Subsequent surgery revealed diffuse pelvic inflammatory disease with bilateral hydropyosalpinx. (**a**) Axial plane T2W image demonstrates multiloculated serpiginous structures (*stars*) in both adnexae with moderately T2-hyperintense content. (**b**) Axial plane T1W image demonstrates hyperintense content of these structures (*stars*) which is suggestive of proteinaceous fluid. (**c**) Note diffuse contrast enhancement in the walls of the dilated fallopian tubes (*arrows*). Axial plane DWI study (**d**) and ADC map (**e**) images showed intense diffusion restriction in the dilated fallopian tubes suggestive of its highly cellular content (*stars* in both figures)

The MR appearance of the abscess may vary depending on its viscosity and content. The abscess content typically shows diffusion restriction with high signal intensity on DW images and decreased signal intensity on ADC maps (Fig. 5.2) [9]. This finding most likely reflects the expected highly viscous content of the TOA. Based on this unique feature of DW-MR imaging, MR may be used as an alternative to contrast-enhanced imaging in selected patients [7].

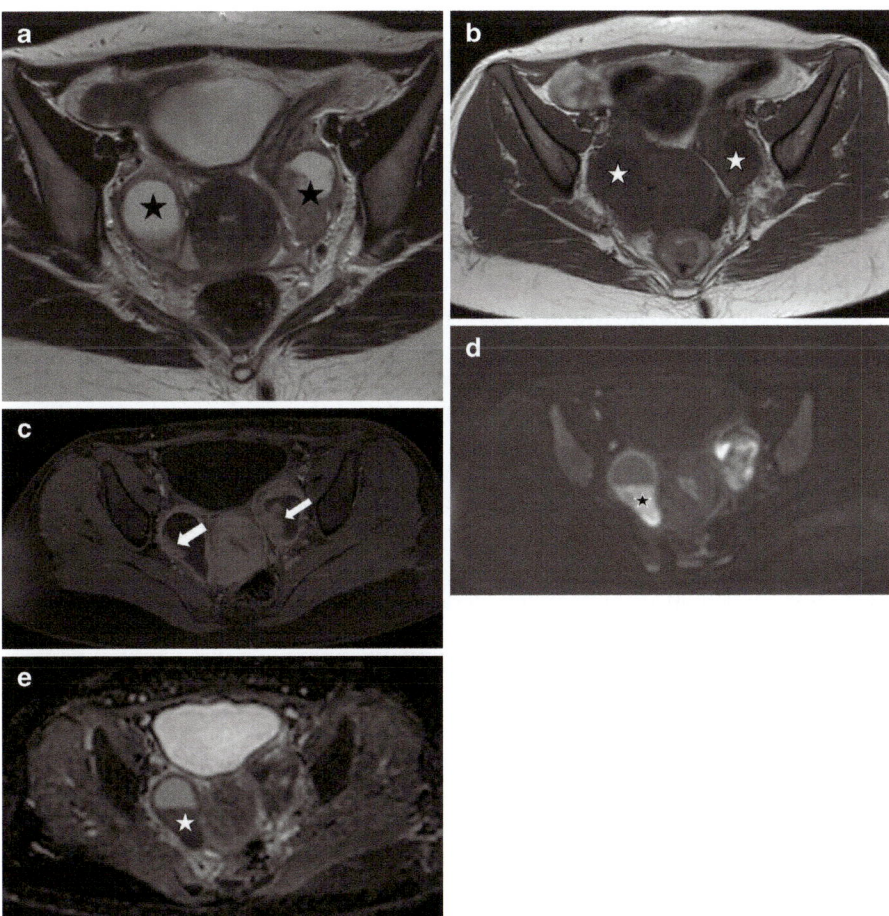

Fig. 5.2 A 45-year-old woman presenting with pelvic pain and mild fever who was finally diagnosed with bilateral oophoritis with abscess formations after surgery. (**a**) Axial plane T2W image demonstrates semi-cystic structures in both ovaries (*stars*), more solid appearing on the left with a fluid debris level in the right ovary. (**b**) On axial plane T1W image, these lesions appear hypointense bilaterally (*stars*). (**c**) Post-contrast fat-sat T1W image demonstrates intense mural enhancement in these cystic structures (*arrows*) mimicking a neoplastic process. Axial plane DWI study (**d**) and ADC map (**e**) images showed intense diffusion restriction in the debris part of the right ovarian lesion demonstrating its high cellularity (*stars* in both figures)

5.4   Use of DWI-MR Imaging in Ovarian Torsion

Ovarian torsion (OT) is a true surgical emergency, which necessitates early diagnosis and prompt surgical intervention. MR is not the first imaging modality employed in this clinical situation; however, in problematic cases, MR can be used as a problem-solving modality. An abnormally thickened fallopian tube usually appears as an amorphous solid mass with a target-like appearance. Multiplanar MR imaging may be very helpful, especially for recognizing the torsed ovarian vascular pedicle (whirlpool sign) in any of the corresponding planes. This mass may also appear as a beak-like protrusion extending from the uterus and partially covering the adnexal mass. Despite the aforementioned imaging findings, prompt diagnosis and differentiation from other ovarian pathologies may sometimes be extremely difficult or even impossible.

There is not much information in the literature regarding the role of DW-MR imaging in the diagnosis of OT. In a study comprised of 11 surgically confirmed patients, inhomogeneous abnormal DW (with the b-values of 0 and 1000 s/mm^2) imaging signal intensity in the thickened fallopian tube was the main finding. This imaging feature was attributed to infarcted tissues and blood clots [10].

As the clots also demonstrate high signal on DW-MR imaging, intracystic clot from adnexal hemorrhage may also show diffusion restriction, if present (Fig. 5.3). However, this finding is not specific for adnexal torsion as mature cystic teratomas and mucinous adenomas may also demonstrate abnormal signal intensity on DW-MR images [7].

5.5   Use of DW-MR Imaging in Endometriosis

There is not much information in the literature evaluating the role of DW-MR imaging in pelvic endometriosis. Endometrial cysts typically contain abundant blood clot as well as hemosiderin which causes shortened T2 with a subsequent decrease in the ADC values [11–15]. Based on the data provided, endometriomas as well as ectopic endometrial gland with hemorrhagic content as seen in endometriosis may demonstrate restricted diffusion on DW-MR images [7]. Endometriotic cysts tend to contain hemoglobin degeneration products, and its viscosity lowers ADC values (Fig. 5.4).

Malignant transformation of the endometriomas is a rare clinical event but should be sought after in the affected patients. Clear cell carcinoma and endometrioid carcinoma are primary ovarian cancers arising from ovarian endometriotic cysts (Fig. 5.5).

5.6   Use of DW-MR Imaging in Ovarian Neoplastic Lesions

US is generally the most commonly used modality in evaluating the ovarian pathologies. However, despite its impressive clinical success, in its routine clinical use, 5–25% of all adnexal lesions will remain indeterminate after US exam [16]. In this group of patients especially at premenopausal age, MR comes into play and serves as the problem-solving modality.

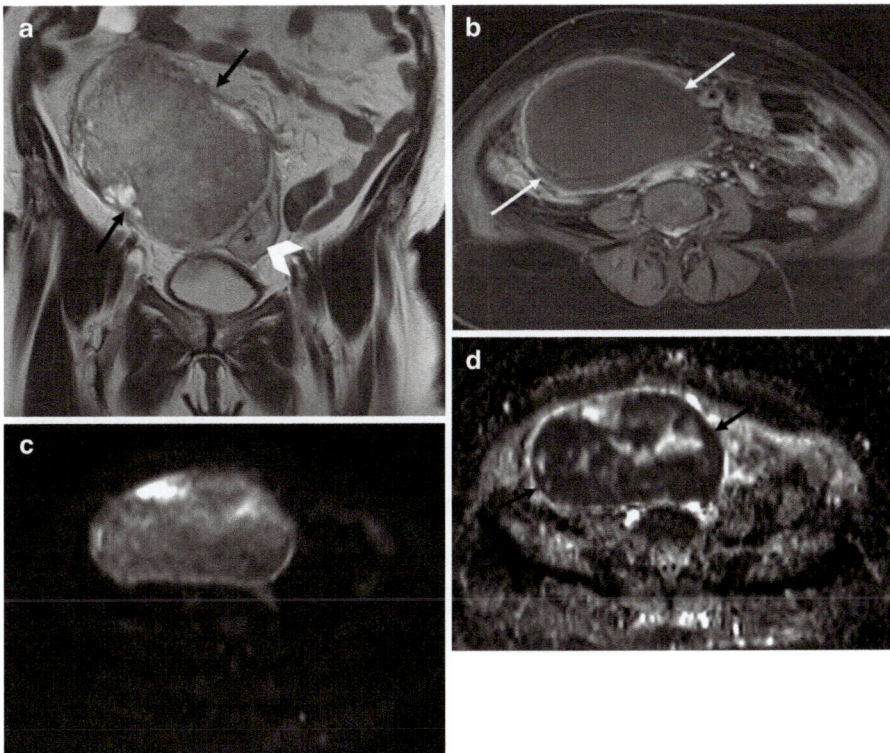

Fig. 5.3 A 29-year-old woman presenting with intense pelvic pain who was referred to MRI after detection of a mass in the right lower quadrant at the US scan. Subsequent surgery and unilateral salpingo-oophorectomy confirmed left ovarian torsion with widespread hemorrhagic necrosis. (**a**) On coronal plane T2W image, there is a large mass located in the right lower quadrant (*arrows*). The whirlpool sign in the salpinx is also revealed on the left adnexa (*white arrow*). This finding is consistent with displaced and torsed left ovary. (**b**) Axial plane post-contrast T1W image demonstrates no obvious internal enhancement of the lesion (*arrows*). Axial plane DWI study (**c**) and ADC map (**d**) images showed intense diffusion restriction manifesting with mild hyperintensity on DW images and significant hypointensity on the ADC map within the internal part of the mass (*arrows*)

Conventional T1 and T2 sequences with and without fat suppression and contrast use are very helpful in evaluating the morphological complexity of ovarian lesions. The enhancing solid components in the wall of cystic lesions as well as heterogeneous enhancement in completely solid lesions are highly suggestive of malignant neoplastic processes; however, it is also well known that there are several overlapping imaging features between benign and malignant ovarian neoplasms.

DW-MR imaging and its quantitative derivative (ADC)—which are displayed as a map or expressed as a value—provide additional data to the MR evaluation of ovarian lesions (Fig. 5.6). There is a controversy whether DW-MR imaging provides information per se or should be used as a complementary tool to morphological MR data. Despite this controversy, there are now several studies in the literature confirming the positive role of DW-MR imaging in evaluating ovarian masses [11, 15, 17–20].

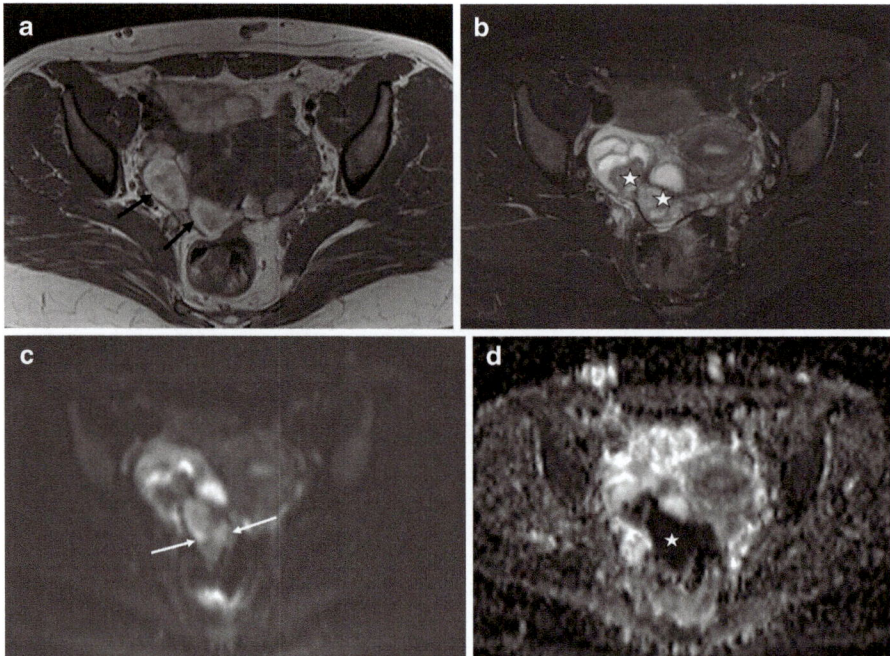

Fig. 5.4 A 27-year-old woman presenting with infertility, bilateral hydrosalpinx, and complex lesion in the right adnexa detected with US. Subsequent laparoscopic surgery confirmed unilateral endometriosis in the right adnexa. (**a**) Axial plane pre-contrast T1W image demonstrates a bilobular lesion in the right adnexa with hyperintense lesion center. (**b**) Axial plane T2W image demonstrates the T1-hyperintense lesion center as hypointense suggestive of hemorrhagic/proteinaceous content. (**c**) DW image demonstrates mild hyperintensity within the lesion (*arrows*). (**d**) Pronounced hypointensity (*star*) within the lesion on the ADC map confirmed diffusion restriction and hypercellularity of this cystic lesion

Generally speaking, malignant ovarian lesions tend to be more cellular which demonstrate diffusion restriction by producing high signal on DW-MR imaging (Fig. 5.6). The signal intensity tends to increase by increasing the b-value and corresponding low signal intensity on ADC mass. In addition to characterization, DW-MR imaging may also increase the lesion conspicuity, and it is particularly helpful in detecting peritoneal metastases and recurrent disease [21, 22].

There are some potential pitfalls to which one should be cautious during the interpretation of DW images. It is of crucial importance to keep in mind that DW images are intrinsically T2 hyperintense and that tissues with slow T2 relaxation rates can also appear bright. T2 shine-through phenomenon refers to persistent hyperintensity detected on high b-value images with a corresponding high ADC value. The high ADC value areas will, therefore, also appear as bright structures on the subsequent ADC maps (Fig. 5.7). This phenomenon can be problematic when it comes to interpretation of the high b-value images in isolation without any reference to corresponding ADC maps (29). Mucinous tumors can show T2 shine through effect and act like simple follicular cysts in DW images. In malignant

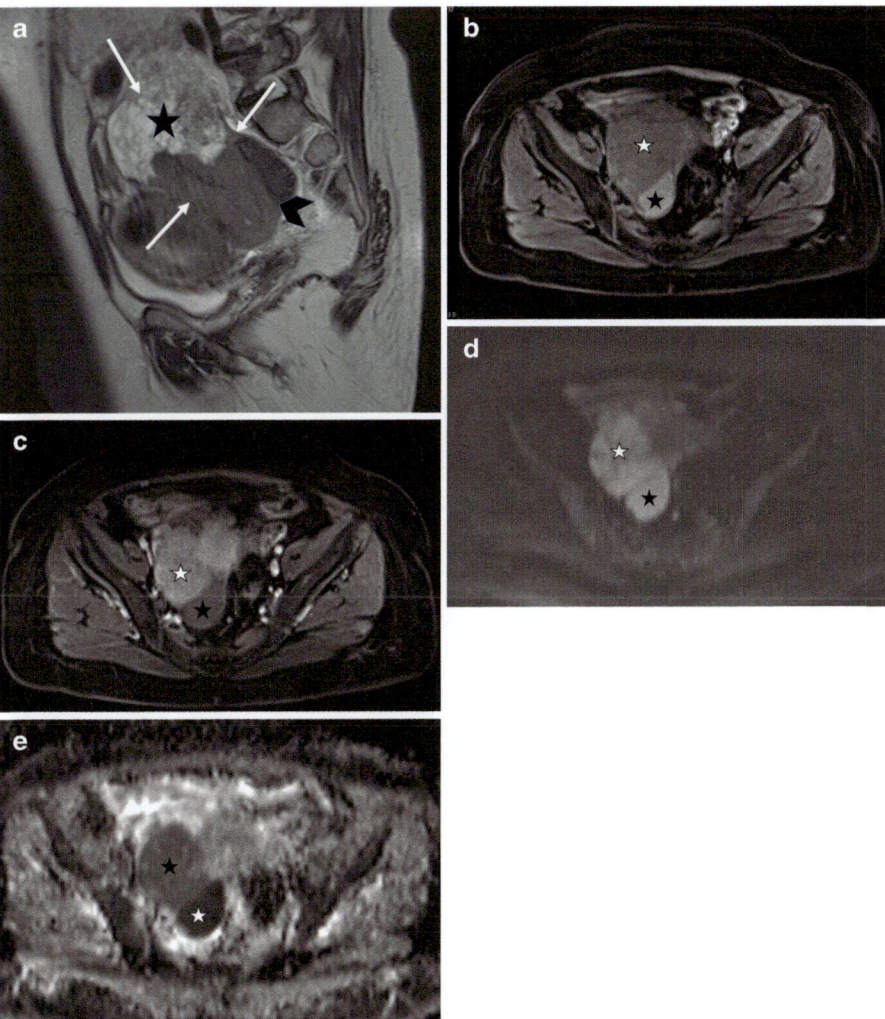

Fig. 5.5 A 34-year-old woman presenting with dull pelvic pain and complex lesion detected in the transvaginal sonographic exam. Subsequent surgery confirmed endometrioid carcinoma in the anterior part of the lesion arising from an endometrioma. The posterior part of the lesion was found to be cystic filled with hemorrhagic elements. (**a**) Sagittal plane T2W image demonstrates a bilobular heterogeneous mass with solid (*black arrowhead*) and cystic (*black star*) components in the right adnexa (*arrows*). The lesion was hyperintense (cystic) in its anterior part while hypointense in the posterior. (**b**) Axial plane pre-contrast T1W image showed the T2-hypointense posterior part as hyperintense (*black star*), whereas the T2-hyperintense anterior part as hypointense (*white star*). The content of the cyst shows high signal intensity on fat-saturated T1-weighted image is another evidence of hemorrhagic material included within an endometriotic cyst. (**c**) On post-contrast axial plane T1W image, there was contrast enhancement in the anterior (solid) part (*white star*) with no obvious enhancement in the posterior part (*black star*). (**d**) DWI demonstrates increased signal in both parts with more hyperintensity in the posterior part (*black star*) compared to its anterior counterpart (*white star*). (**e**) ADC map confirmed marked hypointensity within both parts confirming the diffusion restriction. The restriction was more pronounced in the endometrioma (posterior part, *white arrow*) compared to the anterior solid part (*black star*)

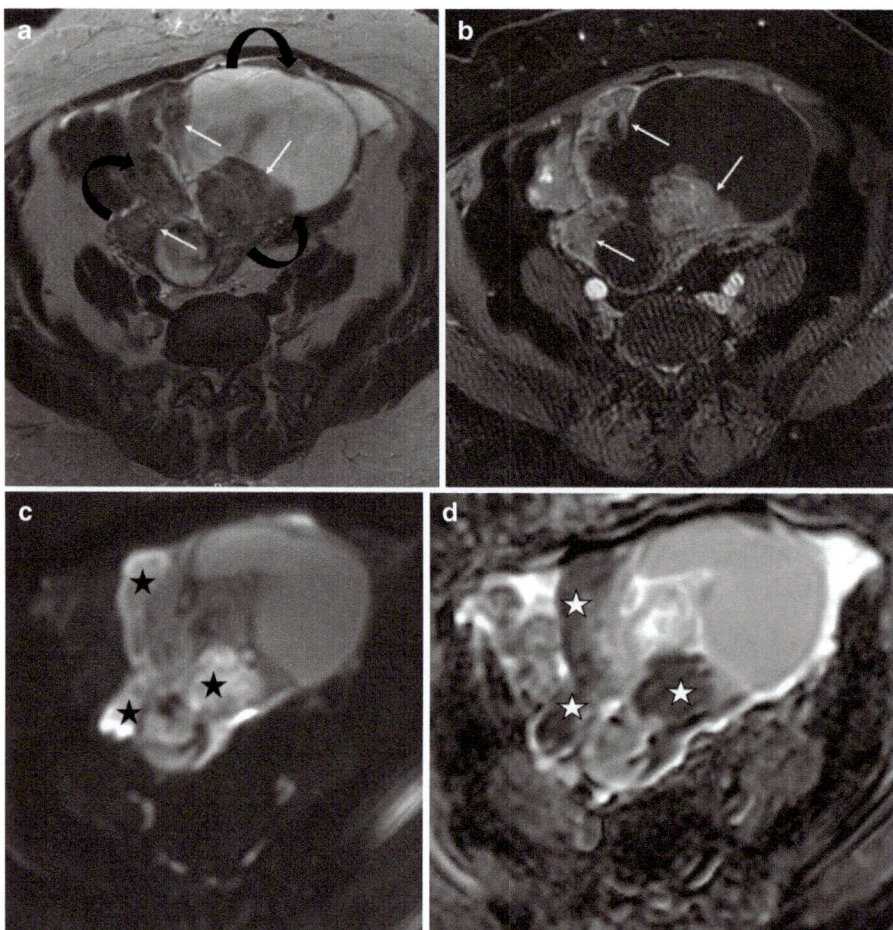

Fig. 5.6 A 65-year-old woman presenting with progressively enlarging abdominal girth and dull pelvic pain. Sonography revealed complex cystic mass in the pelvis. Subsequent surgery revealed serous epithelial ovarian tumor. (**a**) Axial plane T2W image reveals a large predominantly cystic mass (*curved arrows*) with irregular nodularities in its wall (*arrows*). (**b**) Post-contrast axial T1W image demonstrates heterogeneous enhancement in the wall nodularities (*arrows*) confirming their solid and vascular nature. (**c**) DW image demonstrates hyperintensity within the nodular wall lesions (*stars*). (**d**) Pronounced hypointensity (*star*). Corresponding ADC map confirms the diffusion restriction within these nodularities

tumors with low cellularity (eg, well-differentiated adenocarcinomas or ovarian cancers with large cystic components), restriction in the diffusion of water molecules is likely to be much limited and may even not be visible at all in diffusion-weighted images [23].

T2 blackout effect is the term which refers to low signal on ADC map due to lack of enough water protons and not due to restricted diffusion. It is basically the reverse phenomenon of the T2 shine through effect. This phenomenon typically

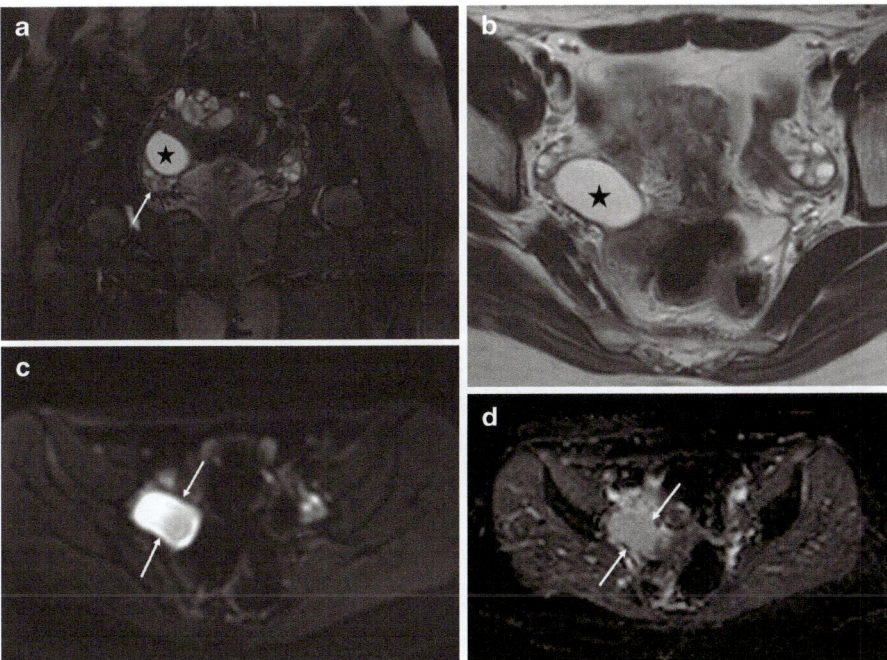

Fig. 5.7 A 26-year-old woman with incidentally diagnosed right adnexal cyst. (**a**) Coronal plane SSFP image shows the cystic structure (*star*) clearly separates from the right ovary (*arrow*) consistent with a paraovarian cyst. (**b**) Axial plane T2W image demonstrates the lesion is purely cystic (*star*) with marked T2 signal. (**c**) Axial plane DW image shows homogeneous hyperintensity of the lesion (*arrows*). (**d**) Corresponding ADC map also shows diffuse hyperintensity confirming the absence of diffusion restriction within the lesion consistent with T2 shine-through phenomenon

occurs when there is low or very low signal intensity of the solid component on T2WI which is mostly due to high collagen content and low cellularity of the lesion [24].

Accordingly, low ADC values may be misinterpreted for a malignant process, and concurrent evaluation with DWI may be necessary. It should be noted that many benign ovarian masses including endometriomas, mature cystic teratomas, and fibrothecomas may also demonstrate restricted diffusion [25]. Because of this overlap, it must be borne in that ADC maps and high *b*-value images should be interpreted in conjunction with anatomic images and morphological clues derived from other conventional MR sequences.

Mature cystic teratomas deserve a specific attention as they have been demonstrated to exhibit lower ADC values, due to their keratinoid epithelium, fat, and calcification content, than any other benign or malignant adnexal lesions. This unique feature may be helpful for correct diagnosis for lesions with a paucity of fat [14, 26]. Low signal on T2-weighted fat-saturated images is the diagnostic sign for T2 blackout. It may be difficult to differentiate mature cystic teratomas from their malignant counterparts, as imaging findings may be similar (Fig. 5.8).

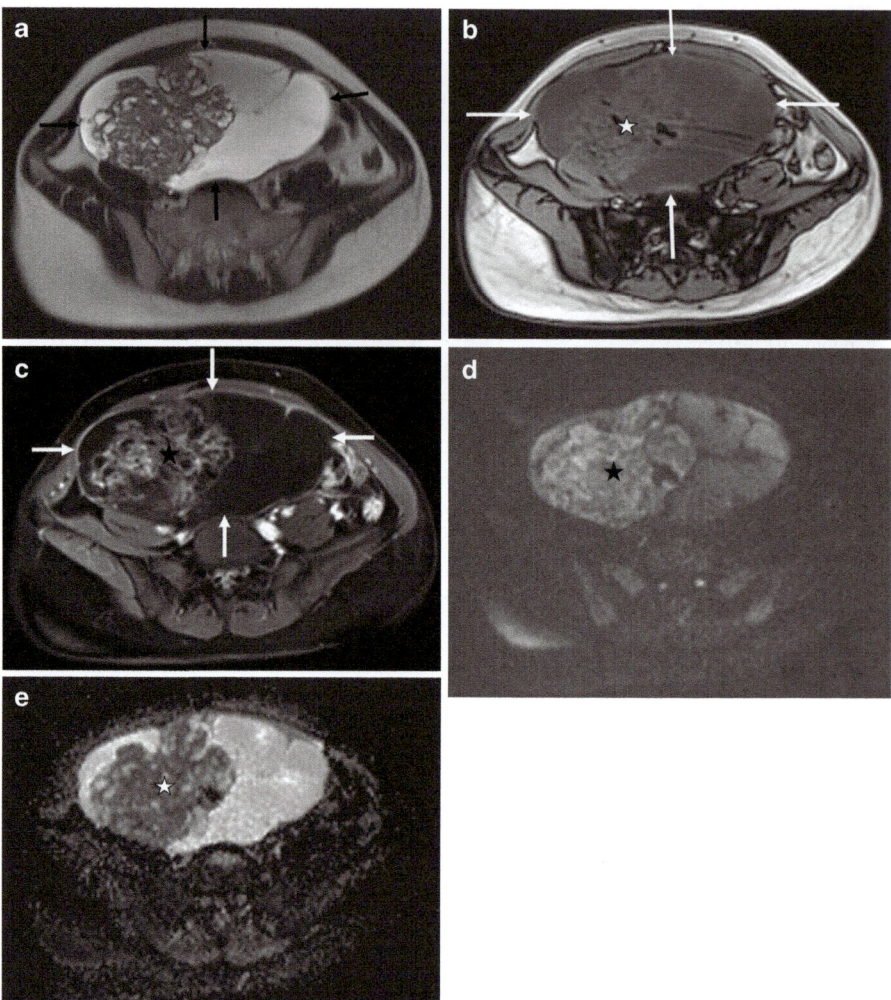

Fig. 5.8 A 35-year-old woman with pelvic pain and recently discovered complex pelvic mass with US. Subsequent surgery revealed immature cystic teratoma as the final diagnosis. (**a**) Axial plane T2W image demonstrates a large cystic mass (*arrows*) with a voluminous solid component (*star*). (**b**) Axial plane T1W pre-contrast image demonstrates the same mass (*arrows*) with the solid component (*star*) appearing predominantly hypointense. (**c**) Axial plane T1W post-contrast image demonstrates avid enhancement of the solid component (*star*). (**d**) Axial plane DW image reveals mild-moderate hyperintensity of the solid component (*star*). (**e**) Corresponding ADC map shows moderate hypointensity of the solid component confirming true diffusion restriction

In the same manner, endometriomas tend to contain hemoglobin degeneration products, and its viscosity lowers ADC values compared to other cystic ovarian lesions [25]. Despite the mentioned clues for differential diagnosis, no significant consistent differences have been demonstrated between the ADC values of benign and malignant cystic ovarian lesions [11, 14, 19, 21, 26].

Table 5.2 Schematic representation of several ovarian benign and malignant diseases on DWI

Diffusion WI	T2 shine-through	T2 blackout	Diffusion restriction (−)	Diffusion restriction (+)
B 0				
B 500–1000				
ADC				
Lesions	Foli cular/simple cysts Mucinous tumors	Endometrioma Fibrous tissue Calcification Cystadenofibroma Brenner tumor Fibrothecoma	Good differentiated tumors Good response to tumor therapy	Blood Fat(teratomas) Melanoma metastasis Necrosis Malignant tumors

Several inflammatory and granulomatous adnexal pathologies may manifest as morphologically solid lesions with restricted water diffusion on MRI. Mucinous adenomas, decidualized endometriomas, and polypoid endometriosis all may show abnormal diffusion signal on MR imaging [21]. These lesions, therefore, may closely mimic a malignant tumor and correct diagnosis and, based on imaging alone, may sometimes be impossible. On the other side, it should also be noted that several malignant ovarian tumors may mimic benign tumors from DWI and morphologic imaging standpoints. Serous adenocarcinomas with associating massive ascites, solid portions of clear cell adenocarcinomas, septal solid components of metastatic appendiceal cancers, and solid parts of endometrioid borderline tumors should all be mentioned among malignant mimickers of benign ovarian tumors. Diffusion-weighted imaging findings of the common benign and malignant lesions are summarized in Table 5.2.

5.7 The Role of DW-MR Imaging in Peritoneal Dissemination of Ovarian Tumors

Peritoneal surfaces are common sites for metastases in patients with ovarian tumors. Accurate and early detection of these peritoneal implants is of crucial importance for staging and surgical planning in these patients.

The sensitivity and specificity of DW-MR imaging was found to be high (90% and 95.5%, respectively) (Fig. 5.9). These implants are typically observed as lesions with moderate to high peritoneal foci when compared to mild intensity of other pelvic organs. The minimum size of the implants detected with DW-MR imaging was reported to be 5 mm [21]. This finding, when compared to several other studies performed with contrast-enhanced CT and MR to detect peritoneal implants [27–29], indicates that DW-MR imaging has equal value to contrast-enhanced cross-sectional modalities for detecting peritoneal implants [21].

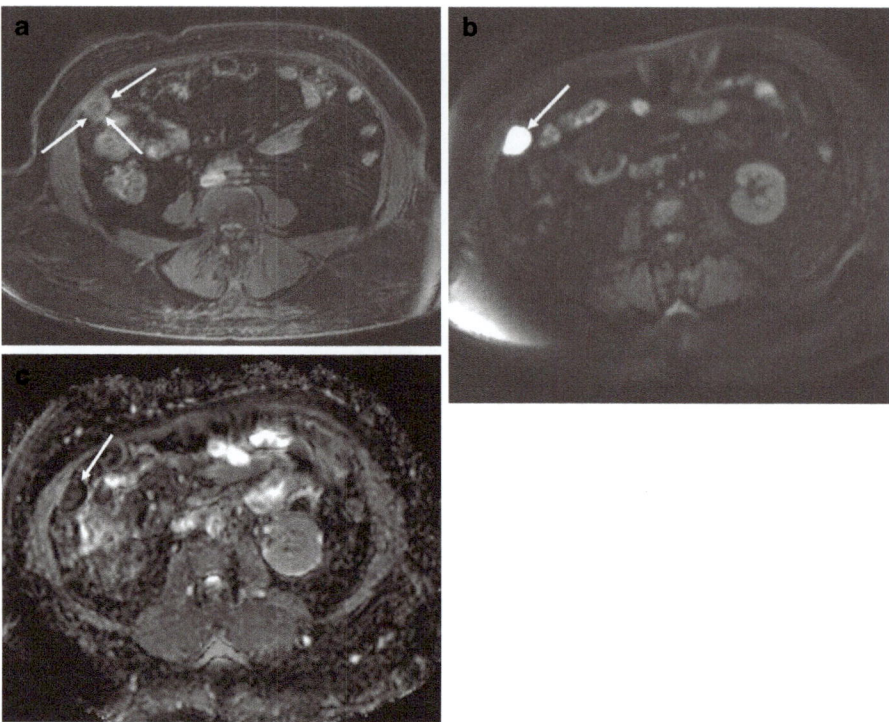

Fig. 5.9 A 67-year-old woman with a history of serous epithelial type ovarian cancer and increased serum CA-125 level 2 years after surgery. (**a**) Axial plane T1-weighted image demonstrates small nodular implant in the right paracolic gutter (*arrows*). (**b**) Axial plane DW image reveals the same lesion as significantly hyperintense (*arrow*). (**c**) The same lesion appears markedly hypointense on ADC map image (*arrow*) confirming the true diffusion restriction

Metastasis to ovaries is also seen as diffusion-restricted masses as other malignant lesions of the ovary; however, it does not have a significant role in differentiating primary ovarian malignancy from the metastatic one (Fig. 5.10).

5.8 The Role of DW-MR Imaging in Detection and Characterization of Pelvic Lymph Nodes

The most commonly used criterion to differentiate benign from malignant pelvic lymph nodes has been fundamentally based on the size of the short-axis axial diameter [7]. However, it is well known that this measure has been a weak indicator in pelvic imaging [29, 30]. The use of ultrasmall superparamagnetic iron oxide

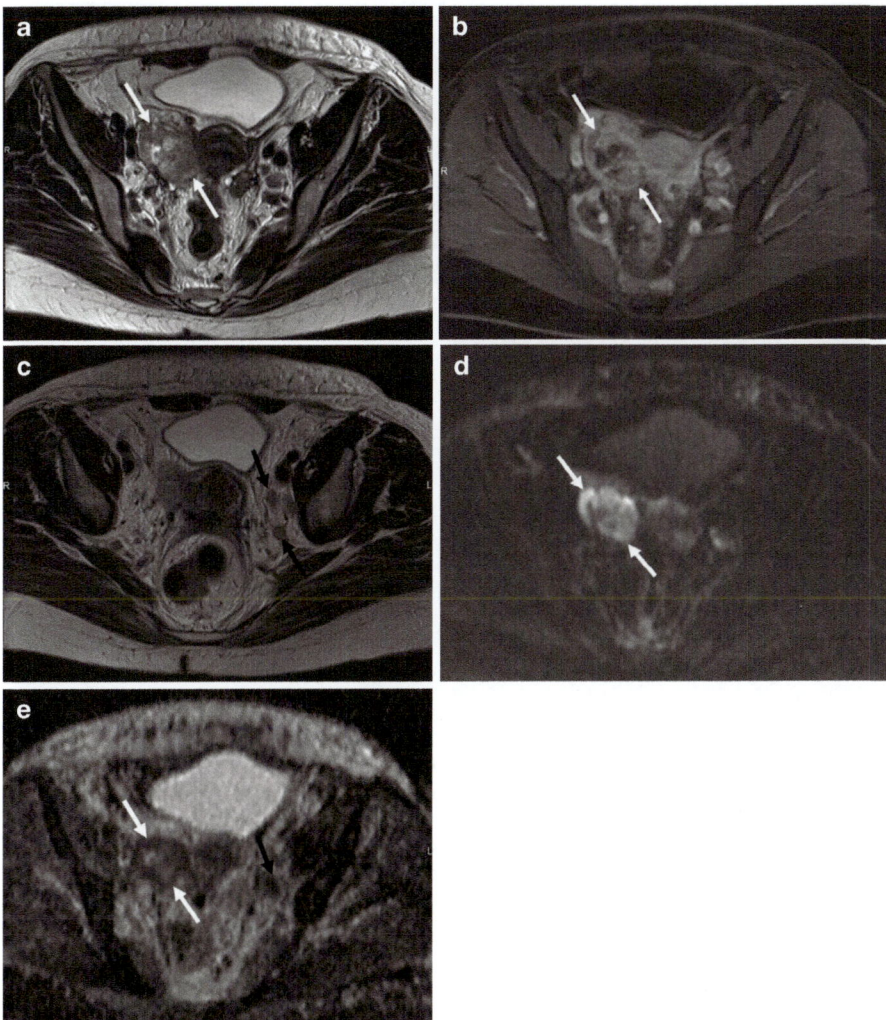

Fig. 5.10 A 53-year-old woman who was on chemotherapy with known history of breast cancer was found to have a new developed complex-appearing solid lesion in the right adnexa on US study and was referred for a pelvic MRI exam. Tumor marker Ca 125 was elevated measuring 325 IU/mL. (**a**) Axial plane T2W image reveals complex mass replacing the right ovary (*arrows*). (**b**) Post-contrast T1W axial plane image shows heterogeneous contrast enhancement within the mass. (**c**) Axial plane T2W image also demonstrates small-size lymph nodes (*black arrows*) with heterogeneous internal texture in the left pelvic sidewall. Axial plane DW image (**d**) and corresponding ADC map image (**e**) reveal significant diffusion restriction within the right ovarian mass (*white arrows*) and the enlarged lymph node (*black arrow*). Both the right ovarian mass and left pelvic sidewall lymph nodes are consistent with metastatic breast cancer

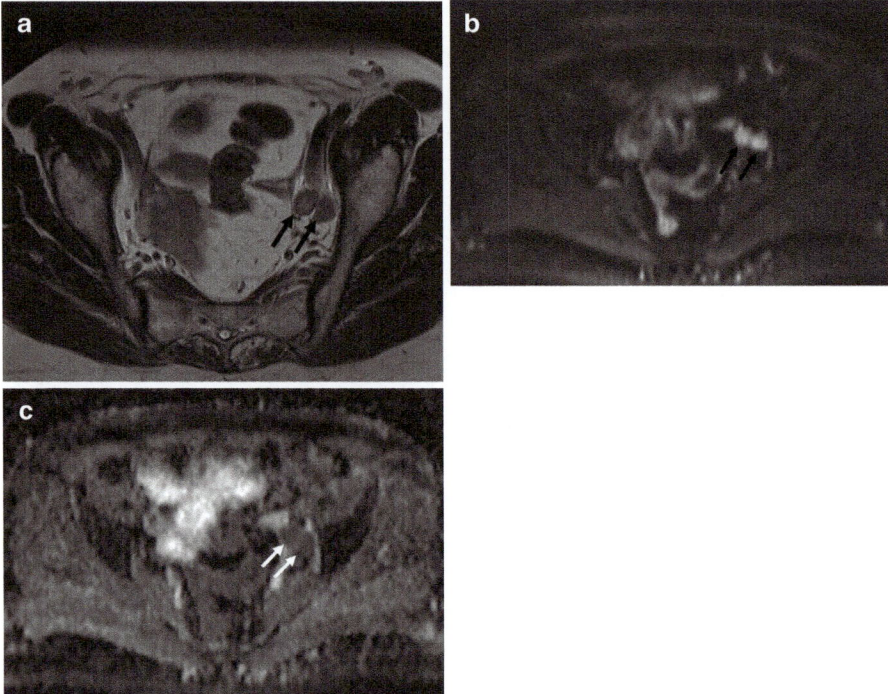

Fig. 5.11 A 71-year-old woman with a history of surgically treated undifferentiated-type ovarian cancer with increasing serum CA-125 levels was found to have two enlarged lymph nodes in the pelvic sidewall on CT exam in an outside center (not shown). Patient was referred to pelvic MRI in our institute which confirmed the findings of prior CT. Pathologic exam after surgical excision confirmed tumor involvement in both lymph nodes. (**a**) Axial plane T2W image shows two mildly enlarged lymph nodes (*arrows*) in the left pelvic sidewall. (**b**) Axial plane DW image shows increased signal in these enlarged lymph nodes (*arrows*). (**c**) Corresponding ADC map image confirmed diffusion restriction

particles was presented as a new technique to improve performance of MR. However, this technique has not gained wide acceptance in imaging society [7].

There are only few papers discussing the role of DW-MR imaging in discriminating malignant from benign pelvic lymph nodes, and the results of these studies were discrepant [31–33]. A different study using DW-MR imaging with b-values of 0 and 1000 s/mm^2 concluded that the addition of DW-MR imaging to morphological sequences was useful in identifying small lymph nodes [34] (Fig. 5.11). In this study, all lymph nodes demonstrated high signal intensity on DW-MR images, allowing them to be clearly identified against the low intensity surrounding pelvic structures. However, the ADC values of these lymph nodes did not improve the differentiation of metastatically involved lymph nodes from the noninvolved ones.

5.9   Limitations of DW-MR Imaging in Ovarian Lesions

As mentioned above, there are a lot of overlapping points in DW-MR imaging findings of benign and malignant ovarian lesions. This aforementioned fact underlines the importance of morphological findings and, if ever used, the contrast enhancement pattern. The use of DW-MR imaging ($b = 1000$ s/mm^2) in conjunction with T2-weighted images may help to differentiate benign from malignant neoplasms. Complex adnexal lesions with a solid component that is hypointense on both T2-weighted and DW-MR images ($b = 1000$ s/mm^2) were reported to be benign ($P < 0.0001$), while adnexal lesions that were hyperintense on diffusion-weighted images ($b = 1000$ s/mm^2) and intermediate signal intensity on T2-weighted images were found to be most likely malignant ($P < 0.0001$) [19]. In poorly differentiated malignant tumors, the extracellular space is characterized by increased tortuosity, with a resultant decrease in ADC values, whereas well-differentiated malignant tumors (particularly adenocarcinomas) may not show high signal intensity on DWI or low ADC values [24].

The combination of conventional MR imaging and time-signal intensity curves derived from dynamic contrast-enhanced MR imaging in association with DW-MR imaging was demonstrated to improve characterization of adnexal lesions [20]. In the same paper, a solid adnexal mass with restricted diffusion in addition to intermediate signal intensity on T2-weighted images and early rapid enhancement after IV contrast injection was found to be a strong indicator of malignancy.

Conclusion

No imaging modality, including MRI, may definitively differentiate benign ovarian neoplasms from the malignant ones. Borderline lesions of the ovaries are also another confounder in the classification of ovarian neoplasms, a situation which also cannot be confidently diagnosed with imaging.

DW-MR imaging, with its easy acquisition without the need for IV gadolinium contrast, may be an important contributor to MR imaging with its unique ability for tissue characterization. However, it should be noted that DW-MR imaging findings may appear to be most useful when the data from this sequence are combined with information coming from conventional morphological MR images. Further studies are needed to optimally combine the conventional morphological MR images with the novel functional MR sequences, including DW-MR imaging, in order to maximize the information derived from MR studies. The optimum combination of these morphological and functional MR sequences, without compromising their unique strengths, is of paramount importance for accurate diagnosis. Only by doing that, we can develop the practical approach to better characterization of adnexal lesions with accurate results. Translation of advanced MR imaging techniques into daily clinical radiology practice will most likely open new dimensions in pelvic imaging in the, not very distant, future.

References

1. Ackerman S, Irshad A, Lewis M, Anis M. Ovarian cystic lesions: a current approach to diagnosis and management. Radiol Clin N Am. 2013;51(6):1067–85.
2. Spencer JA, Ghattamaneni S. MR imaging of the sonographically indeterminate adnexal mass. Radiology. 2010;256(3):677–94.
3. Outwater EK, Mitchell DG. Magnetic resonance imaging techniques in the pelvis. Magn Reson Imaging Clin N Am. 1994;2(2):161–88.
4. Troiano RN, McCarthy S. Magnetic resonance imaging evaluation of adnexal masses. Semin Ultrasound CT MR. 1994;15(1):38–48.
5. Woodward PJ, Gilfeather M. Magnetic resonance imaging of the female pelvis. Semin Ultrasound CT MR. 1998;19(1):90–103.
6. Koh DM, Collins DJ. Diffusion-weighted MRI in the body: applications and challenges in oncology. AJR Am J Roentgenol. 2007;188(6):1622–35.
7. Coutinho AC Jr, Krishnaraj A, Pires CE, Bittencourt LK, Guimaraes AR. Pelvic applications of diffusion magnetic resonance images. Magn Reson Imaging Clin N Am. 2011;19(1):133–57.
8. Kim SH, Kim SH, Yang DM, Kim KA. Unusual causes of tubo-ovarian abscess: CT and MR imaging findings. Radiographics. 2004;24(6):1575–89.
9. Heverhagen JT, Klose KJ. MR imaging for acute lower abdominal and pelvic pain. Radiographics. 2009;29(6):1781–96.
10. Fujii S, Kaneda S, Kakite S, Kanasaki Y, Matsusue E, Harada T, et al. Diffusion-weighted imaging findings of adnexal torsion: initial results. Eur J Radiol. 2011;77(2):330–4.
11. Fujii S, Kakite S, Nishihara K, Kanasaki Y, Harada T, Kigawa J, et al. Diagnostic accuracy of diffusion-weighted imaging in differentiating benign from malignant ovarian lesions. J Magn Reson Imaging. 2008;28(5):1149–56.
12. Katayama M, Masui T, Kobayashi S, Ito T, Sakahara H, Nozaki A, et al. Diffusion-weighted echo planar imaging of ovarian tumors: is it useful to measure apparent diffusion coefficients? J Comput Assist Tomogr. 2002;26(2):250–6.
13. Moteki T, Ishizaka H. Diffusion-weighted EPI of cystic ovarian lesions: evaluation of cystic contents using apparent diffusion coefficients. J Magn Reson Imaging. 2000;12(6):1014–9.
14. Nakayama T, Yoshimitsu K, Irie H, Aibe H, Tajima T, Nishie A, et al. Diffusion-weighted echo-planar MR imaging and ADC mapping in the differential diagnosis of ovarian cystic masses: usefulness of detecting keratinoid substances in mature cystic teratomas. J Magn Reson Imaging. 2005;22(2):271–8.
15. Namimoto T, Awai K, Nakaura T, Yanaga Y, Hirai T, Yamashita Y. Role of diffusion-weighted imaging in the diagnosis of gynecological diseases. Eur Radiol. 2009;19(3):745–60.
16. Forstner R, Thomassin-Naggara I, Cunha TM, Kinkel K, Masselli G, Kubik-Huch R, et al. ESUR recommendations for MR imaging of the sonographically indeterminate adnexal mass: an update. Eur Radiol. 2017;27(6):2248–57.
17. Chung BM, Park SB, Lee JB, Park HJ, Kim YS, Oh YJ. Magnetic resonance imaging features of ovarian fibroma, fibrothecoma, and thecoma. Abdom Imaging. 2015;40(5):1263–72.
18. Kierans AS, Bennett GL, Mussi TC, Babb JS, Rusinek H, Melamed J, et al. Characterization of malignancy of adnexal lesions using ADC entropy: comparison with mean ADC and qualitative DWI assessment. J Magn Reson Imaging. 2013;37(1):164–71.
19. Thomassin-Naggara I, Darai E, Cuenod CA, Fournier L, Toussaint I, Marsault C, et al. Contribution of diffusion-weighted MR imaging for predicting benignity of complex adnexal masses. Eur Radiol. 2009;19(6):1544–52.
20. Thomassin-Naggara I, Toussaint I, Perrot N, Rouzier R, Cuenod CA, Bazot M, et al. Characterization of complex adnexal masses: value of adding perfusion- and diffusion-weighted MR imaging to conventional MR imaging. Radiology. 2011;258(3):793–803.
21. Fujii S, Matsusue E, Kanasaki Y, Kanamori Y, Nakanishi J, Sugihara S, et al. Detection of peritoneal dissemination in gynecological malignancy: evaluation by diffusion-weighted MR imaging. Eur Radiol. 2008;18(1):18–23.

22. Sala E, Priest AN, Kataoka M, Graves MJ, McLean MA, Joubert I, et al. Apparent diffusion coefficient and vascular signal fraction measurements with magnetic resonance imaging: feasibility in metastatic ovarian cancer at 3 Tesla: technical development. Eur Radiol. 2010;20(2):491–6.
23. Whittaker CS, Coady A, Culver L, Rustin G, Padwick M, Padhani AR. Diffusion-weighted MR imaging of female pelvic tumors: a pictorial review. Radiographics. 2009;29(3):759–74; discussion 74–8.
24. Motoshima S, Irie H, Nakazono T, Kamura T, Kudo S. Diffusion-weighted MR imaging in gynecologic cancers. J Gynecol Oncol. 2011;22(4):275–87.
25. Mohaghegh P, Rockall AG. Imaging strategy for early ovarian cancer: characterization of adnexal masses with conventional and advanced imaging techniques. Radiographics. 2012;32(6):1751–73.
26. Chilla B, Hauser N, Singer G, Trippel M, Froehlich JM, Kubik-Huch RA. Indeterminate adnexal masses at ultrasound: effect of MRI imaging findings on diagnostic thinking and therapeutic decisions. Eur Radiol. 2011;21(6):1301–10.
27. Coakley FV, Choi PH, Gougoutas CA, Pothuri B, Venkatraman E, Chi D, et al. Peritoneal metastases: detection with spiral CT in patients with ovarian cancer. Radiology. 2002;223(2):495–9.
28. Ricke J, Sehouli J, Hach C, Hanninen EL, Lichtenegger W, Felix R. Prospective evaluation of contrast-enhanced MRI in the depiction of peritoneal spread in primary or recurrent ovarian cancer. Eur Radiol. 2003;13(5):943–9.
29. Tempany CM, Zou KH, Silverman SG, Brown DL, Kurtz AB, McNeil BJ. Staging of advanced ovarian cancer: comparison of imaging modalities—report from the Radiological Diagnostic Oncology Group. Radiology. 2000;215(3):761–7.
30. Tangjitgamol S, Manusirivithaya S, Jesadapatarakul S, Leelahakorn S, Thawaramara T. Lymph node size in uterine cancer: a revisit. Int J Gynecol Cancer. 2006;16(5):1880–4.
31. Kim JH, Beets GL, Kim MJ, Kessels AG, Beets-Tan RG. High-resolution MR imaging for nodal staging in rectal cancer: are there any criteria in addition to the size? Eur J Radiol. 2004;52(1):78–83.
32. Lin G, Ho KC, Wang JJ, Ng KK, Wai YY, Chen YT, et al. Detection of lymph node metastasis in cervical and uterine cancers by diffusion-weighted magnetic resonance imaging at 3T. J Magn Reson Imaging. 2008;28(1):128–35.
33. Nakai G, Matsuki M, Inada Y, Tatsugami F, Tanikake M, Narabayashi I, et al. Detection and evaluation of pelvic lymph nodes in patients with gynecologic malignancies using body diffusion-weighted magnetic resonance imaging. J Comput Assist Tomogr. 2008;32(5):764–8.
34. Roy C, Bierry G, Matau A, Bazille G, Pasquali R. Value of diffusion-weighted imaging to detect small malignant pelvic lymph nodes at 3 T. Eur Radiol. 2010;20(8):1803–11.

Cervical Masses

6

João Lopes Dias and Teresa Margarida Cunha

Abbreviations

ADC	Apparent diffusion coefficient
BEM	Bi-exponential models
CRT	Chemoradiotherapy
D	Pure molecular diffusion (D)
D^*	Pseudo-diffusion coefficient
DCE	Dynamic contrast enhanced
DWI	Diffusion-weighted imaging
DWIBS	Diffusion-weighted whole-body imaging with background body signal suppression
f	Perfusion fraction
FIGO	International Federation of Gynaecology and Obstetrics
LN	Lymph nodes
MEM	Mono-exponential model
MRI	Magnetic resonance imaging
PMI	Parametrial invasion
SEM	Stretched exponential model
T1WI	T1-weighted imaging
T2WI	T2-weighted imaging

J.L. Dias (✉)
Centro Hospitalar de Lisboa Central, Hospital dos Lusíadas de Lisboa, NOVA Medical School, Lisbon, Portugal
e-mail: joaolopesdias85@gmail.com

T.M. Cunha
Department of Radiology, Instituto Português de Oncologia de Lisboa Francisco Gentil, Lisbon, Portugal
e-mail: tmargarida@gmail.com

© Springer International Publishing AG 2018
D. Akata, N. Papanikolaou (eds.), *Diffusion Weighted Imaging of the Genitourinary System*, https://doi.org/10.1007/978-3-319-69575-4_6

Key Points
- DWI is useful for detection, staging of malignancy and assessment of treatment response in cervical cancer.
- ADC quantification has been studied for prediction of response to neoadjuvant therapy and disease-free survival.
- Some benign conditions like cellular leiomyomas and actinomycosis may show restriction on DWI.
- Distinguishing typical squamous cell carcinoma from other cervical malignancies is not possible regarding only DWI features.

6.1   Introduction

In regard to the uterine cervix, diffusion-weighted imaging (DWI) has been used for detection and staging of malignancy, as well as for assessing treatment response. However, other promising applications have been studied, namely, the prediction of response to neoadjuvant therapy and disease-free survival. Besides emphasizing its role in the detection and characterization of cervical malignancy, this chapter also reviews the typical appearance of the normal cervix and the most common cervical benign conditions on DWI.

6.2   Normal Cervix

Data in the literature concerning the normal appearance of the uterine cervix on DWI is scarce. In a recent study regarding the utility of DWI in cervical cancer, Chen et al. [1] included 20 control patients and identified three different layers: a hyperintense inner zone (endocervix), which is contiguous to the endocervical canal, a hypointense intermediate zone (cervical stroma) and a slightly hyperintense outer zone (myocervix) (Fig. 6.1).

The zonal anatomy of the uterus depends on the hormonal status, so age-related and iatrogenic variations should be considered while evaluating both morphological and functional sequences on magnetic resonance imaging (MRI). However, these variations seem to be more significant in the uterine body, which grows significantly under hormonal stimulation at puberty and atrophies after menopause. Moreover, cervical zonal anatomy does not show significant changes throughout menstrual cycle [2]. In an interesting study, Messiou et al. [3] showed that the use of oral contraceptives is unlikely to have a significant effect on the use of DWI for detection and staging of cervical cancer. However, it seems to have an effect on the apparent diffusion coefficient (ADC) and should be taken into account while evaluating endometrial cancer with DWI.

6.3   Benign Conditions

The cervix is susceptible to a variety of benign conditions, ranging from simple Nabothian cysts to cervicitis and solid epithelial and non-epithelial masses. Nabothian cysts are very common and typically easy to recognize. Like any other

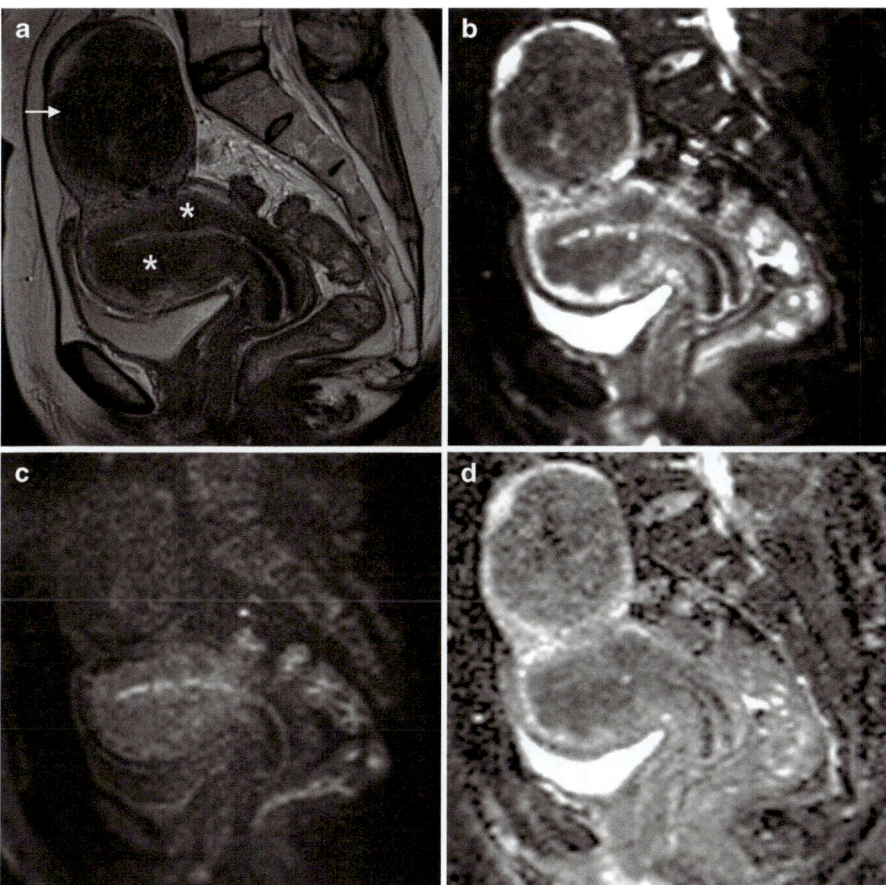

Fig. 6.1 A 74-year-old female imaged for other purposes. Sagittal T2WI depicting the normal zonal anatomy of the cervix, as well as a huge subserosal leiomyoma (*arrow*) and adenomyosis (*asterisks*) (**a**). Sagittal b0, b1000 and ADC map showing the normal stratification of the cervix. The hyperintense endocervix, hypointense stroma and slightly hyperintense myocervix are clearly depicted at b0 (**b**), becoming less conspicuous at b1000 (**c**) and on the ADC map (**d**)

cyst, their signal depends on the protein content, but they are typically hypointense on T1-weighted imaging (T1WI), hyperintense on T2-weighted imaging (T2WI), non-enhancing and non-restrictive on DWI [4].

Benign endocervical polyps are focal, hyperplastic protrusions of endocervical folds that rarely develop into dysplasia or carcinoma. They may be recognized on T2WI as hypointense lesions surrounded by hyperintense fluid or large multicystic masses. On DWI, endocervical polyps usually do not show restriction [4].

Cervical leiomyomas are uncommon, accounting for 8–10% of all leiomyomas. These well-defined, pseudocapsulated masses are histologically similar to those of the uterine body and are usually hypointense on both T1WI and T2WI, except if degeneration occurs. On DWI, cervical leiomyomas typically do not show restriction, unless they are cellular (Figs. 6.2 and 6.3). However, data in the literature is limited in regard to this issue [4, 5].

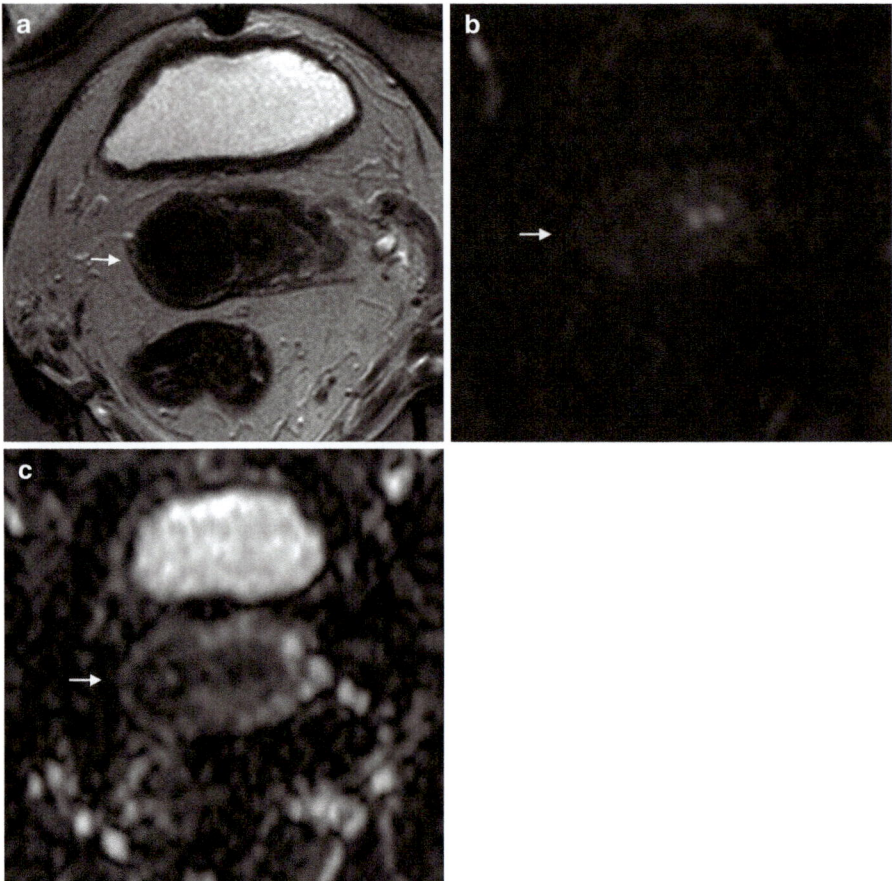

Fig. 6.2 Cervical leiomyoma in a 74-year-old female. Axial T2WI showing a solid, exophytic, well-defined, hypointense mass, occupying the right half of the cervical stroma (*arrow*) (**a**). Axial b1000 and ADC map showing no restriction to diffusion, both with low signal (*arrows*) (**b, c**)

Cervicitis may be difficult to distinguish from other conditions like glandular hyperplasia or adenoma malignum. It usually appears as centrally located, multicystic lesions with high signal on T2WI and typically no solid enhancing components. It is not expected to show restriction on DWI, unless complicated infection occurs [4]. Necrotizing cervical infections and abscesses are uncommon but have already been reported in the setting of puerperal sepsis or complicated caesareans. Like in other locations, cervical abscesses may show restriction on DWI [6, 7].

Actinomycosis is an invasive infection that may involve the cervix and parametria, despite the ovaries and fallopian tubes are most commonly affected. It

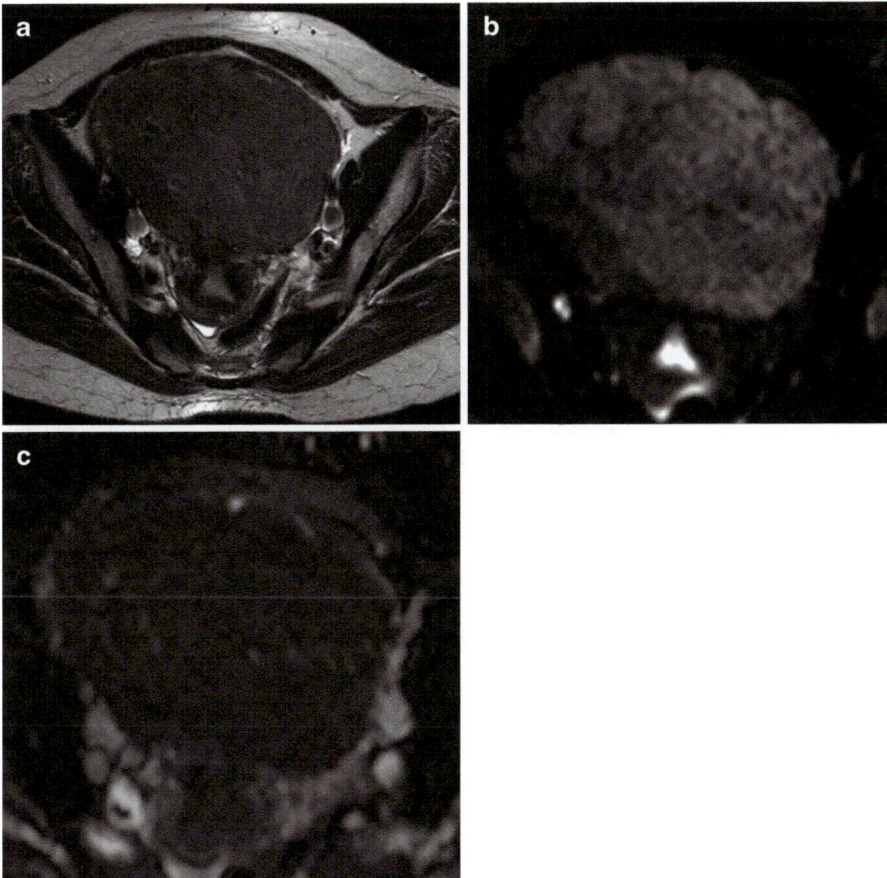

Fig. 6.3 Cervical leiomyoma with high cellularity in a 47-year-old female. Axial T2WI showing a huge, solid, exophytic, hypointense mass, originated from the anterior portion of the cervix (**a**). Axial b1000 and ADC map showing restriction to diffusion, the first with high signal intensity and the last displaying low signal intensity (**b, c**)

mimics malignancy not only clinically but also in imaging studies. Compared with the more typical tubo-ovarian abscesses, actinomycosis shows larger solid components that usually enhance after intravenous contrast administration. Moreover, due to the presence of prominent fibrotic tissue, both the solid parts and the inflammatory surrounding stranding tend to display intermediate to low signal intensity on T2WI. The solid component may be restrictive on DWI, showing high signal intensity at high b-values and low ADCs. The surrounding inflammation may not show prominent restriction if oedema predominates over cytotoxic content [8] (Fig. 6.4).

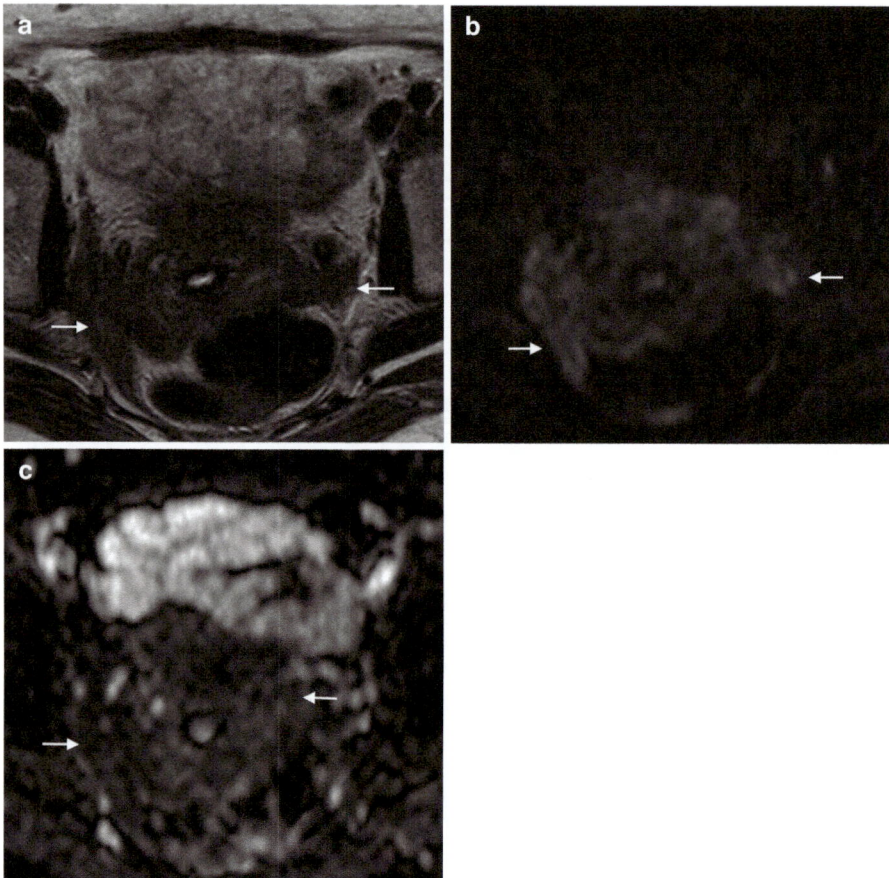

Fig. 6.4 Actinomycosis with cervical involvement in a 51-year-old female. Axial T2WI showing cervical enlargement, surrounded by solid, speculated, hypointense tissue that protrudes into the parametria (*arrows*) (**a**). Axial b1000 and ADC map showing restriction to diffusion within the parametria, with high and low signal intensity, respectively (*arrows*) (**b, c**)

6.4   Cervical Carcinoma

6.4.1   Detection and Staging

MRI is now considered an accurate method for both detection and staging of cervical cancer. On T2WI, tumours tend to appear hyperintense and are easily recognizable from the hypointense stroma. The sagittal plane is preferable to evaluate tumour extension into the body of the uterus and vagina, while the axial oblique T2WI perpendicular to the long axis of the cervix is essential to detect parametrial invasion. On T1WI, tumours are usually isointense to the normal cervix. Dynamic contrast-enhanced MRI (DCE-MRI) does not improve staging accuracy when compared to T2WI alone, so it is usually excluded from the protocol [9].

DWI has been considered very helpful in the detection of cervical cancer [10–12]. Several studies have been published regarding this issue, for instance, Naganawa et al. [13], who found a significant difference for median ADC between cervical cancer and normal cervix before treatment. Using a 1.5-T magnet, the mean ADC value of cervical cancer lesions was 1.09 (±0.20) × 10^{-3} mm^2/s, and that of normal cervix tissue was 1.79 (±0.24) × 10^{-3} mm^2/s. Later, a meta-analysis from Hou et al. [14], which included 645 tumour tissues and 504 normal tissues, confirmed this significant difference. In other study, Hoogendam et al. [15] showed that the difference on ADC values between benign and malignant cervical tissues does not depend on the used b-value combinations. However, it should be emphasized that ADC values vary considerably between institutions, which makes it difficult to establish ADC cut-offs for the daily clinical practice. Differences in scanner hardware and sequence parameters are likely to explain this variability [12].

Chen et al. [1] reported high sensitivity (100%) and specificity (84.8%) levels of DWI for tumour detection. However, some questions need to be considered in regard to the clinical application of DWI in cervical cancer. Is it really important to use DWI for cancer detection? And if so, which patients are the best candidates? Since the diagnosis of cervical cancer is usually performed at a screening cytology or biopsy, the main role of MRI remains in the local staging of known cervical cancers. And what about staging? Is DWI useful? Actually, more studies have to be developed in order to get stronger conclusions. These and other questions will be answered throughout this chapter. In order to discuss it, the 2009 revised International Federation of Gynaecology and Obstetrics (FIGO) staging system for cervical carcinoma should be remembered [16].

By definition, stage IA tumours are clinically imperceptible and not visible on imaging studies. Stage IB tumours are clinically visible lesions limited to the cervix. Its further differentiation depends on the size, so IB1 tumours have 4.0 cm or less in greatest dimension, while IB2 tumours have more than 4.0 cm in greatest dimension. The FIGO staging system encourages the use of MRI to assess the size of the primary tumour [16]. As previously stated, T2WI is usually enough to delimitate the tumour, which tend to be surrounded by the hypointense stroma. However, some isointense tumours or early cervical cancers are difficult to recognize on T2WI and may be better assessed on DWI. This is particularly valid in young patients, who may show moderate intense cervical stroma on T2WI. Moreover, some authors state that DWI is not only able to detect cancer but also allows to precisely identify the tumour limits without significantly overestimating its volume, which may occur in T2WI, where both oedema and tumour show increased signal intensity comparing to the normal cervical stroma (Fig. 6.5) [10, 17].

Accurate delimitation is also needed to subdivide IIA tumours into IIA1 (≤4.0 cm in greatest dimension) and IIA2 stages (>4.0 cm in greatest dimension). These tumours invade beyond the uterus, without invading the parametria, the pelvic wall or the lower third of the vagina. By its turn, IIB tumours invade

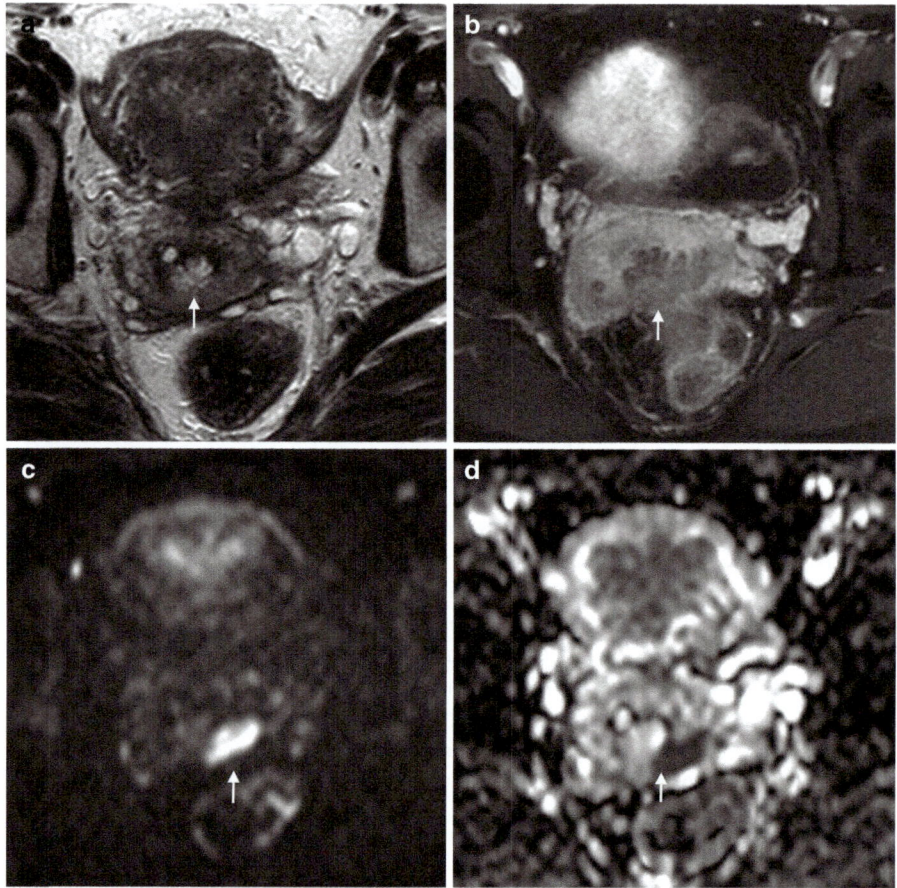

Fig. 6.5 IB1 stage cervical squamous cell carcinoma in a 47-year-old female. Axial T2WI depicting a partial, posterior interruption of the hypointense cervical stroma (*arrow*), without a well-defined nodule (**a**). Axial DCE-MRI showing a hypovascular lesion in the posterior portion of the cervix (*arrow*) (**b**). Axial b1000 and ADC map showing a restrictive lesion without parametrial invasion (*arrows*) (**c, d**)

the parametria, but not the pelvic wall or the lower third of the vagina (Fig. 6.6). An accurate prediction of the presence or absence of parametrial invasion (PMI) is critical for treatment planning. The majority of studies evaluate T2WI alone with no mention to DWI, but new data has appeared concerning this issue. According to Park et al. [18], DWI may provide useful additional information in predicting PMI. The authors found that tumour ADC and PMI signs on T2WI are independent predictors of pathologic PMI in early-stage cervical cancer. Moreover, they stated that the combination of both predictors improved the diagnostic performance of MRI for the identification of patients at low risk of PMI. One year later, Park et al. [19] showed that fusion of T2WI with the recently developed diffusion-weighted whole-body imaging with background body signal suppression (DWIBS), which

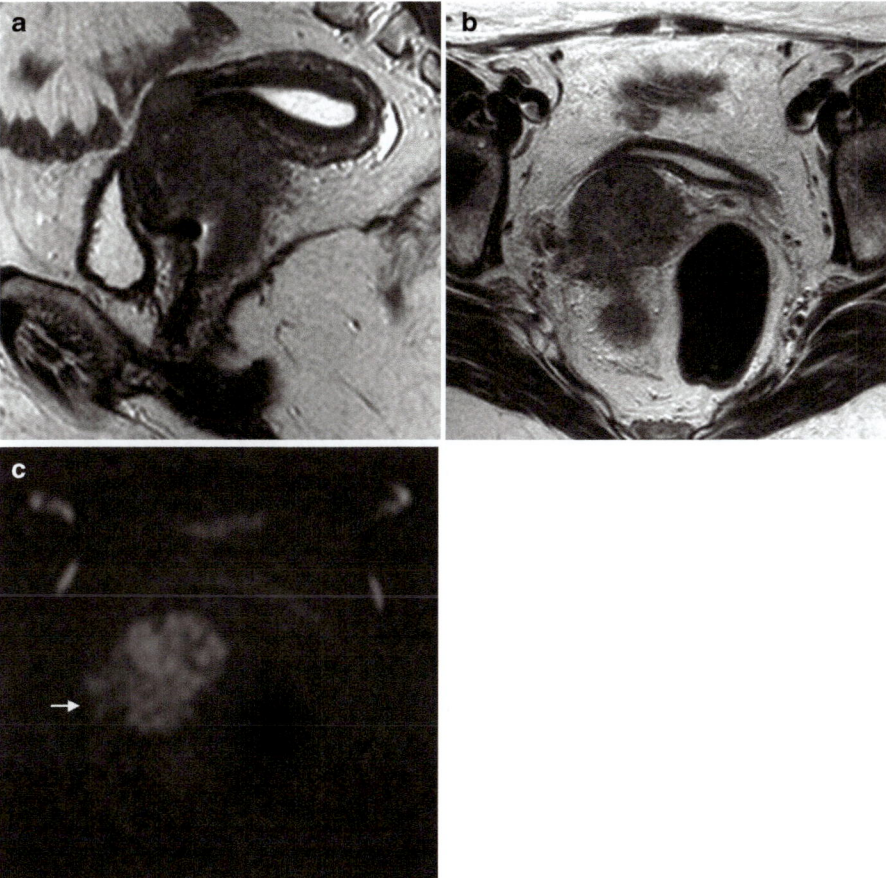

Fig. 6.6 IIB stage cervical squamous cell carcinoma in a 60-year-old female. Sagittal and axial T2WI showing a huge cervical tumour invading the parametria laterally and posteriorly (**a**, **b**). Axial b1000 showing a restrictive tumour with some speculated projections into the parametria, essentially at the right side (*arrow*) (**c**)

provides high contrast-to-noise ratio, can improve the diagnostic performance of MRI in the detection of parametrial invasion in cervical cancer compared to T2WI alone. Accuracy of fused T2WI-DWIBS, combined T2WI and fused T2WI-DWIBS and T2WI alone was 90.1%, 93.4% and 85.5%, respectively.

IIIA tumours involve the lower third of the vagina, with no extension to the pelvic wall, while IIIB tumours extend to the pelvic wall and/or present with hydronephrosis or non-functioning kidney. DWI may recognize these advanced stages by finding restrictive tissue within the involved structures. However, this nonquantitative evaluation may be hampered due to lack of anatomical references at high *b*-value images, which is possible to overcome by acquiring T2WI-DWI fusion images. Quantitative evaluation regarding these particular features has not yet been studied [17].

In stage IVA, the tumour invades the mucosa of the bladder or rectum. MRI is able to exclude it with a negative predictive value of 100%, which makes cystoscopy and sigmoidoscopy unneeded [17, 20]. Reported sensitivity and specificity values vary in different studies, ranging from 71% to 100% and 88% to 91%, respectively. However, these values account only for morphological sequences, so the real utility of DWI in this stage is not reported. It is expectable to find restrictive tumour within the lumen of the bladder or the rectum, but once again lack of anatomical references may hamper this evaluation. In this particular setting, the interpretation of T2WI-DWI fusion images should be done carefully, since both the bladder and rectum may change its position during examination due to urinary filling and peristaltic movements. In regard to the bladder, another condition should be emphasized: bullous oedema (Fig. 6.7). It may mimic tumour involvement by

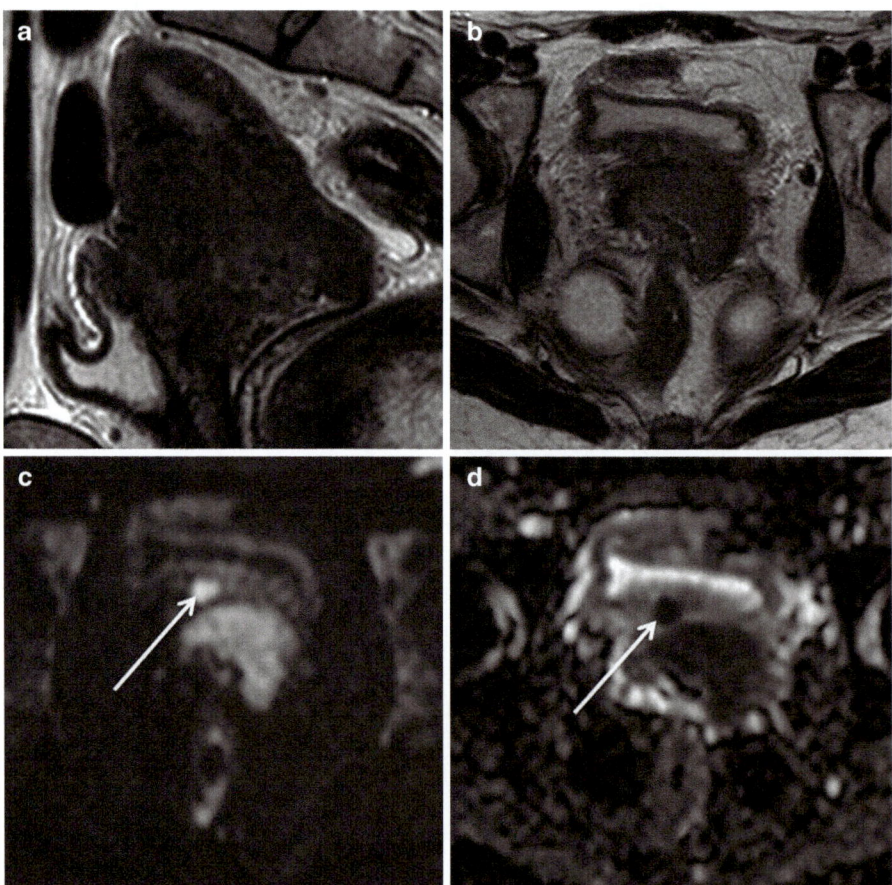

Fig. 6.7 IIB stage cervical squamous cell carcinoma in a 49-year-old female. Sagittal and axial of the cervix T2WI showing a huge cervical tumour (**a**, **b**). Axial b1000 and ADC map showing the tumour invading the bladder wall, but not the bladder mucosa (*arrow*) (**c**, **d**). We can also detect the presence of bullous oedema

showing high-signal-intensity thickening of the bladder wall on T2WI, due to reactive inflammation. The absence of restriction on DWI makes the wall thickening unlikely to represent tumour invasion.

Stage IVB is characterized by tumour spread to distant organs, including the para-aortic and inguinal lymph nodes, lung, liver and bone. Like in other malignancies, it is expected to find metastases as hyperintense foci at high b-value images and concomitant low signal on the ADC map.

Determining the histological type of cervical cancer based on ADC values is not feasible due to considerable overlap between the most common types [11]. However, in a study of Liu et al. [21], squamous cell carcinoma showed lower ADC values compared to adenocarcinoma. The same study suggests that DWI may give rise to a new method for evaluating the pathologic grading of tumour. Actually, it is known that the ADC values of high-grade tumours tend to be lower if the cellular density is also high. However, some high-grade tumours have necrotic areas that may show high ADC values.

6.4.2 Node Metastases

The standard evaluation of lymph nodes (LN) includes only morphological features. The short axis diameter remains the most consensual parameter. A threshold of 10 mm for detecting nodal metastases is the most commonly used, but sensitivity remains low. If a lower threshold is used (namely, 8 mm), sensitivity increases, but specificity decreases [9]. DWI is a promising noninvasive technique in the assessment of lymph node metastases, which appears to increase sensitivity levels when compared to MRI morphological sequences and computed tomography [12].

Replacing standard surgical LN assessment might be beneficial for patients with cervical cancer by avoiding unnecessary treatment and consequent immediate and delayed complications. Several studies have been published regarding node metastases with variable results [22, 23]. A meta-analysis from Shen et al. [24], which included 15 studies and 1021 patients, concluded that DWI is useful for differentiation between metastatic and benign LN in patients with uterine cervical cancer. Despite the heterogeneity between those studies, there was no evidence for threshold effect and publication bias, and the pooled sensitivity and specificity achieved 0.86 and 0.84, respectively. In other study, Schob et al. [25] reported significant differences in ADC-derived histogram parameters comparing nodal-negative and nodal-positive cervical cancer. The same study showed that ADC entropy might become an imaging biomarker for tumour heterogeneity and molecular changes like loss of p53 expression.

6.4.3 Post-treatment Evaluation

The added value of DWI in the assessment of treatment response in patients undergoing surgery and/or chemoradiotherapy (CRT) has been recognized in several studies [26]. Lucas et al. [27] showed that the addition of DWI to T2W sequences considerably improves the diagnostic ability of MRI in the assessment of cervical cancer recurrence and recommend leaving DCE sequences as an option for uncertain cases. It can be assessed both qualitatively by checking signal intensity on high b-value images and quantitatively with ADC measurements. Both persistence and recurrence tend to appear hyperintense at high b-values and hypointense on the ADC map (Figs. 6.8 and 6.9). After radical surgery, the vaginal vault may be difficult to assess on DWI, so morphological correlation using T2WI or T2WI-DWI fusion images is mandatory.

Tumour size is the standard parameter to compare between examinations in patients with advanced cervical cancer undergoing CRT, but other non-volumetric

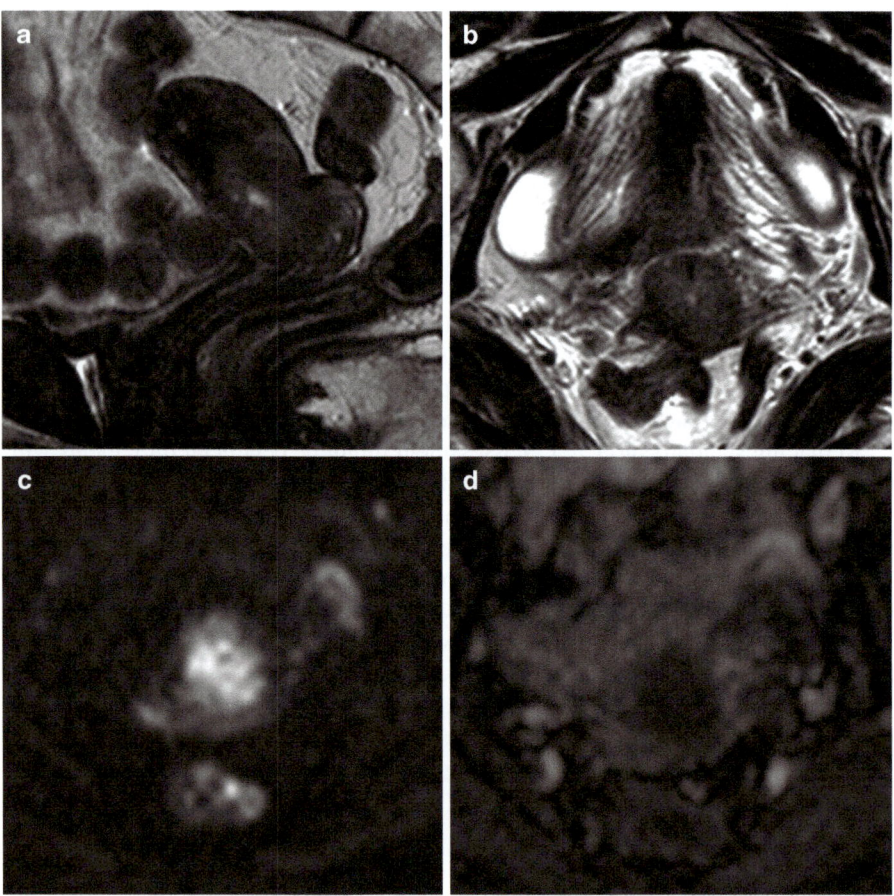

Fig. 6.8 Pre- and post-CRT cervical squamous cell carcinoma in a 61-year-old female. Sagittal and axial T2WI showing a huge cervical tumour invading the upper third of the vagina (**a, b**). Axial b1000 and ADC map depicting a cervical restrictive tumour (**c, d**). Sagittal and axial T2WI showing a narrow, hypointense cervix after CRT (**e, f**). Axial b1000 and ADC map showing no restrictive tissue within the cervix (**g, h**)

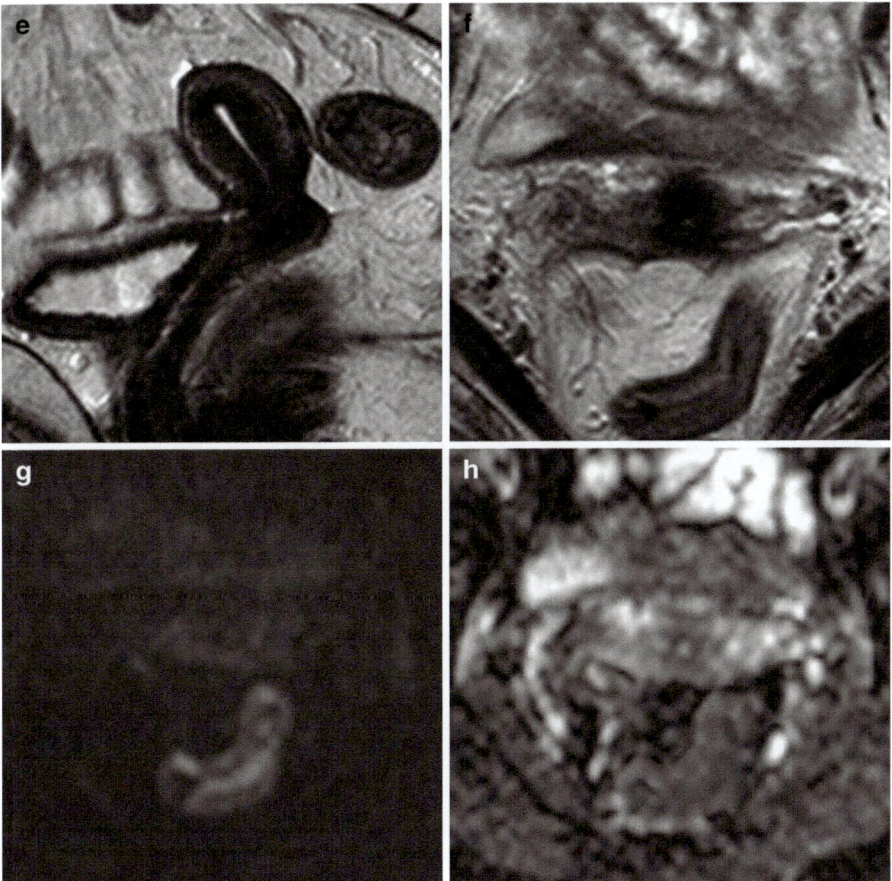

Fig. 6.8 (continued)

features are being studied. DWI appears to be able to assess early tumour response to CRT even before volumetric changes are seen [28]. The measurement of ADC provides an early and reproducible indicator of tumour response, which may ultimately allow for the development of individualized regimens. By inducing necrosis and apoptosis, extracellular space increases and thus water diffusion increases too. Therefore, higher post-treatment ADC values suggest a positive response and may be related to tumour lysis. Actually, once therapy is started, ADC may rapidly decrease over several hours due to cell swelling, but it is followed by an increase over several days after cell death [29]. In a systematic review including 9 studies with 231 patients, Schreuder et al. [30] concluded that DWI can be used for monitoring treatment response after CRT by comparing baseline ADC values to the ADC values after treatment, but not for early monitoring treatment response. For clinical practice, it matters to know that high increases of ADC values from pretreatment baseline to mid-therapy MRI reflect response to non-surgical therapies [31].

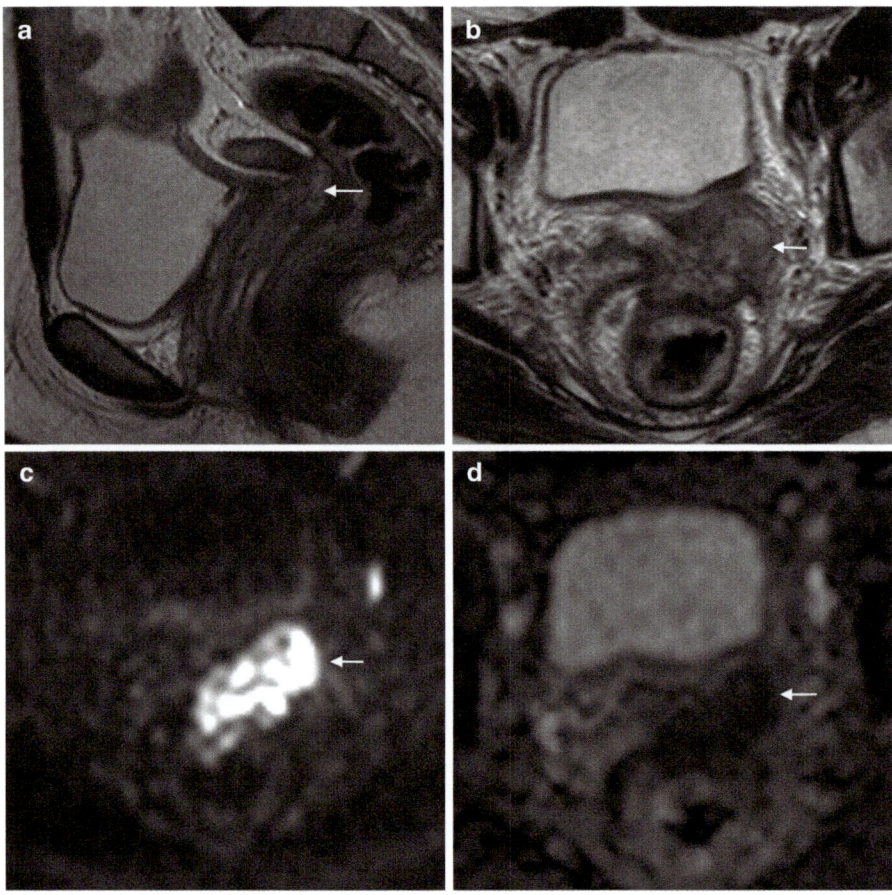

Fig. 6.9 Post-surgical persistence of cervical squamous cell carcinoma in a 41-year-old female. Sagittal and axial T2WI revealing tumour persistence in the upper third and vault of the vagina a huge cervical tumour invading the upper third of the vagina (*arrows*) (**a, b**). Axial b1000 and ADC map clearly delimitating the persistence (*arrows*) (**c, d**)

ADC histogram analysis appears to provide more detailed information when compared to common ADC parameters [25]. Meng et al. [32] found significant changes in some ADC histogram parameters like ADC mean, mode and percentiles at the early stage of CRT, which may reveal their potential in monitoring early tumour response to therapy. In other study, Erbay et al. [33] concluded that ADC75, ADC90 and ADC95 of the primary tumour were significant predictors of disease recurrence in cervical cancer patients treated with definitive CRT. More studies are warranted to confirm these preliminary findings regarding ADC histogram and to identify the best parameters for tumour prognosis.

The prediction of response to neoadjuvant therapy and disease-free survival is one of the most promising fields regarding DWI. Some studies have been performed, for instance, Ho et al. [34] showed that the mean ADC of the primary tumour may be a significant predictor of disease-free survival in cervical cancer patients treated with CRT. Other study of Onal et al. [35] showed that the pretreatment mean ADC value is an independent prognostic factor for disease-free survival and overall survival. A meta-analysis from Wang et al. [36], which included 9 studies involving a total of 796 patients, revealed that DWI may be a predictor of recurrence in patients with cervical cancer. Additionally, Bae et al. [37] showed that tumour ADC changes between pretreatment and 4 weeks after initiating therapy might be a useful clinical prognostic biomarker for the prediction of cervical cancer recurrence after CRT.

Jalaguier-Coudray et al. [38] reported an eightfold higher probability of earlier recurrence in patients with a mean ADC of 1.4×10^{-3} mm^2/s or less on a 1.5-T unit. However, it may not be true regarding response to treatment. We should remember that some tumours with high pretreatment ADC values may be necrotic and hypoxic, which tends to make them less responsive to CRT [10].

6.4.4 Chemoradiotherapy Toxicity

Concurrent CRT is the standard treatment for locally advanced cervical cancer, so haematological toxicity, pelvic skeletal changes and proctopathy are potential complications that should be aware of. Recent advances, as presented by Lee et al. [39], showed that intravoxel incoherent motion is able to detect early cellular environment changes in the pelvic bone marrow. Regarding acute radiation proctopathy, ADC measurement appears to be useful in the identification of poor-prognosis patients, which are those that may develop into chronic disease. As stated by Li et al. [40], ADC tends to be higher in poor-prognosis groups. These findings may serve as an important basis for proper timely adjustment of radiotherapy in order to maximally reduce the radiation injury of rectum.

6.5 Cervical Stroma Invasion

In a chapter dedicated to cervical masses, a word is missing in regard to cervical stroma invasion by endometrial cancer. The updated 2009 FIGO staging system specified cervical stromal invasion as stage II disease, which is known to increase the risk of lymph nodal spread and to be a poor prognostic factor. Recent studies like that of Lin et al. [41] suggest that DWI is a reasonable alternative to DCE-MRI for assessing cervical stromal invasion (Fig. 6.10). Sagittal images may be helpful for this evaluation.

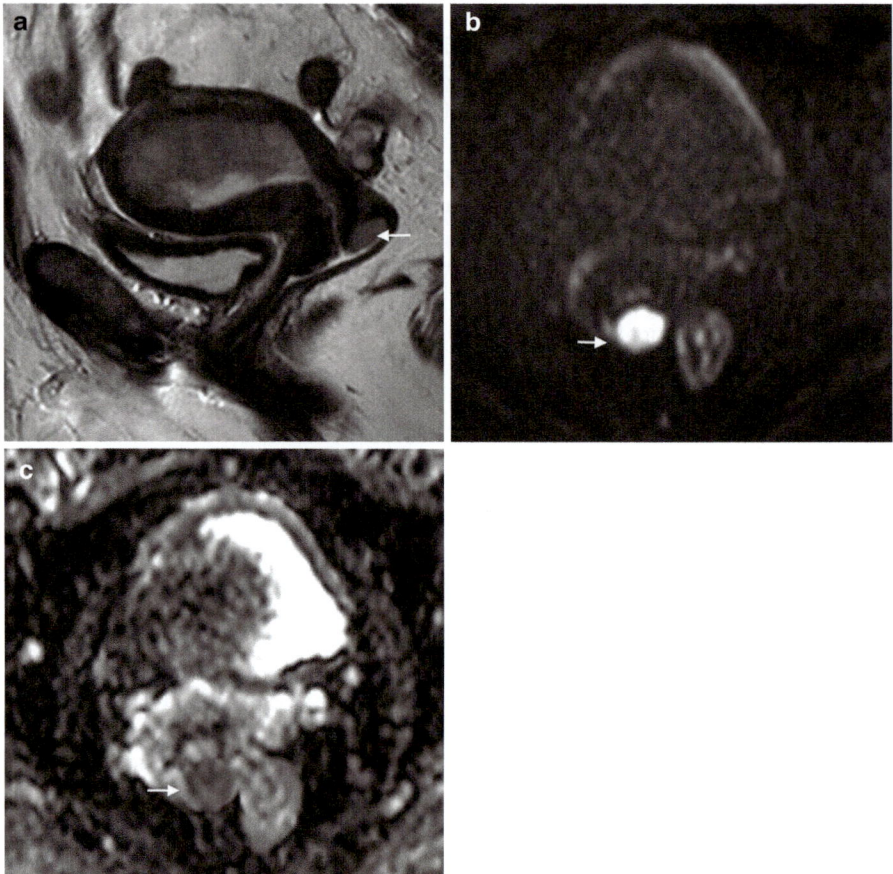

Fig. 6.10 Cervical metastasis of a serous endometrial carcinoma in a 66-year-old female. Sagittal T2WI showing a huge endometrial tumour without invasion of the exterior myometrium (not shown) and a skip metastasis in the posterior lip of the cervix (*arrow*) (**a**). Axial b1000 and ADC map also depicting a restrictive skip lesion (*arrows*) (**b, c**)

6.6   Other Malignant Masses

Imaging findings of rare cervical malignant tumours are similar to those of squamous cell carcinoma, so histological differentiation is not possible regarding only MRI features, even if ADC measurement is used. For daily practice, the most important point is that malignant tumours are likely to be restrictive regardless the histology. Neuroendocrine tumours, malignant melanoma, lymphoma or even sarcoma may occur within the cervix and does not show distinctive features on DWI.

Small cell carcinoma, the most common cervical neuroendocrine tumour, is generally very aggressive and tends to be diagnosed in advanced FIGO stages, so highly restrictive tissues and low ADCs are likely to be found, unless necrotic tissue is present [4, 42]. Malignant melanoma may show distinctive features on morphological sequences (Fig. 6.11). Probably due to the paramagnetic effects of stable free radicals within melanin granules and haemorrhage, some cases have been reported with high signal intensity on both T1WI and T2WI. However, no particular findings are reported regarding DWI [4]. By its turn, cervical lymphomas tend to be large and non-necrotic masses and usually do not infiltrate surrounding structures. The visualization of an intact mucosa seems to be distinctive feature of lymphomas. Their typical hypercellular environment makes lymphomas usually restrictive, but once again with no distinctive features [4] (Fig. 6.12).

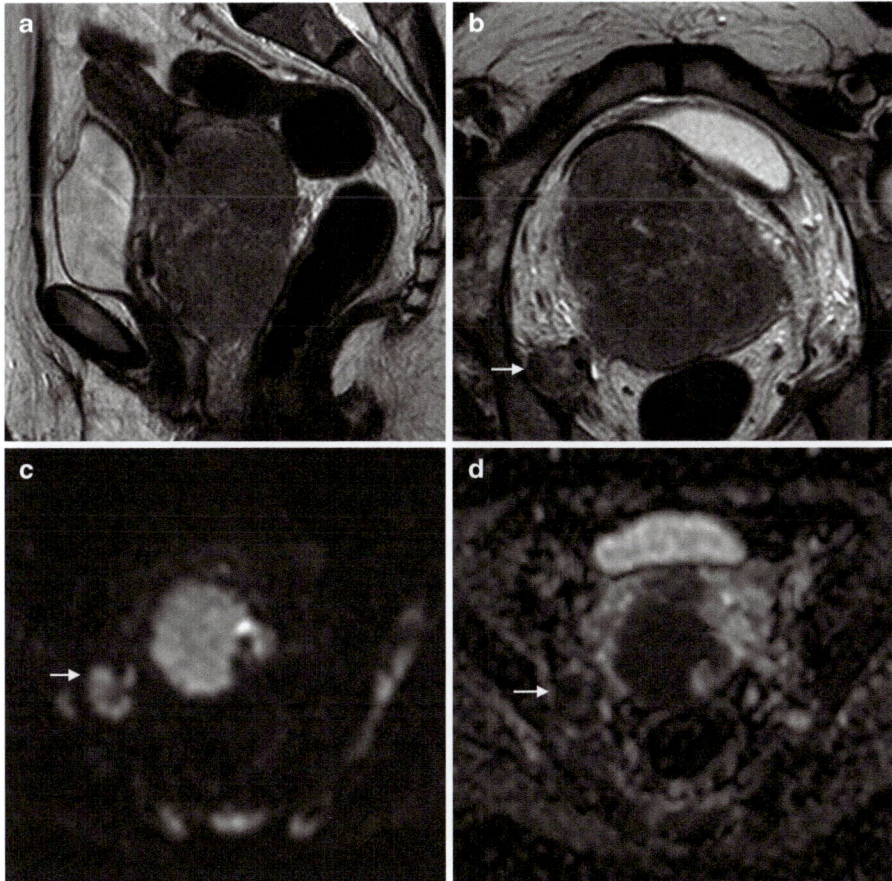

Fig. 6.11 Malignant melanoma of the cervix in a 41-year-old female. Sagittal and axial T2WI showing a huge tumour of the posterior lip of the cervix invading the upper two thirds of the vagina (**a**), as well as a right obturator node metastasis (*arrow*) (**b**). Axial b1000 and ADC map showing a strongly restrictive tumour, as well as the right obturator node metastasis (*arrow*) and multiple bone restrictive lesions representing metastases (**c**, **d**)

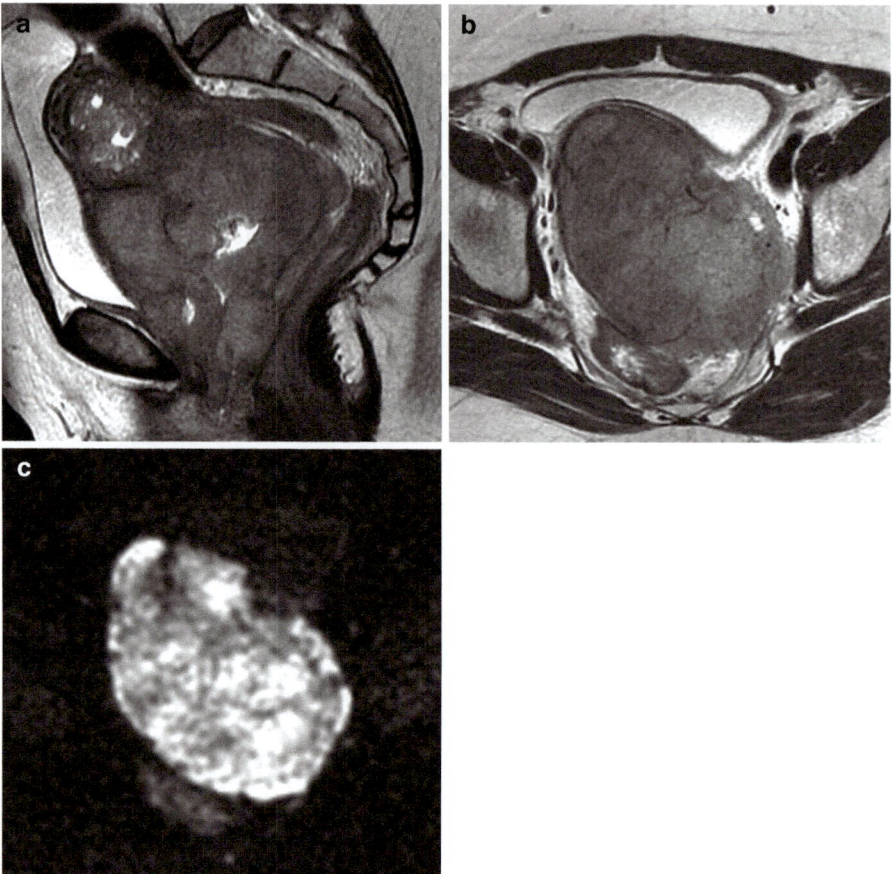

Fig. 6.12 Cervical primary lymphoma in a 47-year-old female. Sagittal and axial T2WI showing a huge cervical mass, extending to the body of the uterus and the vagina (**a, b**). Axial b1000 showing a strongly hyperintense mass (**c**)

6.7   Beyond Mono-exponential DWI

The mono-exponential model (MEM) of DWI is the most commonly assessed and usually uses the apparent diffusion coefficient (ADC) as a quantifying parameter. However, this common evaluation misses information regarding capillary microcirculation. When bi-exponential models (BEM) are applied, blood perfusion and true diffusion effects are separated, thus allowing for assessing other parameters like pure molecular diffusion (D), pseudo-diffusion coefficient (D^*) and perfusion fraction (f). While D is a diffusion-related parameter, D^* and f are perfusion-related parameters and appear to be correlated with DCE-MR parameters [43]. Some studies have concluded that the BEM-derived metrics might be superior to ADC in tumour diagnosis and pathological grade prediction [44].

The stretched exponential model (SEM) aims to evaluate diffusion and intra-voxel heterogeneity, as represented by distributed diffusion coefficient (DDC) and water diffusion heterogeneity index (alpha) [44]. Lin et al. [44] investigated the use of these three DWI models—MEM, BEM and SEM—in cervical carcinoma, concluding that supplementary BEM and SEM parameters showed reliability and feasibility in clinical use in addition to the ADC from MEM.

A recent study of Winfield et al. [45] shows that parameters from non-mono-exponential models are related to different aspects of tumour microstructure. The authors achieved this conclusion by reporting that α from the stretched exponential model, K from the kurtosis model and f and D^* from the bi-exponential model were significantly different between squamous cell carcinomas and adenocarcinomas. The potential use of these parameters to characterize the tumour phenotype and thus give information in respect to prognosis and disease progression is a challenging field.

References

1. Chen J, Zhang Y, Liang B, Yang Z. The utility of diffusion-weighted MR imaging in cervical cancer. Eur J Radiol. 2010;74(3):e101–6.
2. Well D, Yang H, Houseni M, Iruvuri S, Alzeair S, Sansovini M, et al. Age-related structural and metabolic changes in the pelvic reproductive end organs. Semin Nucl Med. 2007;37(3):173–84.
3. Messiou C, Morgan VA, De Silva SS, Ind TE, deSouza NM. Diffusion weighted imaging of the uterus: regional ADC variation with oral contraceptive usage and comparison with cervical cancer. Acta Radiol. 2009;50(6):696–701.
4. Okamoto Y, Tanaka YO, Nishida M, Tsunoda H, Yoshikawa H, Itai Y. MR imaging of the uterine cervix: imaging-pathologic correlation. Radiographics. 2003;23(2):425–45.
5. Deshmukh SP, Gonsalves CF, Guglielmo FF, Mitchell DG. Role of MR imaging of uterine leiomyomas before and after embolization. Radiographics. 2012;32(6):E251–81.
6. Castagnola DE, Hoffman MK, Carlson J, Flynn C. Necrotizing cervical and uterine infection in the postpartum period caused by group A streptococcus. Obstet Gynecol. 2008;111(2 Pt 2):533–5.
7. Chou C-Y, Liang P-C, Chen C-A, Lee C-N. Cervical abscess with vaginal fistula after extra-peritoneal cesarean section. J Formos Med Assoc. 2007;106(12):1048–51.
8. Heo SH, Shin SS, Kim JW, Lim HS, Seon HJ, Jung S-I, et al. Imaging of actinomycosis in various organs: a comprehensive review. Radiographics. 2014;34(1):19–33.
9. Sala E, Rockall A, Rangarajan D, Kubik-Huch RA. The role of dynamic contrast-enhanced and diffusion weighted magnetic resonance imaging in the female pelvis. Eur J Radiol [Internet]. 2014;76(3):367–85.
10. Manoharan D, Das CJ, Aggarwal A, Gupta AK. Diffusion weighted imaging in gynecological malignancies—present and future. World J Radiol. 2016;8(3):288–97.
11. McVeigh PZ, Syed AM, Milosevic M, Fyles A, Haider MA. Diffusion-weighted MRI in cervical cancer. Eur Radiol. 2008;18(5):1058–64.
12. Punwani S. Diffusion weighted imaging of female pelvic cancers: concepts and clinical applications. Eur J Radiol. 2014;78(1):21–9.
13. Naganawa S, Sato C, Kumada H, Ishigaki T, Miura S, Takizawa O. Apparent diffusion coefficient in cervical cancer of the uterus: comparison with the normal uterine cervix. Eur Radiol. 2005;15(1):71–8.
14. Hou B, Xiang S-F, Yao G-D, Yang S-J, Wang Y-F, Zhang Y-X, et al. Diagnostic significance of diffusion-weighted MRI in patients with cervical cancer: a meta-analysis. Tumour Biol. 2014;35(12):11761–9.

15. Hoogendam JP, Klerkx WM, de Kort GAP, Bipat S, Zweemer RP, Sie-Go DMDS, et al. The influence of the b-value combination on apparent diffusion coefficient based differentiation between malignant and benign tissue in cervical cancer. J Magn Reson Imaging. 2010;32(2):376–82.
16. Pecorelli S. Revised FIGO staging for carcinoma of the vulva, cervix, and endometrium. Int J Gynaecol Obstet. 2009;105(2):103–4.
17. Freeman SJ, Aly AM, Kataoka MY, Addley HC, Reinhold C, Sala E. The revised FIGO staging system for uterine malignancies: implications for MR imaging. Radiographics. 2012;32:1805–27.
18. Park JJ, Kim CK, Park SY, Park BK, Kim B. Value of diffusion-weighted imaging in predicting parametrial invasion in stage IA2-IIA cervical cancer. Eur Radiol. 2014;24(5):1081–8.
19. Park JJ, Kim CK, Park SY, Park BK. Parametrial invasion in cervical cancer: fused T2-weighted imaging and high-b-value diffusion-weighted imaging with background body signal suppression at 3T. Radiology. 2015;274(3):734–41.
20. Rockall AG, Ghosh S, Alexander-Sefre F, Babar S, Younis MTS, Naz S, et al. Can MRI rule out bladder and rectal invasion in cervical cancer to help select patients for limited EUA? Gynecol Oncol. 2006;101(2):244–9.
21. Liu Y, Bai R, Sun H, Liu H, Wang D. Diffusion-weighted magnetic resonance imaging of uterine cervical cancer. J Comput Assist Tomogr. 2009;33(6):858–62.
22. Park SO, Kim JK, Kim KA, Park B-W, Kim N, Cho G, et al. Relative apparent diffusion coefficient: determination of reference site and validation of benefit for detecting metastatic lymph nodes in uterine cervical cancer. J Magn Reson Imaging. 2009;29(2):383–90.
23. Kim JK, Kim KA, Park B-W, Kim N, Cho K-S. Feasibility of diffusion-weighted imaging in the differentiation of metastatic from nonmetastatic lymph nodes: early experience. J Magn Reson Imaging. 2008;28(3):714–9.
24. Shen G, Zhou H, Jia Z, Deng H. Diagnostic performance of diffusion-weighted MRI for detection of pelvic metastatic lymph nodes in patients with cervical cancer: a systematic review and meta-analysis. Br J Radiol. 2015;88(1052):20150063.
25. Schob S, Meyer HJ, Pazaitis N, Schramm D, Bremicker K, Exner M, et al. ADC histogram analysis of cervical cancer aids detecting lymphatic metastases-a preliminary study. Mol Imaging Biol. 2017;19(6):953–62.
26. Kitajima K, Tanaka U, Ueno Y, Maeda T, Suenaga Y, Takahashi S, et al. Role of diffusion weighted imaging and contrast-enhanced MRI in the evaluation of intrapelvic recurrence of gynecological malignant tumor. PLoS One. 2015;10(1):e0117411.
27. Lucas R, Lopes Dias J, Cunha TM. Added value of diffusion-weighted MRI in detection of cervical cancer recurrence: comparison with morphologic and dynamic contrast-enhanced MRI sequences. Diagn Interv Radiol. 2015;21(5):368–75.
28. Whittaker CS, Coady A, Culver L, Rustin G, Padwick M, Padhani AR. Diffusion-weighted MR imaging of female pelvic tumors: a pictorial review. Radiographics. 2009;29(3):758–9.
29. Harry VN, Semple SI, Gilbert FJ, Parkin DE. Diffusion-weighted magnetic resonance imaging in the early detection of response to chemoradiation in cervical cancer. Gynecol Oncol. 2008;111(2):213–20.
30. Schreuder SM, Lensing R, Stoker J, Bipat S. Monitoring treatment response in patients undergoing chemoradiotherapy for locally advanced uterine cervical cancer by additional diffusion-weighted imaging: a systematic review. J Magn Reson Imaging. 2015;42(3):572–94.
31. Rizzo S, Buscarino V, Origgi D, Summers P, Raimondi S, Lazzari R, et al. Evaluation of diffusion-weighted imaging (DWI) and MR spectroscopy (MRS) as early response biomarkers in cervical cancer patients. Radiol Med. 2016;121(11):838–46.
32. Meng J, Zhu L, Zhu L, Ge Y, He J, Zhou Z, et al. Histogram analysis of apparent diffusion coefficient for monitoring early response in patients with advanced cervical cancers undergoing concurrent chemo-radiotherapy. Acta Radiol. 2017;58(11):1400–8.
33. Erbay G, Onal C, Karadeli E, Guler OC, Arica S, Koc Z. Predicting tumor recurrence in patients with cervical carcinoma treated with definitive chemoradiotherapy: value of quantitative histogram analysis on diffusion-weighted MR images. Acta Radiol. 2017;58(4):481–8.

34. Ho JC, Allen PK, Bhosale PR, Rauch GM, Fuller CD, Mohamed ASR, et al. Diffusion-weighted magnetic resonance imaging as a predictor of outcome in cervical cancer after chemoradiation. Int J Radiat Oncol Biol Phys. 2017;97(3):546–53.
35. Onal C, Erbay G, Guler OC. Treatment response evaluation using the mean apparent diffusion coefficient in cervical cancer patients treated with definitive chemoradiotherapy. J Magn Reson Imaging. 2016;44(4):1010–9.
36. Wang Y-T, Li Y-C, Yin L-L, Pu H. Can diffusion-weighted magnetic resonance imaging predict survival in patients with cervical cancer? A meta-analysis. Eur J Radiol. 2016;85(12):2174–81.
37. Bae JM, Kim CK, Park JJ, Park BK. Can diffusion-weighted magnetic resonance imaging predict tumor recurrence of uterine cervical cancer after concurrent chemoradiotherapy? Abdom Radiol (New York). 2016;41(8):1604–10.
38. Jalaguier-Coudray A, Villard-Mahjoub R, Delouche A, Delarbre B, Lambaudie E, Houvenaeghel G, et al. Value of dynamic contrast-enhanced and diffusion-weighted MR imaging in the detection of pathologic complete response in cervical cancer after Neoadjuvant therapy: a retrospective observational study. Radiology. 2017;284(2):432–42.
39. Lee EYP, Perucho JAU, Vardhanabhuti V, He J, Siu SWK, Ngu SF, et al. Intravoxel incoherent motion MRI assessment of chemoradiation-induced pelvic bone marrow changes in cervical cancer and correlation with hematological toxicity. J Magn Reson Imaging. 2017;46(5):1491–8.
40. Li XS, Fang H, Song Y, Li D, Wang Y, Zhu H, et al. The stratification of severity of acute radiation proctopathy after radiotherapy for cervical carcinoma using diffusion-weighted MRI. Eur J Radiol. 2017;87:105–10.
41. Lin G, Huang Y-T, Chao A, Lin Y-C, Yang L-Y, Wu R-C, et al. Endometrial cancer with cervical stromal invasion: diagnostic accuracy of diffusion-weighted and dynamic contrast enhanced MR imaging at 3T. Eur Radiol. 2017;27(5):1867–76.
42. Lopes Dias J, Cunha TM, Gomes FV, Calle C, Felix A. Neuroendocrine tumours of the female genital tract: a case-based imaging review with pathological correlation. Insights Imaging. 2015;6(1):43–52.
43. Lee EYP, Hui ESK, Chan KKL, Tse KY, Kwong WK, Chang TY, et al. Relationship between intravoxel incoherent motion diffusion-weighted MRI and dynamic contrast-enhanced MRI in tissue perfusion of cervical cancers. J Magn Reson Imaging. 2015;42(2):454–9.
44. Lin M, Yu X, Chen Y, Ouyang H, Wu B, Zheng D, et al. Contribution of mono-exponential, bi-exponential and stretched exponential model-based diffusion-weighted MR imaging in the diagnosis and differentiation of uterine cervical carcinoma. Eur Radiol. 2017;27(6):2400–10.
45. Winfield JM, Orton MR, Collins DJ, Ind TEJ, Attygalle A, Hazell S, et al. Separation of type and grade in cervical tumours using non-mono-exponential models of diffusion-weighted MRI. Eur Radiol. 2017;27(2):627–36.

Added Value of Diffusion-Weighted Imaging in Endometrial Cancer

7

Stephanie Nougaret, Helen Addley, Mariana Horta,
Teresa Margarida Cunha, and Evis Sala

Abbreviations

ADC	Apparent diffusion coefficient
D&C	Dilatation and curettage
DCE-MRI	Dynamic multiphase contrast-enhanced imaging
DWI	Diffusion-weighted imaging
ESMO	European Society of Medical Oncology
FIGO	International Federation of Gynecology and Obstetrics
FOV	Field of view
MRI	Magnetic resonance imaging
NCCN	National Comprehensive Cancer Network
SLN	Sentinel nodes mapping

S. Nougaret, M.D. Ph.D. (✉)
Department of Radiology, Institut Régional du Cancer de Montpellier, Montpellier, France

IRCM, Institut de Recherche en Cancérologie de Montpellier, INSERM, U1194,
Montpellier, France
e-mail: stephanienougaret@free.fr

H. Addley
Department of Radiology, Addenbrokes Hospital, Cambridge, UK
e-mail: helenclareaddley@hotmail.co.uk

M. Horta • T.M. Cunha
Department of Radiology, Instituto Português de Oncologia de Lisboa Francisco Gentil,
Lisbon, Portugal

E. Sala
Department of Radiology, Memorial Sloan Kettering Cancer Center, New York, NY, USA
e-mail: salae@mskcc.org

© Springer International Publishing AG 2018
D. Akata, N. Papanikolaou (eds.), *Diffusion Weighted Imaging of the Genitourinary System*, https://doi.org/10.1007/978-3-319-69575-4_7

Key Points
- MRI is recognized as the gold standard imaging modality for endometrial cancer staging.
- The combination of T2-weighted imaging, dynamic contrast-enhanced MRI, and diffusion-weighted imaging (DWI) enables to accurately assess deep myometrial invasion.
- T2 and DWI sequences most be angled perpendicularly to the uterus axis to better evaluated deep myometrial invasion.

7.1 Introduction

Endometrial cancer is the most common gynecological malignancy in developed countries [1]. Its incidence is rising, mainly due to increased life expectancy and obesity [1, 2]. Endometrial cancer affects predominantly postmenopausal women, and most of them are diagnosed at an early stage (80% stage I) [3].

Magnetic resonance imaging (MRI) is the imaging modality of choice to preoperatively determine the depth of myometrial invasion. The depth of tumor invasion into the myometrium is the most important factor to assess on MRI as it correlates with tumor grade, lymph node metastases, and patient survival [4, 5]. Recently diffusion-weighted imaging (DWI) has been shown to increase accuracy of assessing depth of myometrial invasion [6–9].

In the following text, the advantages and challenges of MRI staging of endometrial cancer will be discussed with a particular focus on the MRI acquisition protocol and the role of DWI.

7.2 Epidemiology

7.2.1 Incidence, Risk Factors, and Pathogenesis

Endometrial cancer mainly affects postmenopausal women in their sixth/seventh decades [5, 6]. Classical risk factors are summarized in Table 7.1.

Endometrial carcinomas are divided into two subtypes based on their prognosis (Table 7.2). Briefly, type 1 endometrial carcinomas are estrogen-dependent tumors. They include FIGO grades 1 and 2 endometrioid adenocarcinomas. Type 1 accounts for approximately 90% of endometrial cancers. They are associated with prolonged unopposed estrogen exposure such as estrogen replacement therapy, tamoxifen treatment, polycystic ovary syndrome, estrogen-producing ovarian tumors, obesity, diabetes, early menarche, late menopause, and nulliparity.

Type 2 endometrial carcinomas include serous papillary, clear cell adenocarcinomas, carcinosarcomas, and FIGO grade 3 endometrioid adenocarcinomas. Type 2 tumors are not driven by estrogen and tend to present at a higher stage and behave more aggressively.

Table 7.1 Risk factors for endometrial cancer

Risk factors for endometrial cancer
Excess estrogen exposure
• Endogenous estrogen
– Obesity
– Early menarche and late menopause
– Chronic anovulation
Estrogen secreting tumors
• Exogenous estrogen or estrogen agonists
– Unopposed estrogen therapy
– Tamoxifen
– Estrogen-progestin postmenopausal hormone therapy
Age
Family history of Lynch syndrome
Associated factors
Diabetes and hypertension
Nulliparity and infertility
Breast cancer
Tubal ligation

Table 7.2 Endometrial cancer types

	Type 1 endometrial carcinoma	Type 2 endometrial carcinoma
Hormone dependency	*Estrogen* dependent	Non-*estrogen* dependent
Percentage	80–85%	10–15%
Age at diagnosis	Pre- to perimenopausal patient	Postmenopausal patient
Risk factors	• Obesity • Unopposed estrogen exposure • Nulliparity and infertility (polycystic ovary syndrome)	None
Histologic features	• Low-grade tumor • Endometrioid G1–G2 • Endometrioid with squamous differentiation • Mucinous	• High-grade tumor • Endometrioid G3 • Clear cell • Serous • Undifferentiated • Carcinosarcoma
Clinical course	• Early initial stage • Slow growing • Local recurrence	• Advanced initial stage • Rapid progression • Aggressive behavior with poor prognosis
5-year survival	80%	40%

7.2.2   Diagnosis

Vaginal bleeding is abnormal in postmenopausal patient, and it is the most common symptom presented by patient with endometrial cancer. The initial standard evaluation includes pelvic ultrasound. Several thresholds of endometrial thickness have been evaluated; a cutoff value of 4 or 5 mm has been proposed to detect cancer with a sensitivity of up to 95% and specificity of 77% [10] and therefore stratify patients accordingly for further assessment with hysteroscopy.

7.3   The Role of MRI in Endometrial Cancer Management

7.3.1   Conservative Fertility-Sparing Management

Although endometrial cancer predominantly occurs in postmenopausal women, a significant proportion (15–25%) of patients will be diagnosed with this disease before menopause [1]. Progestogen treatment may be an alternative for women who want to preserve their fertility provided they have disease limited to the endometrium. In this small cohort of patients, response evaluation to medical treatment alone is performed at 6–9 months with repeat D&C and MR imaging. After pregnancy, surgery is advised due to high risk of recurrence.

Eligibility criteria for fertility-sparing treatment are strict, and only patients with FIGO IA grade 1 endometrioid adenocarcinoma confined to the endometrium (no myometrial invasion) can be considered.

7.3.2   Standard Treatment

Standard therapy for endometrial cancer includes total hysterectomy, bilateral salpingo-oophorectomy with peritoneal washings, and pelvic and para-aortic lymph node dissection. However, systematic lymphadenectomy in all patients regardless their FIGO staging is under debate. Lymphadenectomy increases the risk of lymphocele and lymphedema. It increases the anesthesia and operating time which is associated with increased morbidity [11]. Recently, two clinical trials showed no survival benefit of lymphadenectomy in patients with FIGO grade 1 or 2 stage IA endometrial cancer. Therefore, sentinel nodes mapping (SLN) has been proposed by several surgical teams prior to lymphadenectomy in order to select the patient who would benefit from lymph nodes dissection [12–17]. The role of SLN mapping is still debated but has already been included recently in the American National Comprehensive Cancer Network (NCCN) guidelines [18]. Which recommend SLN for "apparent uterine-confined malignancy when there is no metastasis demonstrated by imaging studies or no obvious extrauterine disease at exploration." In this setting, MRI plays an important role by distinguishing patients who may benefit from this technique from those with more advanced stage who will undergo systematic lymphadenectomy.

In the meantime, European guidelines from the European Society of Medical Oncology (ESMO) have endorsed a risk stratification algorithm that aggregates multiple prognostic factors of recurrence risk [19–23]. Indeed, ESMO guidelines propose to subdivide stage I cancer into four risk categories [24, 25] and do not recommend lymphadenectomy in the low-risk group corresponding to stage I endometrioid type, grade 1 or grade 2, with <50% myometrial invasion and without lymphovascular invasion [24, 25]. Other more advanced groups are referred for lymphadenectomy. Consequently, preoperative information about depth of myometrial invasion and histological grade is essential to tailor the surgical approach for patients with endometrial cancer.

MRI can accurately predict the depth of myometrial invasion; histological grade can be determined with endometrial sampling. However, the histologic grade of endometrial carcinoma on histology obtained from biopsy may be subject to sampling error [26–28]. Several studies have demonstrated an association between low ADC values and high-grade tumor [8, 29–31], while others did not find differences [6, 9]. As such, the results of the added value of ADC to predict tumor grade are yet inconclusive [6–9, 29–34].

7.4   MRI Protocol

7.4.1   Patient Preparation

To diminish artifacts due to peristalsis, patients are instructed to fast for 4–6 h prior to MRI, and an antiperistaltic agent is administered intramuscularly or intravenously at the beginning of the examination. An empty urinary bladder is also recommended to decrease artifacts related to bladder motion and filling [35].

7.4.2   MRI Protocol

7.4.2.1 Conventional Sequences

The conventional protocol includes small field of view (FOV) high-resolution axial and sagittal T2WI of the pelvis and large FOV axial T1 of the pelvis extended up to aortic bifurcation. A high-resolution small FOV axial oblique T2WI angled perpendicularly to the endometrial cavity is critical to assess the depth of myometrial invasion [35].

7.4.2.2 Functional MRI

Diffusion-Weighted Imaging (DWI)
Protocol should include DWI in at least one or two planes (axial oblique same as axial oblique T2WI and sagittal plane) with a minimum two b values (e.g., $b = 400$, $b = 800$). Acquiring T2WI and DWI on the same plane allows image fusion and optimizes anatomical correlation. Indeed, it is really critical to always read DWI in conjunction with morphological images.

Dynamic Multiphase Contrast-Enhanced Imaging (DCE-MRI)
Dynamic contrast-enhanced MR images are obtained with a three-dimensional gradient echo T1W fat-saturated sequence after the administration of 0.1 mmol/kg of gadolinium at a rate of 2 mL/s. Images are acquired prior to contrast medium injection and then during multiple phases of enhancement in sagittal planes at 25 s and 1 and 2 min after injection; a delayed sequence may be added and acquired on axial oblique 4 min after injection:

- Early phase images (25 s–1 min after injection) are optimal for the detection of subendometrial enhancement.
- Equilibrium phase images (2–3 min after injection) are best for the evaluation of deep myometrium invasion.
- Delayed phase images (4–5 min after injection) are optional to detect cervical stroma invasion.

7.5   MRI Interpretation

7.5.1   Cancer Findings on MRI

- On T2WI, the tumor traditionally demonstrates intermediate to low T2 signal intensity relative to the hyperintense normal endometrium [35] (Fig. 7.1).
- On DWI, tumors appear hyperintense on the high b-value DWI image with corresponding hypointense signal on the ADC map (Fig. 7.1).
- On DCE-MRI, small tumors may enhance early compared to the normal endometrium.

Added Value of DWI
In case of early stage, small tumors may not be associated with endometrial thickening. In those cases, diffusion may be particularly helpful to detect small tumor among the normal non-distended endometrial cavity. Indeed, studies have demonstrated the added value of DWI as a tool to differentiate endometrial cancer from normal endometrium [6, 9, 30, 36, 37]. ADC values of endometrial cancers are significantly lower than those of endometrial polyps and normal endometrium [6, 9, 30, 36, 37]. Multiple ADC thresholds have been proposed ranging from 1.05 to 1.28 to distinguish malignant from benign lesions with range of sensitivity of 60.1–87% and specificity of 100% [6, 34, 36, 38]. Using DWI as a tool to depict endometrial cancer may be particularly helpful when endometrial sampling is not possible.
   Pitfalls
   Blood product retention also demonstrates low ADC and high signal intensity on DWI sequence. T1W sequence can help to confirm presence of blood products. To avoid this pitfall, it is really critical to always read DWI in conjunction with morphological images.

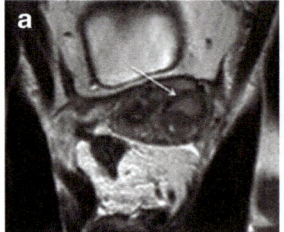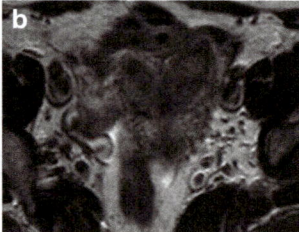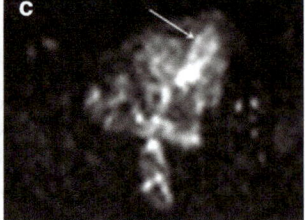

Fig. 7.1 Axial oblique (**a**) and coronal oblique T2-weighted images (**b**) show a septate uterus. The left "pseudo horn" demonstrates endometrial thickening without extension within the myometrium (*arrow*) in keeping with FIGO MR 1A. DWI coronal oblique sequence (**c**) helps to better delineate the tumor as a hyperintense mass within the endometrial cavity (*arrow*)

7.5.2   MRI Cancer Staging

7.5.2.1 Stage I

Stage IA tumors invade less than 50% of the myometrial thickness (Fig. 7.1); stage IB tumors involve more than 50% of the myometrial thickness (Fig. 7.2).

The depth of myometrial invasion is based on the maximal point of tumor extension within the myometrium.

An intact low signal intensity junctional zone on T2WI almost completely excludes myometrial invasion (Fig. 7.1).

However, the evaluation of tumor depth extension within the myometrium may be difficult in various situations: distended endometrial cavity by cancer (Fig. 7.3),

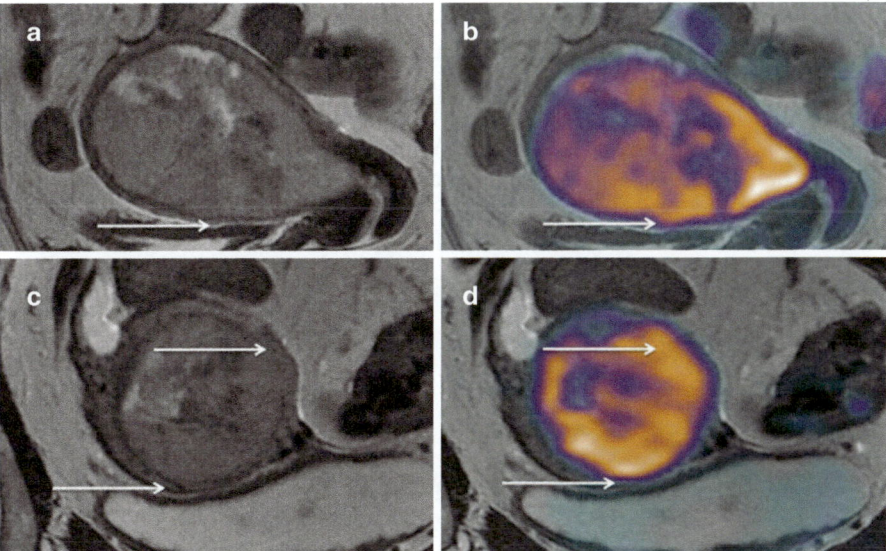

Fig. 7.2   Sagittal (**a**), fused sagittal DWI-T2 (**b**), axial oblique T2-weighted images (**c**), and fused axial oblique DWI-T2 (**d**) demonstrate a large polypoidal soft tissue mass in the endometrial cavity extending into the outer half of the myometrium in keeping with FIGO MR IB disease (*arrows*)

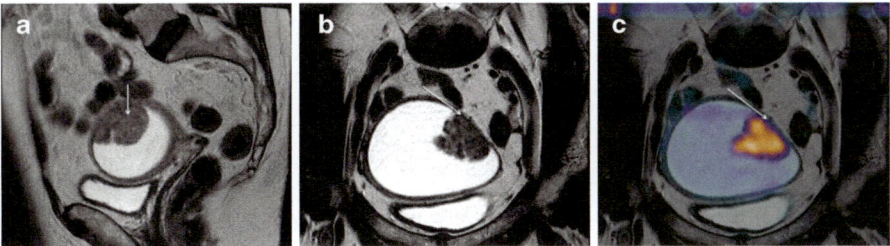

Fig. 7.3   (**a**) Sagittal T2-weighted images show an endometrial tumor largely distending the uterine cavity and compressing the myometrium; (**b**) axial oblique T2 sequence demonstrates no deep myometrial invasion (*arrow*) which is confirmed by the fused axial oblique DWI-T2 (**c**) (*arrow*)

cornua location of tumor (Fig. 7.4), presence of leiomyomas (Fig. 7.5) or coexistent adenomyosis (Figs. 7.6 and 7.7), isointense tumor to the myometrium, and poor definition of the zonal anatomy in postmenopausal patient. In these cases, DCE-MR and DWI-MR play an important role when combined with T2-weighted images.

On DCE, deep myometrial invasion is best depicted at equilibrium phase (2 min 30). In this phase there is more pronounced contrast-to-noise ratio between the myometrium, which is markedly hyperintense, and the endometrial tumor, which is usually hypointense. This is particularly useful when there is a poor difference JZ/myometrium.

Added Value of DWI

Recently, studies have demonstrated the added value of DWI for the evaluation of myometrial invasion [8, 9, 40–46]. DWI is now widely used in combination with T2WI and DCE-MRI in routine clinical practice [47]. It is still under debate whether the combination of T2WI + DWI is superior to DCE-MR [42]. The potential superiority of DWI in assessing myometrial invasion might be explained by its increased accuracy in difficult MRI staging cases, i.e., in the presence of leiomyomas (Fig. 7.5), adenomyosis (Figs. 7.6 and 7.7), poor tumor to myometrium contrast, and corneal tumor extension (Fig. 7.4) [46].

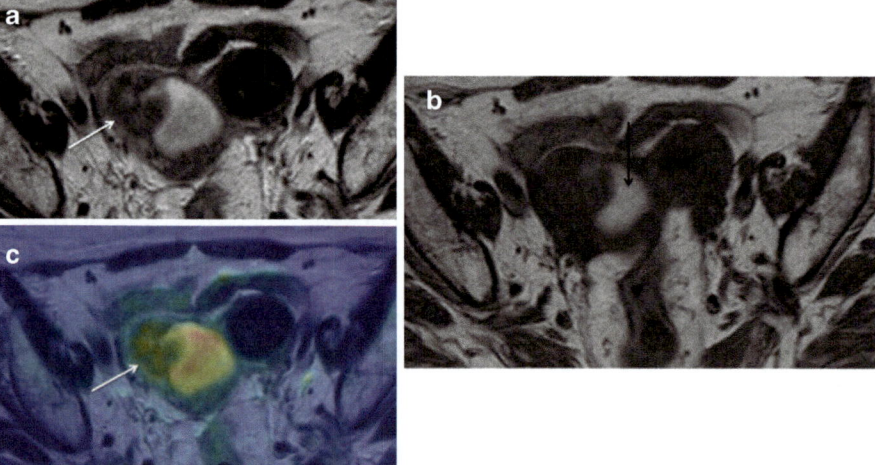

Fig. 7.4 Axial oblique T2-weighted image (**a**) shows a large soft tissue mass at the level of the right cornua and a distended endometrial cavity. Corresponding T1WI shows T1 (**b**) hyperintense signal within the endometrial cavity in keeping with hematometra (*black arrow*). Fused axial T2WI-DWI (**c**) helps better tumor delineation and shows tumor extending into the outer half of the myometrium in keeping with FIGO MR IB disease (*white arrow*)

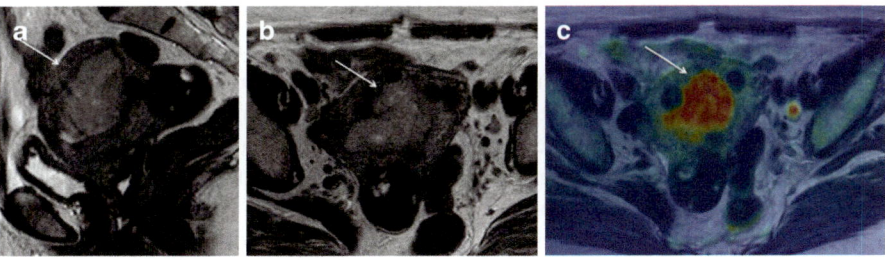

Fig. 7.5 (**a**) Sagittal T2WI shows a large tumor distending the tumor cavity (*white arrow*). (**b**) Axial oblique T2WI demonstrates multiple leiomyomas. (**c**) Fused axial oblique DWI-T2 helps tumor delineation and demonstrates deep myometrial invasion in keeping with FIGO MR IB disease (*white arrow*)

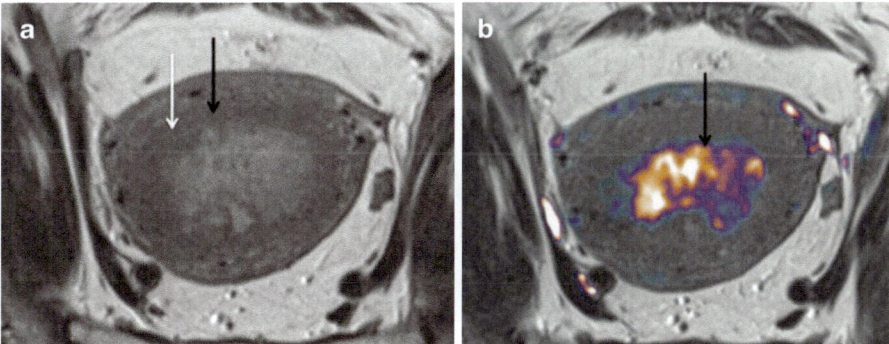

Fig. 7.6 (**a**) Axial oblique T2WI demonstrates a thick junctional zone consistent with adenomyosis (*white arrow*) and a poor tumor to myometrium interface. The tumor extension is difficult to assess on T2WI (*black arrow*). (**b**) Fused T2WI-DWI doesn't demonstrate deep myometrial invasion (*black arrow*) in keeping with FIGO MR IA stage. DWI helps tumor staging in case of adenomyosis

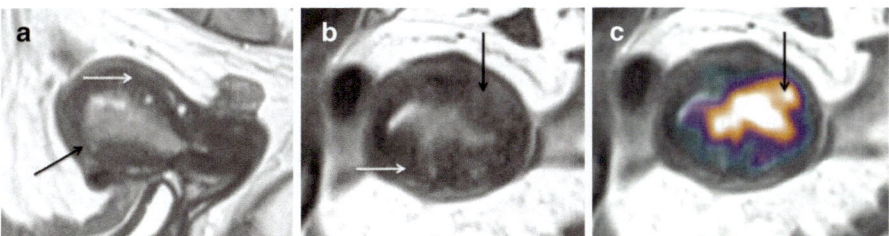

Fig. 7.7 (**a**) Sagittal and (**b**) axial oblique T2WI demonstrates a thick junctional zone consistent with adenomyosis (*white arrow*) and a poor tumor to myometrium interface (*black arrow*). The tumor extension is difficult to assess on T2WI (*black arrow*) due to adenomyosis. (**c**) Fused axial oblique T2WI-DWI demonstrates deep myometrial invasion (*arrow*) in keeping with FIGO MR IB stage. DWI helps tumor staging in case of adenomyosis

7.5.2.2 Stage II

Stage II endometrial cancer corresponds to cervical stromal invasion.

Invasion of the cervical stroma is associated with higher risk of lymphovascular space invasion, which directly correlates with the risk for lymph node metastases.

Cervical stroma invasion is best detected on sagittal and axial oblique T2WI and corresponds to the disruption of the normal low signal intensity of the cervical stroma by the intermediate tumor signal (Figs. 7.8 and 7.9).

On DWI, presence of a high signal intensity on DWI disrupting the cervical stroma is consistent with cervical stroma invasion (Fig. 7.9).

Added Value of DWI

- DWI has been evaluated in cervical stroma invasion [39, 40]. A study demonstrated a higher diagnostic performance of DWI compared to DCE-MRI [41]. Interestingly, the authors pointed out that cervical canal widening was a cause of false negative on DCE-MRI and T2WI but not on DWI.

  Pitfalls

- Nabothian cysts in the cervix may result in hyperintense signal on DWI due to T2 shine-through effect. However, no restriction on ADC map is seen in case of Nabothian cysts which enables to differentiate them from tumor extension within the cervix.

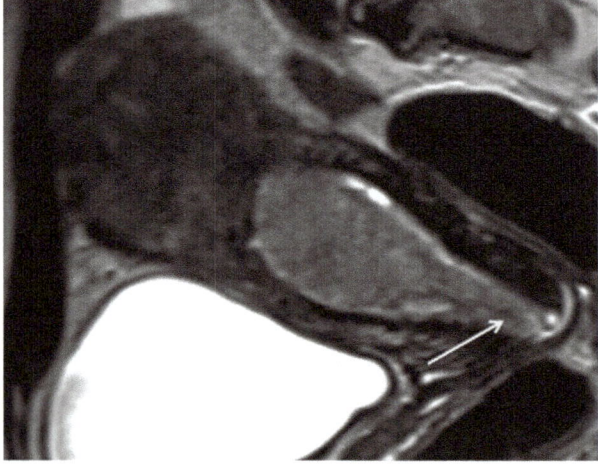

Fig. 7.8 Sagittal T2WI shows widening of the cervical canal. The preservation of a normal hypointense cervical stroma interface with the tumor excludes stroma invasion (*arrow*)

7.5.2.3 Stage III

- *Stage IIIA* refers to tumor extending within the uterine serosa. On MRI, tumor disrupting the normal smooth contour of the outer myometrium suggests serosal involvement (Fig. 7.10). Stage IIIA refers as well to direct tumor spread to the adnexa or ovarian metastases (Fig. 7.11). DWI is particularly helpful to detect small ovarian metastases.

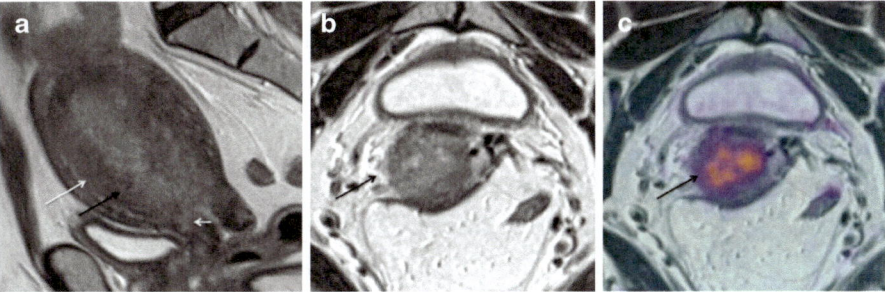

Fig. 7.9 (**a**) Sagittal T2WI demonstrates a thick junctional zone (*white arrow*) in keeping with adenomyosis and a poor tumor to myometrium interface (*black arrow*). Tumor extension into the cervix is hardly seen (*small white arrow*). Tumor extension within the cervix is easily depicted on axial oblique T2WI (**b**) and (**c**) fused axial oblique T2WI (*black arrows*)

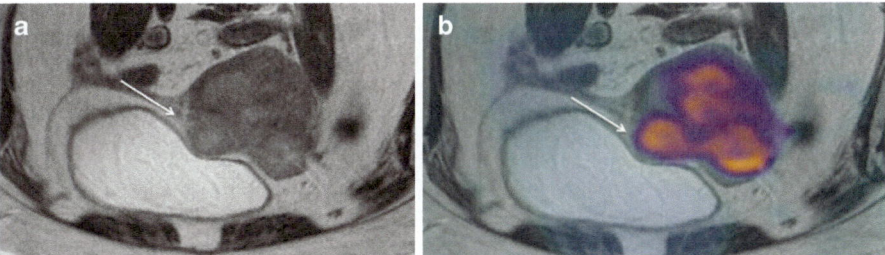

Fig. 7.10 (**a**) Axial oblique T2WI and (**b**) fused axial oblique T2WI-DWI show tumor extension beyond the serosa (*arrows*) in keeping with a FIGO MR IIIA disease

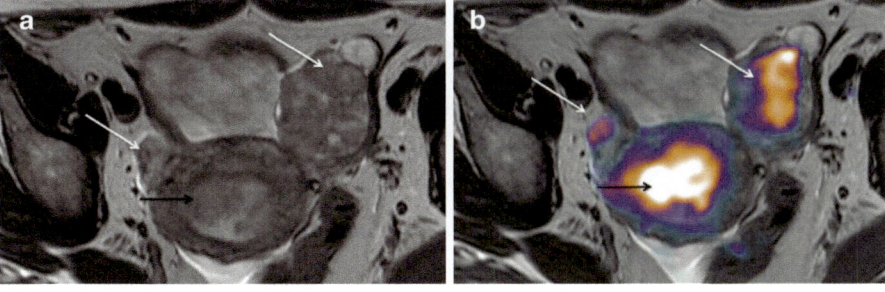

Fig. 7.11 (**a**) Axial oblique T2WI and (**b**) fused axial oblique DWI-T2WI demonstrate two heterogeneous masses (*arrow*) within the ovaries compatible with metastases of an endometrial cancer (*black arrows*) (FIGO MR IIIA disease)

– *Stage IIIB* corresponds to the involvement of vagina, either by direct invasion or metastatic spread (Fig. 7.12). DWI is particularly helpful to detect small cervical and vaginal tumor implants (Fig. 7.12).
– *Stage IIIC* refers to lymph node metastases (stage IIIC1, pelvic; stage IIIC2, para-aortic metastatic lymphadenopathy) (Fig. 7.13). Lymph node measurement of >1 cm in short axis is very specific for nodal metastases but with a very poor sensitivity (range 36–89.5%) [42–44]. DWI has been evaluated for the assessment of lymph node metastases. However, due to a considerable overlap in ADC values, none of the published studies have been able to distinguish benign from malignant lymph nodes.

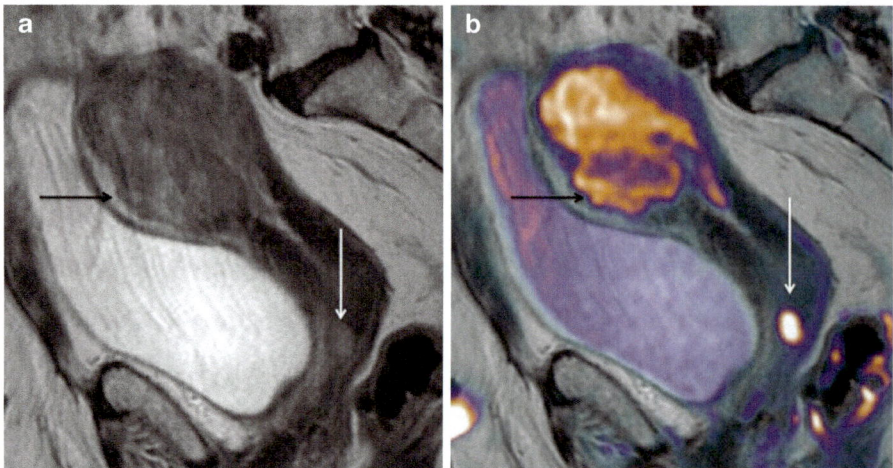

Fig. 7.12 (**a**) Sagittal T2WI and (**b**) fused sagittal T2WI-DWI show tumor extension beyond the serosa (*black arrow*) and a small vaginal implant (*white arrow*) consistent with MR FIGO IIIB. DWI helps better detection of small vaginal deposit

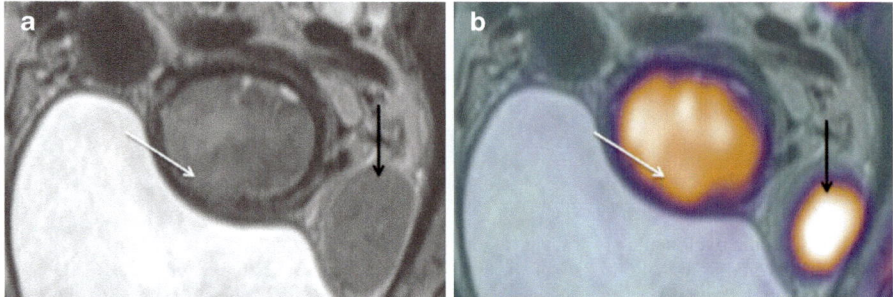

Fig. 7.13 (**a**) Axial oblique T2WI and (**b**) Fused T2WI-DWI demonstrate a large tumor within the endometrial cavity with deep myometrial extension (*white arrow*). An abnormal left external iliac lymph node (*black arrow*) has the same signal characteristics as the primary tumor in keeping with metastatic nodal involvement and stage IIIC1 disease

7.5.2.4 Stage IV

Stage IVA disease represents direct invasion of the bladder or rectal mucosa.

On T2WI, transmural tumor extension into the bladder or rectum must be depicted to assess bladder or rectal invasion. Presence of bladder mucosal edema is not an indicator of mucosal invasion.

Stage IVB disease refers to distant metastases, including suprarenal para-aortic and inguinal lymphadenopathy [54]. DWI helps detection of small peritoneal deposits (Fig. 7.14) [45].

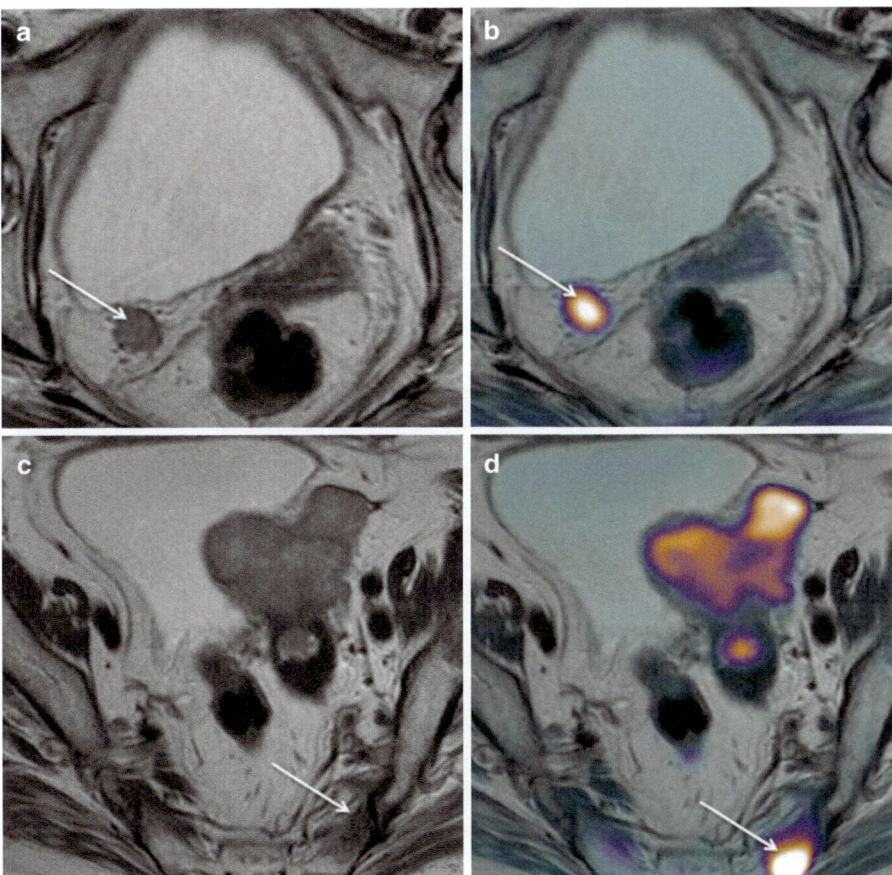

Fig. 7.14 In addition to the primary tumor extending into the serosa, the fused T2D-WI image (**b, d**) clearly depicts restricted diffusion in a soft tissue deposit (**b**) and within the left side of the sacrum (**d**) with corresponding T2WI (**a, c**) in keeping with stage IVB disease. CT imaging also confirmed further metastatic disease in the lungs

7.6   Tumor Recurrence

Approximately 13% of women with endometrial cancer will develop recurrent disease [46]. Recurrence risk varies according to well-defined risk factors such as age, histological type, high tumor grade, the degree of myometrial stromal infiltration, cervical stromal invasion, lymphovascular space invasion, lymph node metastasis, and the presence of peritoneal disease [47].

Most of relapses are symptomatic and will occur in high-risk patients within the first 3 years (80%) [46, 48, 49]. The most frequent sites of recurrent disease in cross-sectional image are the vagina, lymph nodes, peritoneum, and lungs (Figs. 7.15, 7.16, 7.17, 7.18 and 7.19) [50, 51].

Endometrial cancer follow-up protocol usually consists of clinical and gynecological examinations. Radiological exams are indicated if there is clinical suspicion of recurrence [25].

There is limited evidence on the survival benefits of intensive follow-up with routine diagnostic testing when compared to non-intensive follow-up schedules. It is not also established what is the impact of imaging follow-up on the management of these patients [48].

There are very few studies that address the role of DWI in predicting endometrial cancer recurrence. Nakamura et al. correlated the preoperative minimum ADC

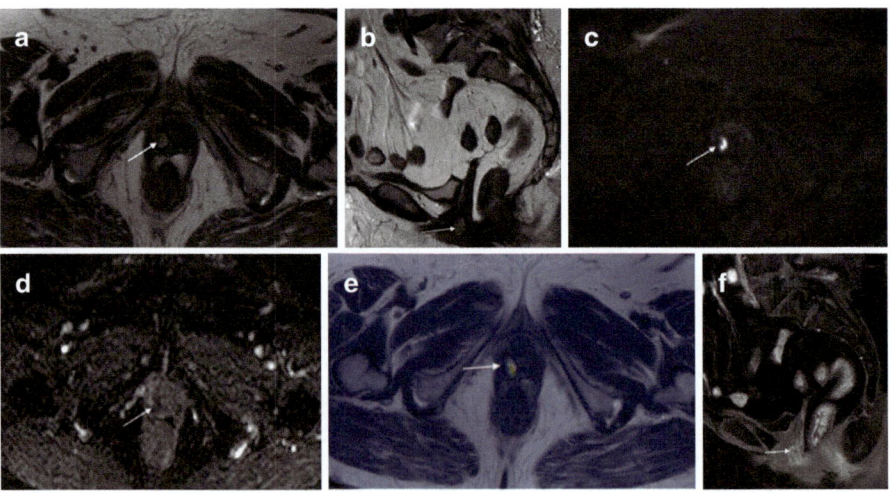

Fig. 7.15 (**a**) Axial T2-weighted image; (**b**) sagittal T2-weighted images. T2-weighted images show a small nodule in the lower third of the vagina that displays intermediate to high signal. With morphologic sequences alone, this nodule could be easily misdiagnosed as a Bartholin's cyst. Diffusion-weighted image ($b = 1000$ mm/s^2) (**c**) and the respective ADC map (**d**) show typical high cellularity restricted diffusion that is very suspicious for tumor recurrence. Fused DWI image ($b = 1000$ mm/s^2) with T2-weighted image further highlights the endometrial cancer recurrence in the vagina (**e**). Sagittal 3D fat-suppressed T1-weighted sequence after the administration of gadolinium also confirms the solid nature of the nodule (**f**)

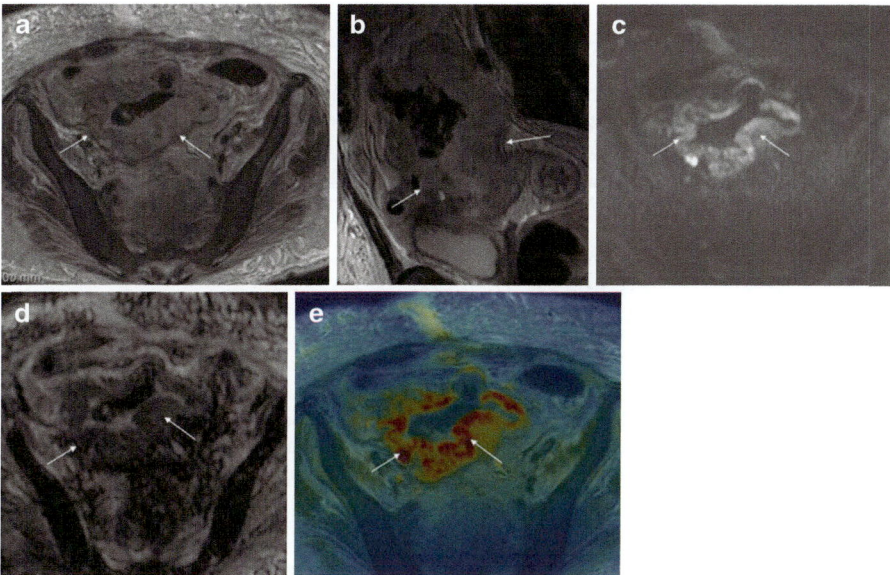

Fig. 7.16 Axial T2-weighted image (**a**) and sagittal T2-weighted image (**b**) show a heterogeneously hyperintense ill-defined mass adherent to the sigmoid colon and to the bowel loops. The colon shows a complete loss of the normal hypointensity of its walls which indicates infiltration; diffusion-weighted image ($b = 1000$ mm/s^2) (**c**) and ADC map (**d**). The mass displays high signal on $b = 1000$ mm/s^2, and it appears markedly hypointense on the ADC map indicating high cellularity typical of tumoral restricted diffusion; (**e**) fused DWI image ($b = 1000$ mm/s^2) with T2-weighted image highlights the endometrial cancer recurrence invading the sigmoid colon and the intestinal loops

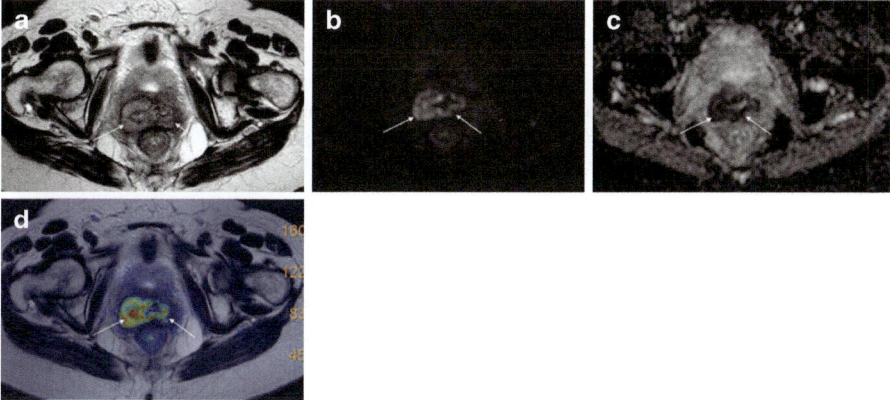

Fig. 7.17 Axial T2-weighted image shows a hyperintense, well-defined lobulated mass at the top of the vaginal vault (**a**). Diffusion-weighted image ($b = 1000$ mm/s^2) (**b**) and ADC map (**c**) show typical restricted diffusion of tumor recurrence. Fused DWI image ($b = 1000$ mm/s^2) with T2-weighted image highlights the endometrial cancer recurrence in the vaginal cuff (**d**)

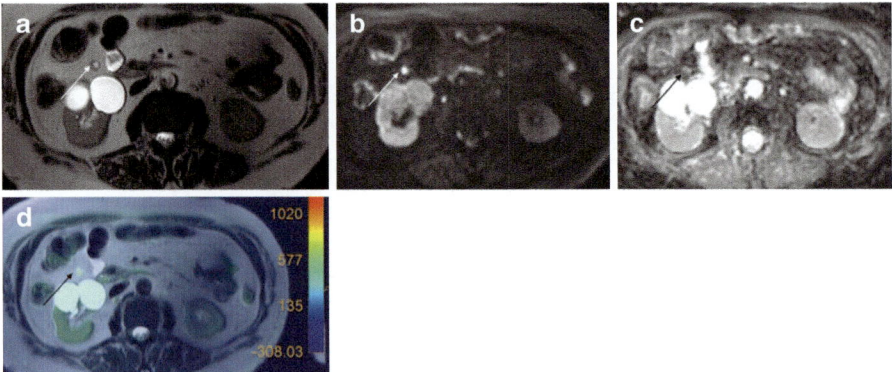

Fig. 7.18 Axial T2-weighted image shows a small mesenteric nodule in front of the right kidney (**a**). Diffusion-weighted image ($b = 1000$ mm/s^2) (**b**) and ADC map (**c**) reveal restricted diffusion which is very suspicious for peritoneal recurrence, typical of this histological type of tumor. Fused DWI image ($b = 1000$ mm/s^2) with T2-weighted image highlights the peritoneal recurrence (**d**)

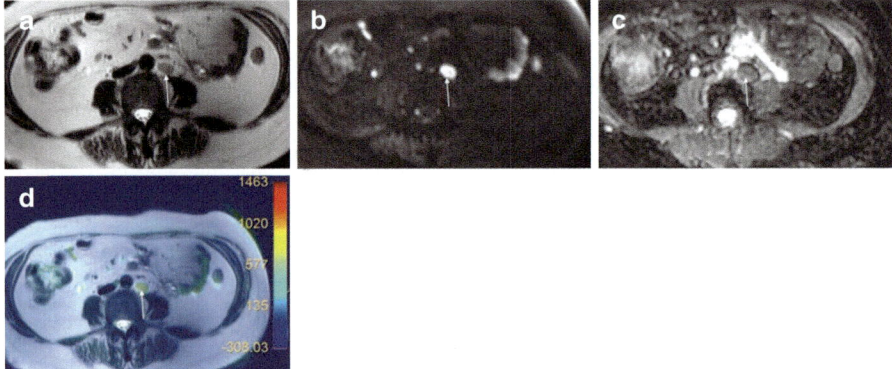

Fig. 7.19 Axial T2-weighted image (**a**); diffusion-weighted image ($b = 1000$ mm/s^2) (**b**) and ADC map (**c**); (**d**) fused DWI image ($b = 1000$ mm/s^2) with T2-weighted image. T2-weighted image shows a left para-aortic lymphadenopathy that shows significant restricted diffusion representing tumor recurrence

(ADCmin) of the primary endometrial tumor of 111 patients with the clinical characteristics and prognosis of these patients. Authors concluded that an endometrial tumor low ADCmin was associated with patient disease-free survival and as such could help for identifying patients at risk of recurrence. Nonetheless, a low ADCmin was not associated with the overall survival rates of these patients [52].

Due to its high soft tissue resolution, MR imaging is very helpful in detecting pelvic recurrences and in assessing their surgical resectability.

Relapses in the vagina display the same signal features of the primary tumor. On T2-weighted images, they present as a hyperintense mass that disrupts the hypointense signal of the vaginal wall (Figs. 7.15 and 7.17).

Central pelvic recurrences can occasionally invade the adjacent pelvic organs, such as the bladder, the rectum, the sigmoid colon, and the bowel loops (Fig. 7.16). Invasion of such organs can be suspected when there is loss of the T2 hypointense signal in their wall and diagnosed if there is tumor inside their lumens (Fig. 7.16). Fistulous tracts can sometimes be seen. Central pelvic recurrences may also invade pelvic side walls, impeding surgical resectability. This should be suspected if the tumor lies within 3 mm of the pelvic side wall or if it distorts or surrounds the iliac vessels [53].

DW images are very helpful in detecting and highlighting pelvic recurrences, improving the degree of diagnostic confidence. DWI along with T2-weighted images is useful in distinguishing posttreatment fibrosis from tumor relapse or persistent disease, the former appearing as a T2, DWI, and ADC map hypointense tissue. DWI is also valuable in differentiating tumor tissue from inflammatory changes, especially in early posttreatment period, when both can show intense radiotracer uptake on PET-CT scans. Low ADC values are more likely to represent active tumoral cells, whereas high ADC values are suggestive of edema and inflammation [54].

Fused T2-weighted images with DW images have shown to outperform conventional T2-weighted and DW images and to have a similar diagnostic performance to DCE fat-suppressed T1-weighted images in the detection of locally recurrent pelvic malignancies [55]. In a study by Kitajima et al., the diagnostic performance of the combination of DWI and T2-weighted images was also comparable to that of DCE-MRI for the assessment of intrapelvic recurrence of gynecological malignant tumors [56].

Peritoneal recurrences are usually present in serous and clear cell endometrial cancers that typically behave as epithelial ovarian cancer (Fig. 7.18). DWI has shown to be very useful in highlighting small cellular peritoneal implants, which typically show high signal on high b-value DWI that contrasts to the generally suppressed background noise (Fig. 7.18) [57]. In one study, the performance of DWI was as high as of contrast-enhanced images for the diagnosis of intrapelvic peritoneal implants in gynecological cancer relapse [56].

There is limited literature on the value of DWI in the detection of lymph node recurrences of endometrial cancer, possibly due to the lack of histopathological correlation (Fig. 7.19).

In conclusion, MRI plays a critical role in stratifying patients with endometrial cancer as it is highly accurate in the assessment of myometrial invasion. The use of DWI in conjunction with morphological sequences offers improved accuracy for endometrial cancer staging and should be added to the routine MRI protocol.

References

1. Siegel RL, Miller KD, Jemal A. Cancer statistics, 2016. CA Cancer J Clin. 2016;66(1):7–30.
2. Chen X, Xiang YB, Long JR, et al. Genetic polymorphisms in obesity-related genes and endometrial cancer risk. Cancer. 2012;118(13):3356–64.
3. Cramer DW. The epidemiology of endometrial and ovarian cancer. Hematol Oncol Clin North Am. 2012;26(1):1–12.
4. Kinkel K, Forstner R, Danza FM, et al. Staging of endometrial cancer with MRI: guidelines of the European Society of Urogenital Imaging. Eur Radiol. 2009;19(7):1565–74.

5. Ben-Shachar I, Vitellas KM, Cohn DE. The role of MRI in the conservative management of endometrial cancer. Gynecol Oncol. 2004;93(1):233–7.
6. Bharwani N, Miquel ME, Sahdev A, et al. Diffusion-weighted imaging in the assessment of tumour grade in endometrial cancer. Br J Radiol. 2011;84(1007):997–1004.
7. Kishimoto K, Tajima S, Maeda I, et al. Endometrial cancer: correlation of apparent diffusion coefficient (ADC) with tumor cellularity and tumor grade. Acta Radiol. 2016;57(8):1021–8.
8. Nougaret S, Reinhold C, Alsharif SS, et al. Endometrial cancer: combined MR volumetry and diffusion-weighted imaging for assessment of myometrial and lymphovascular invasion and tumor grade. Radiology. 2015;276(3):797–808.
9. Rechichi G, Galimberti S, Signorelli M, et al. Endometrial cancer: correlation of apparent diffusion coefficient with tumor grade, depth of myometrial invasion, and presence of lymph node metastases. AJR Am J Roentgenol. 2011;197(1):256–62.
10. Smith-Bindman R, Kerlikowske K, Feldstein VA, et al. Endovaginal ultrasound to exclude endometrial cancer and other endometrial abnormalities. JAMA. 1998;280(17):1510–7.
11. Ghezzi F, Uccella S, Cromi A, et al. Lymphoceles, lymphorrhea, and lymphedema after laparoscopic and open endometrial cancer staging. Ann Surg Oncol. 2012;19(1):259–67.
12. Ferraioli D, Chopin N, Beurrier F, Carrabin N, Buenerd A, Mathevet P. The incidence and clinical significance of the micrometastases in the sentinel lymph nodes during surgical staging for early endometrial cancer. Int J Gynecol Cancer. 2015;25(4):673–80.
13. Rossi EC, Jackson A, Ivanova A, Boggess JF. Detection of sentinel nodes for endometrial cancer with robotic assisted fluorescence imaging: cervical versus hysteroscopic injection. Int J Gynecol Cancer. 2013;23(9):1704–11.
14. Holloway RW, Bravo RA, Rakowski JA, et al. Detection of sentinel lymph nodes in patients with endometrial cancer undergoing robotic-assisted staging: a comparison of colorimetric and fluorescence imaging. Gynecol Oncol. 2012;126(1):25–9.
15. Barlin JN, Khoury-Collado F, Kim CH, et al. The importance of applying a sentinel lymph node mapping algorithm in endometrial cancer staging: beyond removal of blue nodes. Gynecol Oncol. 2012;125(3):531–5.
16. Khoury-Collado F, Murray MP, Hensley ML, et al. Sentinel lymph node mapping for endometrial cancer improves the detection of metastatic disease to regional lymph nodes. Gynecol Oncol. 2011;122(2):251–4.
17. Frimer M, Khoury-Collado F, Murray MP, Barakat RR, Abu-Rustum NR. Micrometastasis of endometrial cancer to sentinel lymph nodes: is it an artifact of uterine manipulation? Gynecol Oncol. 2010;119(3):496–9.
18. Koh WJ, Greer BE, Abu-Rustum NR, et al. Uterine neoplasms, version 1.2014. J Natl Compr Cancer Netw. 2014;12(2):248–80.
19. Imai K, Kato H, Katayama K, et al. A preoperative risk-scoring system to predict lymph node metastasis in endometrial cancer and stratify patients for lymphadenectomy. Gynecol Oncol. 2016;142(2):273–7.
20. Holloway RW, Gupta S, Stavitzski NM, et al. Sentinel lymph node mapping with staging lymphadenectomy for patients with endometrial cancer increases the detection of metastasis. Gynecol Oncol. 2016;141(2):206–10.
21. Sadowski EA, Robbins JB, Guite K, et al. Preoperative pelvic MRI and serum cancer antigen-125: selecting women with grade 1 endometrial cancer for lymphadenectomy. AJR Am J Roentgenol. 2015;205(5):W556–64.
22. Frost JA, Webster KE, Bryant A, Morrison J. Lymphadenectomy for the management of endometrial cancer. Cochrane Database Syst Rev 2015;(9):CD007585.
23. Todo Y, Watari H, Kang S, Sakuragi N. Tailoring lymphadenectomy according to the risk of lymph node metastasis in endometrial cancer. J Obstet Gynaecol Res. 2014;40(2):317–21.
24. Colombo N, Creutzberg C, Amant F, et al. ESMO-ESGO-ESTRO consensus conference on endometrial cancer: diagnosis, treatment and follow-up. Ann Oncol. 2016;27(1):16–41.
25. Colombo N, Preti E, Landoni F, et al. Endometrial cancer: ESMO clinical practice guidelines for diagnosis, treatment and follow-up. Ann Oncol. 2013;24(Suppl 6):vi33–8.

26. Batista TP, Cavalcanti CL, Tejo AA, Bezerra AL. Accuracy of preoperative endometrial sampling diagnosis for predicting the final pathology grading in uterine endometrioid carcinoma. Eur J Surg Oncol. 2016;42(9):1367–71.
27. Williams AR, Brechin S, Porter AJ, Warner P, Critchley HO. Factors affecting adequacy of Pipelle and Tao brush endometrial sampling. BJOG. 2008;115(8):1028–36.
28. Dijkhuizen FP, Mol BW, Brolmann HA, Heintz AP. The accuracy of endometrial sampling in the diagnosis of patients with endometrial carcinoma and hyperplasia: a meta-analysis. Cancer. 2000;89(8):1765–72.
29. Inoue C, Fujii S, Kaneda S, et al. Apparent diffusion coefficient (ADC) measurement in endometrial carcinoma: effect of region of interest methods on ADC values. J Magn Reson Imaging. 2014;40(1):157–61.
30. Tamai K, Koyama T, Saga T, et al. Diffusion-weighted MR imaging of uterine endometrial cancer. J Magn Reson Imaging. 2007;26(3):682–7.
31. Woo S, Cho JY, Kim SY, Kim SH. Histogram analysis of apparent diffusion coefficient map of diffusion-weighted MRI in endometrial cancer: a preliminary correlation study with histological grade. Acta Radiol. 2014;55(10):1270–7.
32. Takahashi M, Kozawa E, Tanisaka M, Hasegawa K, Yasuda M, Sakai F. Utility of histogram analysis of apparent diffusion coefficient maps obtained using 3.0T MRI for distinguishing uterine carcinosarcoma from endometrial carcinoma. J Magn Reson Imaging. 2016;43(6):1301–7.
33. Mainenti PP, Pizzuti LM, Segreto S, et al. Diffusion volume (DV) measurement in endometrial and cervical cancer: a new MRI parameter in the evaluation of the tumor grading and the risk classification. Eur J Radiol. 2016;85(1):113–24.
34. Fujii S, Matsusue E, Kigawa J, et al. Diagnostic accuracy of the apparent diffusion coefficient in differentiating benign from malignant uterine endometrial cavity lesions: initial results. Eur Radiol. 2008;18(2):384–9.
35. Horta M, Cunha T. Endometrial cancer. In: Forstner R, Cunha T, Hamm B, editors. MRI and CT of the female pelvis. Berlin: Springer; 2016. p. 1–30.
36. Takeuchi M, Matsuzaki K, Nishitani H. Diffusion-weighted magnetic resonance imaging of endometrial cancer: differentiation from benign endometrial lesions and preoperative assessment of myometrial invasion. Acta Radiol. 2009;50(8):947–53.
37. Inada Y, Matsuki M, Nakai G, et al. Body diffusion-weighted MR imaging of uterine endometrial cancer: is it helpful in the detection of cancer in nonenhanced MR imaging? Eur J Radiol. 2009;70(1):122–7.
38. Kilickesmez O, Bayramoglu S, Inci E, Cimilli T, Kayhan A. Quantitative diffusion-weighted magnetic resonance imaging of normal and diseased uterine zones. Acta Radiol. 2009;50(3):340–7.
39. Koplay M, Dogan NU, Erdogan H, et al. Diagnostic efficacy of diffusion-weighted MRI for pre-operative assessment of myometrial and cervical invasion and pelvic lymph node metastasis in endometrial carcinoma. J Med Imaging Radiat Oncol. 2014;58(5):538–46; quiz 648
40. Hori M, Kim T, Onishi H, et al. Endometrial cancer: preoperative staging using three-dimensional T2-weighted turbo spin-echo and diffusion-weighted MR imaging at 3.0T: a prospective comparative study. Eur Radiol. 2013;23(8):2296–305.
41. Lin G, Huang YT, Chao A, et al. Endometrial cancer with cervical stromal invasion: diagnostic accuracy of diffusion-weighted and dynamic contrast enhanced MR imaging at 3T. Eur Radiol. 2016;27:2400.
42. Kim SH, Kim SC, Choi BI, Han MC. Uterine cervical carcinoma: evaluation of pelvic lymph node metastasis with MR imaging. Radiology. 1994;190(3):807–11.
43. Yang WT, Lam WW, Yu MY, Cheung TH, Metreweli C. Comparison of dynamic helical CT and dynamic MR imaging in the evaluation of pelvic lymph nodes in cervical carcinoma. AJR Am J Roentgenol. 2000;175(3):759–66.
44. Choi HJ, Kim SH, Seo SS, et al. MRI for pretreatment lymph node staging in uterine cervical cancer. AJR Am J Roentgenol. 2006;187(5):W538–43.

45. Fehniger J, Thomas S, Lengyel E, et al. A prospective study evaluating diffusion weighted magnetic resonance imaging (DW-MRI) in the detection of peritoneal carcinomatosis in suspected gynecologic malignancies. Gynecol Oncol. 2016;142(1):169–75.
46. Tjalma WA, van Dam PA, Makar AP, Cruickshank DJ. The clinical value and the cost-effectiveness of follow-up in endometrial cancer patients. Int J Gynecol Cancer. 2004;14(5):931–7.
47. Testa AC, Di Legge A, Virgilio B, et al. Which imaging technique should we use in the follow up of gynaecological cancer? Best Pract Res Clin Obstet Gynaecol. 2014;28(5):769–91.
48. Fung-Kee-Fung M, Dodge J, Elit L, et al. Follow-up after primary therapy for endometrial cancer: a systematic review. Gynecol Oncol. 2006;101(3):520–9.
49. Sartori E, Pasinetti B, Carrara L, Gambino A, Odicino F, Pecorelli S. Pattern of failure and value of follow-up procedures in endometrial and cervical cancer patients. Gynecol Oncol. 2007;107(1 Suppl 1):S241–7.
50. Sohaib SA, Houghton SL, Meroni R, Rockall AG, Blake P, Reznek RH. Recurrent endometrial cancer: patterns of recurrent disease and assessment of prognosis. Clin Radiol. 2007;62(1):28–34; discussion 5–6
51. Tirumani SH, Shanbhogue AK, Prasad SR. Current concepts in the diagnosis and management of endometrial and cervical carcinomas. Radiol Clin N Am. 2013;51(6):1087–110.
52. Nakamura K, Imafuku N, Nishida T, et al. Measurement of the minimum apparent diffusion coefficient (ADCmin) of the primary tumor and CA125 are predictive of disease recurrence for patients with endometrial cancer. Gynecol Oncol. 2012;124(2):335–9.
53. Sala E, Rockall A, Rangarajan D, Kubik-Huch RA. The role of dynamic contrast-enhanced and diffusion weighted magnetic resonance imaging in the female pelvis. Eur J Radiol. 2010;76(3):367–85.
54. Nougaret S, Tirumani SH, Addley H, Pandey H, Sala E, Reinhold C. Pearls and pitfalls in MRI of gynecologic malignancy with diffusion-weighted technique. AJR Am J Roentgenol. 2013;200(2):261–76.
55. Nishie A, Stolpen AH, Obuchi M, Kuehn DM, Dagit A, Andresen K. Evaluation of locally recurrent pelvic malignancy: performance of T2- and diffusion-weighted MRI with image fusion. J Magn Reson Imaging. 2008;28(3):705–13.
56. Kitajima K, Tanaka U, Ueno Y, et al. Role of diffusion weighted imaging and contrast-enhanced MRI in the evaluation of intrapelvic recurrence of gynecological malignant tumor. PLoS One. 2015;10(1):e0117411.
57. Bozkurt M, Doganay S, Kantarci M, et al. Comparison of peritoneal tumor imaging using conventional MR imaging and diffusion-weighted MR imaging with different b values. Eur J Radiol. 2011;80(2):224–8.

Diffusion-Weighted Imaging in Magnetic Resonance Imaging of the Prostate

8

Sherif Mehralivand, Christopher Knaus, Peter L. Choyke, and Baris Turkbey

8.1 Introduction

Magnetic resonance imaging (MRI) of the prostate was first described in the early 1980s in patients who underwent T1-weighted (T1W) and T2-weighted (T2W) pelvic MRI; however the detection ability for prostate cancer with MRI was limited at that time due to inadequate spatial resolution on anatomical images and lack of functional pulse sequences [1, 2]. With advancements in MRI technology and the development of higher magnetic field strengths and functional sequences, prostate cancer lesions can now be delineated and differentiated from benign structures [3].

The combination of the anatomic sequences (T1W and T2W MRI) and functional sequences such as diffusion-weighted imaging (DWI), dynamic contrast-enhanced (DCE) MRI, and MRI spectroscopy (MRS) is often referred to as multiparametric MRI (mpMRI). While MRS and DCE can offer some additional information, DWI is now considered an integral part of mpMRI. Diffusion-weighted imaging in conjunction with T2W especially at b-values higher than 1000 s/mm^2 significantly increases the tumor detection accuracy [4]. Besides, apparent diffusion

S. Mehralivand, M.D.
Department of Urology and Pediatric Urology, University Medical Center, Mainz, Germany

Urologic Oncology Branch, National Cancer Institute, National Institutes of Health, Bethesda, MD, USA

Molecular Imaging Program, National Cancer Institute, National Institutes of Health, Bethesda, MD, USA

C. Knaus, M.D.
Walter-Reed National Medical Center at Bethesda, Bethesda, MD, USA

P.L. Choyke, M.D. • B. Turkbey, M.D. (✉)
Molecular Imaging Program, National Cancer Institute, National Institutes of Health, Bethesda, MD, USA
e-mail: bturkbey@yahoo.com

© Springer International Publishing AG 2018
D. Akata, N. Papanikolaou (eds.), *Diffusion Weighted Imaging of the Genitourinary System*, https://doi.org/10.1007/978-3-319-69575-4_8

167

coefficients (ADC) derived from DWI can correlate with prostate cancer aggressiveness and Gleason scores and can therefore add additional information about lesion biology [5–7].

Since prostate mpMRI research is historically been conducted in various institutions, many different image acquisition techniques, sequence combinations, and reporting protocols exist. To enhance standardization in image acquisition and reporting, the prostate imaging-reporting and data system version 2 (PI-RADSv2) consensus statement was created in 2015 [8]. This guideline is based on a broader consensus compared to version 1 of the document and defines minimum standards for prostate mpMRI.

This chapter discusses the main applications of mpMRI which are detection, localization, and staging of prostate cancer. The enhanced imaging capability of mpMRI for prostate cancer lesions allows for other potential applications like detection of recurrence, metastatic disease, active surveillance, and focal therapy. However, these applications are still considered experimental, and broad consensus is lacking. Since DWI in prostate MRI is almost always used in conjunction with T2W and other sequences, this chapter also focuses on prostate mpMRI.

8.2   Concepts of Diffusion-Weighted Imaging in Prostate Cancer Imaging

Diffusion-weighted imaging determines the Brownian motion of water molecules in a voxel during a certain time. At a molecular level, this movement is completely random and dependent on kinetic energy and temperature. In biological structures, it is additionally influenced by the structure of the underlying tissue. High cellularity, vascularity, and extracellular matrix restrict the free motion of water molecules [9, 10]. Prostate cancer has much higher cellularity and restriction of diffusion than healthy prostate tissue. This translates into a hyperintense signal in DWI and creates a contrast which enables the detection of prostate cancer lesions. By interpreting T2W and DW images together, the diagnostic accuracy for prostate cancer detection on MRI can be significantly improved compared to T2W alone. Although there is no clear definition of an optimal b-value in multiparametric prostate MRI, higher b-values are usually recommended than in other organs. At b-values between 1500 and 2000 s/mm^2, there seems to be the best suppression of the background signal of healthy prostate tissue, thus allowing most optimal contrast [11–13]. However, this comes at the expense of an impact on the signal-to-noise ration and more susceptibility to motion artifacts and magnetic field inhomogeneities.

Apparent diffusion coefficient is another essential component of DWI in multiparametric prostate MRI. It quantifies the movement of water molecules inside a voxel and is expressed in mm^2/s units. It is calculated from at least two scans with different b-values. In prostate cancer detection, b-values between 500 and 800 s/mm^2 are typically used for calculating ADC maps using mono-exponential decay models. Restriction of diffusion inversely correlates with intensity in ADC, and thus prostate cancer appears hypointense [14]. Besides facilitating prostate cancer detection, ADC values also correlate with prostate cancer aggressiveness. Several studies showed an inverse correlation between ADC values and Gleason scores. However, prediction of Gleason scores is not possible due to overlapping of ADC values among Gleason scores [5, 6, 15–20]. It should be noted that restriction of diffusion is not always specific for prostate cancer. Non-tumor conditions such as benign hyperplasia, post-biopsy hemorrhage, and inflammatory processes and sometimes artifacts can also appear as diffusion-restricted areas [21].Furthermore, ADC values are not reproducible due to lack of standardization among vendors, variations dependent on endorectal coil use, magnetic field strength, and b-values limiting its widespread use [22].

8.3   Image Acquisition and Technical Aspects

Multiparametric MRI has historically been investigated in several centers with different image acquisition and patient preparation techniques. Thus, lack of standardization remains a major drawback of this technique. Although scientific evidence is available for a variety of technical questions, most studies are based on in-house experiences. Multicenter multi-reader prospective randomized trials could clarify the best minimum requirements for high-quality images but are naturally difficult to perform. The PI-RADSv2 guideline defines minimum standards in image acquisition, patient preparation, and image reporting to improve standardization. Although a first step into more standardization, it is solely based on expert consensus [23]. The current section provides an overview on the most common techniques in multiparametric MRI of the prostate that are considered minimum requirements needed for prostate cancer detection.

8.3.1   Magnetic Field Strengths and Use of Endorectal Coil

For prostate cancer detection, images are usually obtained either on 1.5T or 3T scanners. Lower strength magnets are not generally recommended. An endorectal coil (ERC) can be used additionally to a surface coil to increase the signal and improve spatial resolution and resultant lesion detection [24]. With this technique higher-quality DW images can be generated [25]. However, this comes at the expense of higher costs, longer scanning time, and patient discomfort.

The SNR for 3T scanners is theoretically double that of 1.5T devices with lower scanning times. However, detection of prostate cancer is well practicable with both techniques. Utilization of an ERC improves SNR in 1.5T scans and elevates image quality to that of 3T images without ERC [26–29]. Images from newer 1.5T scanners with appropriate surface coil systems can also achieve appropriate images like 1.5T scans with ERC. In 3T scans use of ERC can even improve SNR more as compared to 3T scans without ERC leading to even higher-quality images. Nevertheless, the additional value for prostate cancer detection remains controversial. Due to the various techniques and possible combinations and lack of standardization, internal quality control remains the best way to ensure optimal outcomes.

8.3.2   Patient Preparation

As already mentioned, current accepted standards for patient preparation are missing due to different in-house approaches. Since DWI is susceptible to artifacts caused by motion and magnetic field inhomogeneity, many different approaches have been proposed to optimize patient preparation. Patients are generally recommended to empty the rectum prior to the examination since rectal air can cause artifacts especially in DWI and additionally complicate ERC placement. The use of enemas and spasmolytic agents is part of some protocols, although its benefit remains controversial [30–32] (Fig. 8.1). Their use should be weighed against additional costs and potential side effects. Refraining from sexual intercourse is recommended for a period of 72 h prior to the study to ensure optimal seminal vesicle evaluation specifically for patients older than 60 years of age [33]. However, there is no clear evidence whether this leads to improved detection of seminal vesicle invasion. Most patients referred to an evaluation by multiparametric prostate MRI have a history of prior systematic

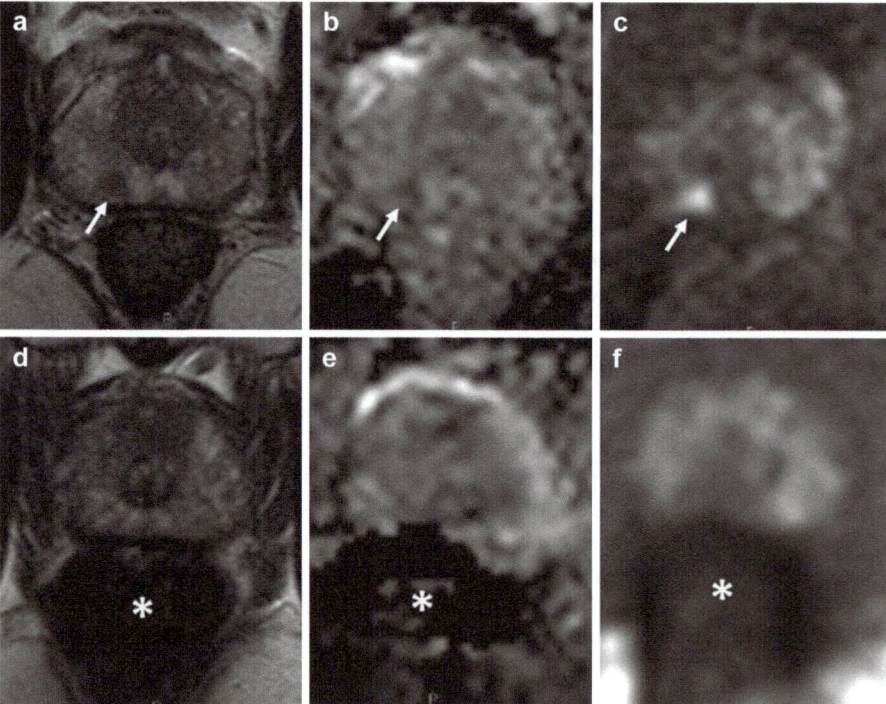

Fig. 8.1 Forty-six-year-old male with PSA of 9.25 ng/mL. Axial T2W MRI shows a subtle lesion in the right apical peripheral zone (*arrow*) (**a**), which also shows restricted diffusion on ADC map (**b**) and b1500 DWI (**c**) (*arrows*). The lesion was biopsied using TRUS/MRI fusion-guided biopsy approach, and histopathology revealed Gleason 3 + 3 prostate cancer. The MRI obtained 1 year ago does not show any lesion in the corresponding slices (**d–f**), which is mainly due to distortion of ADC map and b1500 DWI (**f**) because of rectal gas (*asterix*) (**d–f**). It should be noted that images **a–c** were obtained following fleet enema bowel preparation, whereas no bowel preparation was done prior to acquisition of images **d–f**

prostate biopsies. Post-biopsy hemorrhage can potentially interfere with reading since their hypointensity can obscure prostate cancer lesions. Thus, scans are usually delayed for at least 6 weeks after biopsy [31, 34]. While biopsy-related hemorrhage can be a limitation for intraprostatic lesion detection, it has also been reported that lack of hemorrhage within a focal region of the prostate, which can also be termed as "hemorrhage exclusion sign," may also indicate presence of cancer along with positive findings on DWI and mpMRI. In a retrospective series of 292 patients with two readers, Barrett et al. reported that hemorrhage exclusion sign can occur in about 20% of patients with post-biopsy status and presence of the exclusion sign along with homogeneous hypointense focal signal intensity at T2W within the lesion has a 95% positive predictive value for bearing prostate cancer [35].

8.4 Lesion Detection and Reporting in Multiparametric Prostate MRI

Although the clinical use of multiparametric prostate MRI is expanding, its main application remains as detection and localization of prostate cancer lesions. Until recently, definitive criteria and risk assessment of detected lesions were missing due to different non-standardized in-house criteria. While these systems performed very well in their respective institutions, comparing data among different institutions was challenging. To overcome this, the PI-RADSv2 consensus guideline proposed a five-tier assessment category system in 2015 to improve standardization and interchangeability in MRI lesion detection [8]. These assessment categories reflect the likelihood of clinically significant prostate cancer in detected MRI lesions. To enhance inter-reader reproducibility, the criteria were significantly simplified compared to the previous system. The overall PI-RADSv2 category is now mainly determined by the dominant sequence of the respective zone which is DWI in the peripheral and T2W in the transition zone. Only category 3 lesions in the peripheral zone can be upgraded to category 4 if the DCE sequence shows early enhancement. This sequence plays otherwise a minor role in the current system. Category 3 lesions in the transition zone can only be upgraded if DWI is defined as category 5. Recent validation studies show a relation between higher categories and higher cancer detection rates [36]. However, the inter-reader reproducibility seems to be only moderate [37]. The reason for that is assumed to be due to the lack of quantitative criteria in the current risk category system. More experience from different institutions is needed to define better criteria to optimize risk categorization of detected lesions.

8.5 Clinical Applications

The use of prostate MRI was initially limited to staging of diagnosed prostate cancer patients; however there is an obvious shift in its use from staging to detection of cancer in patients at increased risk. Besides, the ability of mpMRI to localize prostate cancer lesions has the potential to enable detection of cancer recurrence, active surveillance, and focal therapy in the future.

8.5.1   Cancer Detection and Biopsy Guidance

The current main application of multiparametric prostate MRI is detection of cancer in patients with clinical suspicion of prostate cancer due to an elevated PSA or abnormal digital rectal exam. Diffusion-weighted imaging in combination with T2W improves the diagnostic accuracy compared to T2W alone (Figs. 8.2 and 8.3). Thus, prostate cancer lesions can be detected and localized with a high diagnostic accuracy as shown in imaging-histopathology correlation studies with radical pros-tatectomy specimens [38]. However, pathologic confirmation by a biopsy is still needed to diagnose prostate cancer and assess prognostic risk before an appropriate treatment strategy can be recommended. Multiparametric prostate MRI can guide the biopsy to areas with a high risk of prostate cancer. This MRI-targeted biopsy approach can be performed by different techniques. Cognitive fusion uses MRI to manually target lesions in TRUS. In-bore MRI fusion is used to perform the biopsy inside the scanner with MRI monitoring. In MRI/TRUS fusion-guided biopsy, the MRI is fused with TRUS in real time during the biopsy procedure [39]. Although there are only few studies with direct comparisons between all techniques and their results are controversial, it is well known that MRI-guided biopsy improves the detection of clinically significant prostate cancer compared to the standard

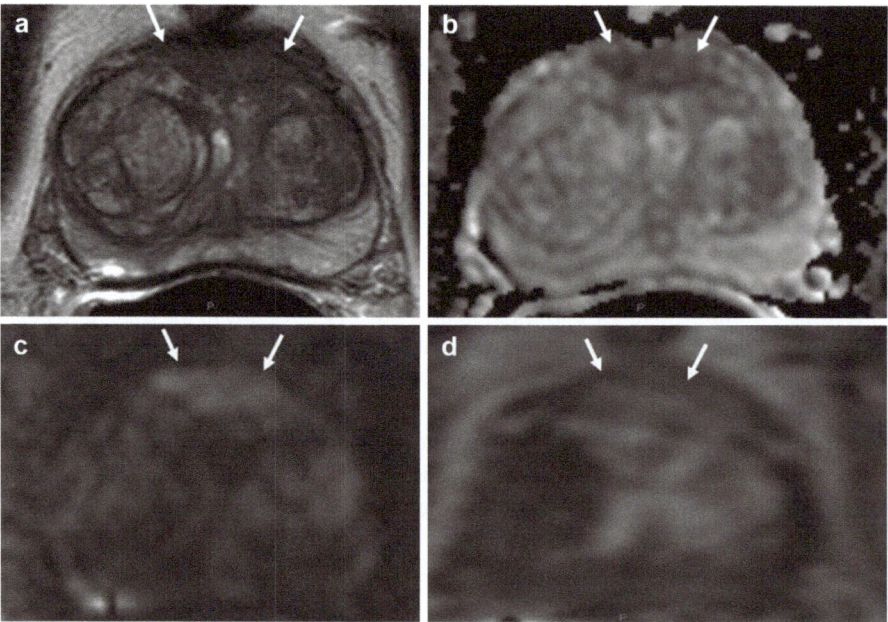

Fig. 8.2 Sixty-year-old man with PSA of 6.19 ng/mL and one prior negative TRUS-guided pros-tate biopsy. Axial T2W MRI shows a lesion in the midline anterior transition zone (*arrows*) (**a**), which has restricted diffusion on ADC map (**b**) and b2000 DWI (**c**) (*arrows*). The lesion demon-strates hypervascularity on DCE MRI (**d**) (*arrow*). TRUS/MRI fusion-guided biopsy of this lesion revealed Gleason 3 + 4 prostate cancer

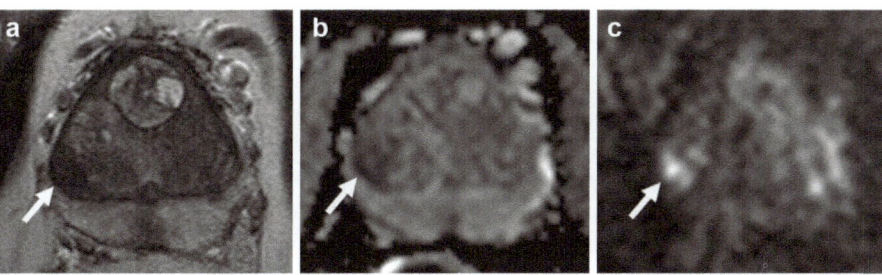

Fig. 8.3 Sixty-eight-year-old male with PSA of 14.78 ng/mL. Axial T2W MRI shows a hypointense indeterminate lesion in the right mid-transition zone (*arrow*) (**a**), which has restricted diffusion on ADC map (**b**) and b1500 DWI (**c**) (*arrows*). TRUS/MRI fusion-guided biopsy of this lesion revealed Gleason 3 + 4 prostate cancer

systematic template biopsy technique. Furthermore, it improves the Gleason score concordance between biopsy and final radical prostatectomy [40]. Since most data is available for patient populations after previous systematic biopsies, current guidelines recommend its use in patients with clinical suspicion of prostate cancer after a previous negative or indeterminate systematic biopsy [41, 42]. Major drawback is the increased complexity of the biopsy procedure since patients must undergo MRI first and then biopsy in a separate session. Furthermore, due to the multi-step nature of this approach, there are more sources of errors which can happen during reading, segmentation of MRI, segmentation of real-time TRUS image, and registration during the biopsy. Finally, increased costs and limited availability restrict its broader application. Despite all this, in theoretical models multiparametric prostate MRI still seems to be more cost-effective than the current paradigm due to better characterization of underlying disease [43].

8.5.2   Prostate Cancer Staging

Correct staging of diagnosed prostate cancer facilitates patient counseling and decision-making before initiating treatment and therefore can lead to optimized clinical outcomes. The presence of extraprostatic extension or seminal vesicle invasion increases the risk for metastasis at the time of diagnosis, making curative treatment less likely to benefit the patient. Traditional parameters such as PSA and DRE have a low diagnostic accuracy in determining the risk for locally advanced disease. Multiparametric MRI can visualize extraprostatic extension and seminal vesicle invasion and improves the accuracy in predicting locally aggressive disease [44, 45]. Large lesion-capsule contact, tumor bulging, irregular and speculated tumor border, obliteration of the recto-prostatic angle, asymmetry or invasion of neurovascular bundles, and direct breach of the capsule or invasion of the bladder wall are indicators of extraprostatic extension [46, 47] (Fig. 8.4). Filling defects with restricted diffusion and increased vascularity, direct invasion of tumor from the base of the prostate, and obliteration of the angle between the prostate and the seminal vesicles

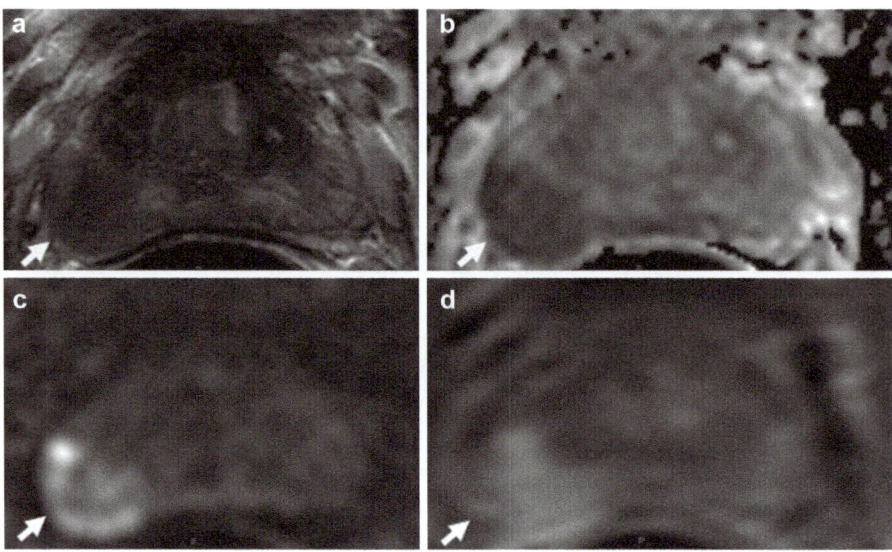

Fig. 8.4 Fifty-one-year-old male with PSA of 11.43 ng/mL and no prior prostate biopsy history. Axial T2W MRI shows a hypointense lesion in the right mid-peripheral zone (*arrow*) (**a**). The lesion shows restricted diffusion on ADC map (**b**) and b = 2000 DW MRI (**c**) (*arrows*) and early contrast enhancement on DCE MRI (**d**) (*arrow*). The lesion has large capsular contact, capsular bulge, and obliteration of the right recto-prostatic angle which suggest extraprostatic extension (**a**). Patient underwent TRUS/MRI fusion-guided biopsy, and histopathology revealed Gleason 3 + 4 prostatic adenocarcinoma

are associated with seminal vesicle invasion. Although local staging mainly relies on anatomic T2W MRI, DWI can also help in both detection and further confirmation of extraprostatic extension and seminal vesicle invasion. A recent meta-analysis showed sensitivity of 57% and specificity of 91% for extraprostatic extension and 58% and 96% for seminal vesical invasion, respectively. The moderate sensitivity is explained by the fact that microscopic invasion cannot be visualized by MRI. Higher magnetic field strengths and the use of DWI can increase the diagnostic accuracy [48]. However, mpMRI cannot rule out locally advanced disease confidently.

8.6   Pitfalls

Although DWI is quite helpful in detection of prostate cancer, several pitfalls can still exist. Some benign anatomic entitites such as exophytic hyperplastic nodules in the peripheral zone (Fig. 8.5) and normal central zone and thickened surgical capsule can also have restricted diffusion and mimic cancer foci [49]. Being familiar with those findings is crucial to avoid false-positive diagnosis on prostate MRI. Although differential diagnosis of abnormal intraprostatic foci on prostate MRI is relatively narrow, some non-tumor pathologies such as acute prostatitis (Fig. 8.6), chronic granulomatous prostatitis (e.g., BCG induced or tuberculous

Fig. 8.5 Fifty-five-year-old male with PSA of 0.6 ng/mL. Axial T2W MRI shows a well-defined lesion in the left apical peripheral zone (*arrow*) (**a**), which shows restricted diffusion on ADC map (**b**) and *b* = 2000 DW MRI (**c**) (*arrows*). The lesion represents an exophytic BPH nodule

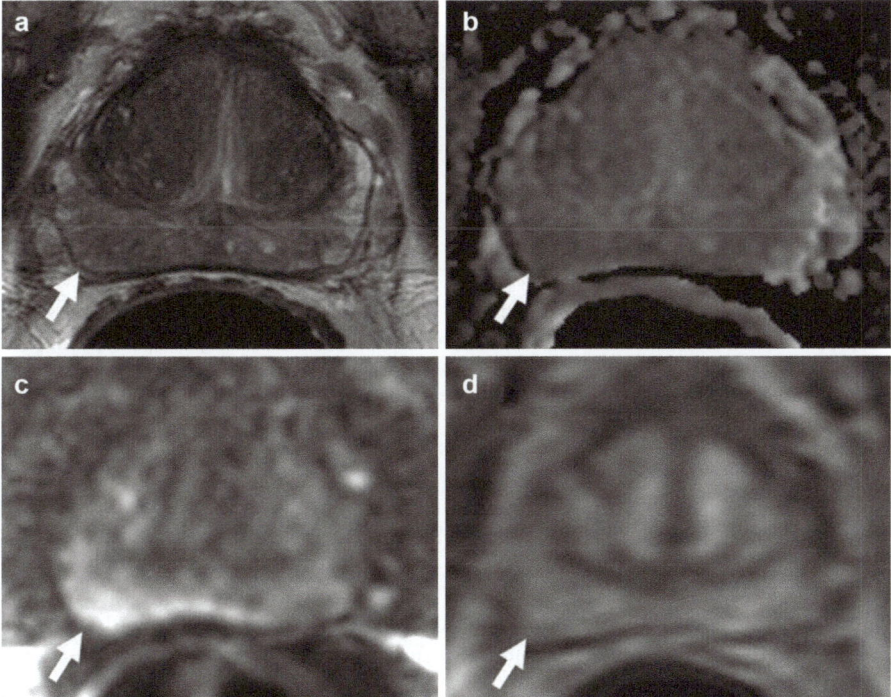

Fig. 8.6 Fifty-year-old male with serum PSA of 4.74 ng/mL. Axial T2W MRI shows diffuse heterogeneous slight hypointense signal pattern in the peripheral zone (more prominently seen on the right compared to the left side) (*arrow*) (**a**), which shows intermediate restricted diffusion on ADC map (**b**) and *b* = 2000 DW MRI (**c**) (*arrows*) with diffuse enhancement on DCE MRI (*arrow*) (**d**). Findings suggest acute prostatitis

related) (Fig. 8.7), prostatic intraepithelial neoplasia, and biopsy-related atrophy and scarring (Fig. 8.8) should also be considered during readouts [49–51]. Accurate distinction of these differential diagnoses from prostate cancer is usually not possible; however having detailed information about patients' past medical history can be quite helpful to reach correct diagnosis.

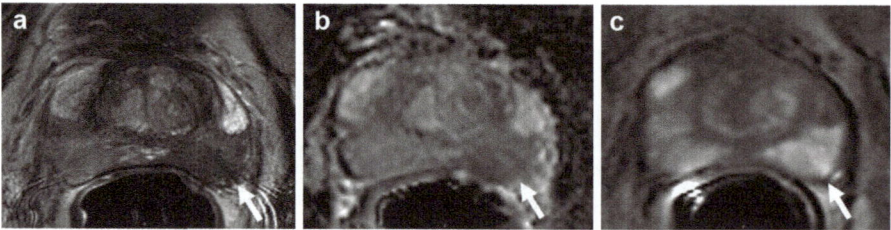

Fig. 8.7 Sixty-year-old male with PSA of 4.06 ng/mL. Axial T2W MRI shows a large hypointense lesion in the left mid-peripheral zone (*arrow*) (**a**) with marked restricted diffusion on ADC map (**b**) and early enhancement on DCE MRI (*arrows*) (**c**). TRUS/MRI fusion-guided targeted biopsy revealed chronic granulomatous prostatitis

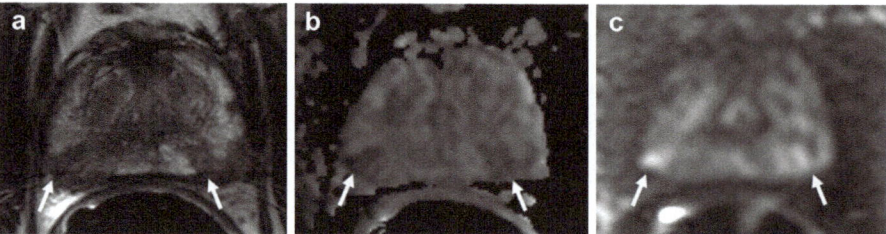

Fig. 8.8 Fifty-eight-year-old male with PSA of 3.58 ng/mL and previous history of multiple prostate biopsies prior to prostate MRI. Axial T2W MRI shows bilateral wedge-shaped hypointense foci in the apical peripheral zone (*arrows*) (**a**), which show restricted diffusion on ADC map (**b**) and b = 2000 DW MRI (*arrows*). These lesions represent biopsy-related scarring

Conclusion

The implementation of DWI into prostate MRI has become an integral part of mpMRI. Currently, DWI plays a major role in lesion detection and PI-RADSv2 scoring of detected lesions. Additionally, ADC maps can aid radiologists in predicting histopathological grading with acceptable limitations. Standardization of DWI acquisition and interpretation will further enhance its acceptance and use.

References

1. Hricak H, et al. Anatomy and pathology of the male pelvis by magnetic resonance imaging. AJR Am J Roentgenol. 1983;141(6):1101–10.
2. Steyn JH, Smith FW. Nuclear magnetic resonance imaging of the prostate. Br J Urol. 1982;54(6):726–8.
3. Turkbey B, et al. Prostate cancer: value of multiparametric MR imaging at 3T for detection—histopathologic correlation. Radiology. 2010;255(1):89–99.
4. Agarwal HK, et al. Optimal high b-value for diffusion weighted MRI in diagnosing high risk prostate cancers in the peripheral zone. J Magn Reson Imaging. 2016.

5. Hambrock T, et al. Relationship between apparent diffusion coefficients at 3.0-T MR imaging and Gleason grade in peripheral zone prostate cancer. Radiology. 2011;259(2):453–61.
6. Oto A, et al. Diffusion-weighted and dynamic contrast-enhanced MRI of prostate cancer: correlation of quantitative MR parameters with Gleason score and tumor angiogenesis. AJR Am J Roentgenol. 2011;197(6):1382–90.
7. Turkbey B, et al. Is apparent diffusion coefficient associated with clinical risk scores for prostate cancers that are visible on 3-T MR images? Radiology. 2011;258(2):488–95.
8. PI-RADS^{tm.} A.C.o.R. Prostate Imaging and Reporting and Data System 2015, version 2; 2015.
9. Le Bihan D, et al. Separation of diffusion and perfusion in intravoxel incoherent motion MR imaging. Radiology. 1988;168(2):497–505.
10. Le Bihan D, et al. MR imaging of intravoxel incoherent motions: application to diffusion and perfusion in neurologic disorders. Radiology. 1986;161(2):401–7.
11. Katahira K, et al. Ultra-high-b-value diffusion-weighted MR imaging for the detection of prostate cancer: evaluation in 201 cases with histopathological correlation. Eur Radiol. 2011;21(1):188–96.
12. Metens T, et al. What is the optimal b value in diffusion-weighted MR imaging to depict prostate cancer at 3T? Eur Radiol. 2012;22(3):703–9.
13. Rosenkrantz AB, et al. Diffusion-weighted imaging of the prostate: Comparison of b1000 and b2000 image sets for index lesion detection. J Magn Reson Imaging. 2013;38(3):694–700.
14. Turkbey B, et al. Multiparametric prostate magnetic resonance imaging in the evaluation of prostate cancer. CA Cancer J Clin. 2016;66(4):326–36.
15. De Cobelli F, et al. Apparent diffusion coefficient value and ratio as noninvasive potential biomarkers to predict prostate cancer grading: comparison with prostate biopsy and radical prostatectomy specimen. AJR Am J Roentgenol. 2015;204(3):550–7.
16. Kim JH, et al. Apparent diffusion coefficient: prostate cancer versus noncancerous tissue according to anatomical region. J Magn Reson Imaging. 2008;28(5):1173–9.
17. Kitajima K, et al. Do apparent diffusion coefficient (ADC) values obtained using high b-values with a 3-T MRI correlate better than a transrectal ultrasound (TRUS)-guided biopsy with true Gleason scores obtained from radical prostatectomy specimens for patients with prostate cancer? Eur J Radiol. 2013;82(8):1219–26.
18. Salami SS, et al. Risk stratification of prostate cancer utilizing apparent diffusion coefficient value and lesion volume on multiparametric MRI. J Magn Reson Imaging. 2017;45(2):610–6.
19. Turkbey B, et al. Is apparent diffusion coefficient associated with clinical risk scores for prostate cancers that are visible on 3-T MR images? Radiology. 2010;258(2):488–95.
20. Woo S, et al. Preoperative evaluation of prostate cancer aggressiveness: using ADC and ADC ratio in determining Gleason score. AJR Am J Roentgenol. 2016;207(1):114–20.
21. Rosenkrantz AB, Taneja SS. Radiologist, be aware: ten pitfalls that confound the interpretation of multiparametric prostate MRI. AJR Am J Roentgenol. 2014;202(1):109–20.
22. Litjens GJ, et al. Interpatient variation in normal peripheral zone apparent diffusion coefficient: effect on the prediction of prostate cancer aggressiveness. Radiology. 2012;265(1):260–6.
23. Barentsz JO, et al. Synopsis of the PI-RADS v2 guidelines for multiparametric prostate magnetic resonance imaging and recommendations for use. Eur Urol. 2016;69(1):41–9.
24. Turkbey B, et al. Comparison of endorectal coil and nonendorectal coil T2W and diffusion-weighted MRI at 3 Tesla for localizing prostate cancer: correlation with whole-mount histopathology. J Magn Reson Imaging. 2014;39(6):1443–8.
25. Gawlitza J, et al. Impact of the use of an endorectal coil for 3T prostate MRI on image quality and cancer detection rate. Sci Rep. 2017;7:40640.
26. Beyersdorff D, et al. MRI of prostate cancer at 1.5 and 3.0T: comparison of image quality in tumor detection and staging. AJR Am J Roentgenol. 2005;185(5):1214–20.
27. Shah ZK, et al. Performance comparison of 1.5-T endorectal coil MRI with 3.0-T nonendorectal coil MRI in patients with prostate cancer. Acad Radiol. 2015;22(4):467–74.
28. Sosna, J., et al., MR imaging of the prostate at 3 Tesla: comparison of an external phased-array coil to imaging with an endorectal coil at 1.5 Tesla. Acad Radiol, 2004. 11(8): p. 857–62.

29. Torricelli P, et al. Comparative evaluation between external phased array coil at 3T and endorectal coil at 1.5T: preliminary results. J Comput Assist Tomogr. 2006;30(3):355–61.
30. Wagner M, et al. Effect of butylscopolamine on image quality in MRI of the prostate. Clin Radiol. 2010;65(6):460–4.
31. Tamada T, et al. Prostate cancer: relationships between postbiopsy hemorrhage and tumor detectability at MR diagnosis. Radiology. 2008;248(2):531–9.
32. Johnson W, et al. The value of hyoscine butylbromide in pelvic MRI. Clin Radiol. 2007;62(11):1087–93.
33. Kabakus IM, et al. Does abstinence from ejaculation before prostate MRI improve evaluation of the seminal vesicles? AJR Am J Roentgenol. 2016;207(6):1205–9.
34. Qayyum A, et al. Organ-confined prostate cancer: effect of prior transrectal biopsy on endorectal MRI and MR spectroscopic imaging. AJR Am J Roentgenol. 2004;183(4):1079–83.
35. Barrett T, et al. Value of the hemorrhage exclusion sign on T1-weighted prostate MR images for the detection of prostate cancer. Radiology. 2012;263(3):751–7.
36. Mehralivand S, et al. Prospective evaluation of prostate imaging-reporting and Data System Version 2 using the International Society of Urological Pathology Prostate Cancer Grade Group System. J Urol. 2017;198(3):583–90.
37. Rosenkrantz AB, et al. Interobserver reproducibility of the PI-RADS Version 2 Lexicon: a multicenter study of six experienced prostate radiologists. Radiology. 2016;280(3):793–804.
38. Turkbey B, et al. Multiparametric 3T prostate magnetic resonance imaging to detect cancer: histopathological correlation using prostatectomy specimens processed in customized magnetic resonance imaging based molds. J Urol. 2011;186(5):1818–24.
39. Brown AM, et al. Recent advances in image-guided targeted prostate biopsy. Abdom Imaging. 2015;40(6):1788–99.
40. Siddiqui MM, et al. Comparison of MR/ultrasound fusion-guided biopsy with ultrasound-guided biopsy for the diagnosis of prostate cancer. JAMA. 2015;313(4):390–7.
41. Rosenkrantz AB, et al. Prostate magnetic resonance imaging and magnetic resonance imaging targeted biopsy in patients with a prior negative biopsy: a consensus statement by AUA and SAR. J Urol. 2016;196(6):1613–8.
42. Mottet N, et al. EAU-ESTRO-SIOG guidelines on prostate cancer. Part 1: screening, diagnosis, and local treatment with curative intent. Eur Urol. 2017;71(4):618–29.
43. de Rooij M, et al. Cost-effectiveness of magnetic resonance (MR) imaging and MR-guided targeted biopsy versus systematic transrectal ultrasound-guided biopsy in diagnosing prostate cancer: a modelling study from a health care perspective. Eur Urol. 2014;66(3):430–6.
44. Gupta RT, et al. Can radiologic staging with multiparametric MRI enhance the accuracy of the partin tables in predicting organ-confined prostate cancer? Am J Roentgenol. 2016;207(1):87–95.
45. Kim CK, et al. Diffusion-weighted MRI as a predictor of extracapsular extension in prostate cancer. AJR Am J Roentgenol. 2014;202(3):W270–6.
46. Baco E, et al. Predictive value of magnetic resonance imaging determined tumor contact length for extracapsular extension of prostate cancer. J Urol. 2015;193(2):466–72.
47. Kongnyuy M, et al. Tumor contact with prostate capsule on magnetic resonance imaging: a potential biomarker for staging and prognosis. Urol Oncol. 2017;35(1):30.e1–8.
48. de Rooij M, et al. Accuracy of magnetic resonance imaging for local staging of prostate cancer: a diagnostic meta-analysis. Eur Urol. 2016;70(2):233–45.
49. Bhowmik NM, et al. Benign causes of diffusion restriction foci in the peripheral zone of the prostate: diagnosis and differential diagnosis. Abdom Radiol (NY). 2016;41(5):910–8.
50. Logan JK, et al. Changes observed in multiparametric prostate magnetic resonance imaging characteristics correlate with histopathological development of chronic granulomatous prostatitis after intravesical Bacillus Calmette-Guerin therapy. J Comput Assist Tomogr. 2014;38(2):274–6.
51. Rais-Bahrami S, et al. Clinical and multiparametric MRI signatures of granulomatous prostatitis. Abdom Radiol (NY). 2017;42(7):1956–62.

GPSR Compliance

The European Union's (EU) General Product Safety Regulation (GPSR)
is a set of rules that requires consumer products to be safe and our
obligations to ensure this.

If you have any concerns about our products, you can contact us on
ProductSafety@springernature.com

In case Publisher is established outside the EU, the EU authorized
representative is:

Springer Nature Customer Service Center GmbH
Europaplatz 3
69115 Heidelberg, Germany

Batch number: 09635427

Printed by Printforce, the Netherlands